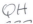

The Ethical Dimensions of the Biological and Health Sciences, 2nd ed.

This is the second edition of an acclaimed textbook on the responsible conduct of biomedical and health sciences research. It is designed for students and faculty in health sciences and biomedical research programs, and is ideal for use in graduate programs funded by National Institutes of Health training grants. Life sciences faculty and administrators in general universities, academic health centers, and graduate schools in the health professions will also find this book a highly useful resource.

The book opens with a comprehensive history of the ethics movement in biological and health sciences, which provides context for the issues to come. The ten subsequent sections address the core ethical issues in research integrity, including the origins of ethics in scientific research, the responsible conduct of research, authorship and publication, research with persons, populations, and animals, data management, and the relationships between science and academia, science and industry, and science and society. Each one begins with an in-depth introductory essay, followed by important primary documents and classic articles from well-known scientists and ethicists, and concludes with questions for discussion and recommendations for supplemental reading. As a new feature in the second edition, the book also includes a series of cases addressing each of the ten key areas and guidelines for conducting case discussion.

Ruth Ellen Bulger is Professor of Anatomy, Physiology, and Genetics at the Uniformed Services University of the Health Sciences, Bethesda, Maryland.

Elizabeth Heitman is Professor of Medicine, Surgery, and Anesthesiology at the University of Mississippi Medical Center, Jackson, Mississippi, and Associate Professor in Management and Policy Sciences at the University of Texas Health Science Center at Houston.

Stanley Joel Reiser is the Griff T. Ross Professor of Humanities and Technology in Health Care at the University of Texas Health Science Center at Houston.

Praise for the first edition:

". . . an outstanding book." *Canadian Philosophical Reviews*

". . . the editors have selected high-quality essays, and the discussion questions that follow are uniformly insightful and provocative." *Isis*

". . . a useful introduction to some of the ethical dilemmas facing research scientists . . . a stimulating resource for anyone involved in biological research." *The Lancet*

"This book will be of great value to all who are responsible for the education of biomedical scientists in the changing world, where the perception of science and scientists has changed." *The Pharos*

"This book is a model of organization and content of a graduate course of ethics in the biological sciences. It is highly recommended not only for the personal library of a scientist or scientist-in-training but also for use in graduate ethics courses for the biological scientist." *Doodv's Health Sciences Book Review Annual*

The Ethical Dimensions of the Biological and Health Sciences

Second Edition

RUTH ELLEN BULGER
Uniformed Services University of the Health Sciences

ELIZABETH HEITMAN
University of Mississippi Medical Center and
University of Texas Health Science Center at Houston

STANLEY JOEL REISER
University of Texas Health Science Center at Houston

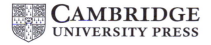
CAMBRIDGE
UNIVERSITY PRESS

PUBLISHED BY THE PRESS SYNDICATE OF THE UNIVERSITY OF CAMBRIDGE
The Pitt Building, Trumpington Street, Cambridge, United Kingdom

CAMBRIDGE UNIVERSITY PRESS
The Edinburgh Building, Cambridge CB2 2RU, UK
40 West 20th Street, New York, NY 10011-4211, USA
477 Williamstown Road, Port Melbourne, VIC 3207, Australia
Ruiz de Alarcón 13, 28014 Madrid, Spain
Dock House, The Waterfront, Cape Town 8001, South Africa

http://www.cambridge.org

First published 2002

Printed in the United States of America

Typeface Times 10/12 pt.   *System* LaTeX 2_ε [TB]

A catalog record for this book is available from the British Library.

Library of Congress Cataloging in Publication data

The ethical dimensions of the biological and health sciences / Ruth Ellen
    Bulger, Elizabeth Heitman, Stanley Joel Reiser. – 2nd ed.
        p.   cm.
    Includes bibliographical references and index.
    ISBN 0-521-81053-1 (hbk.) – ISBN 0-521-00886-7 (pbk.)
    1. Bioethics.   I. Bulger, Ruth Ellen.   II. Heitman, Elizabeth.   III. Reiser, Stanley Joel.
QH332 .E73   2002
174′.957 – dc21   2001043382

ISBN 0 521 81053 1 hardback
ISBN 0 521 00886 7 paperback

We dedicate this book to

Roger J. Bulger, M.D.
R.W. Butcher, Ph.D.,
and
to the memory of the late
Thomas F. Burks, Ph.D.

Their help was vital to
initiating and sustaining
our work in scientific ethics
and creating an ethos of
ethical concern as university
administrators and scholars.

Contents

Preface

Biological and health research have become a public enterprise. While discoveries in this area continue to be a product of private and group work in laboratory and research centers, the social and economic effects of these discoveries have drawn the attention of powerful public constituencies – government, industry, legislatures, and the population at large – whose support is crucial to maintaining the scientific endeavor.

This new position of biomedical science was epitomized by a 1991 issue of *Time* magazine, which portrayed science as "under a microscope" and "under siege." The review outlined a "crisis" brought on by "a budget squeeze and bureaucratic demands, internal squabbling, harassment by activists, embarrassing cases of fraud and failure, and the growing alienation of Congress and the public."[1] That the topic could generate sufficient public interest to warrant an eight-page feature in an international magazine is itself a large part of the story.

As the discoveries of bioscience foster profound changes in our view of ourselves and our ability to overcome threats to human health and create enormous investment opportunities for entrepreneurs, bioscience is increasingly perceived as an essential social enterprise that requires both the support and decision-making involvement of those outside of the scientific community. For students and professional researchers to live in this new environment successfully, they need the knowledge necessary to understand it.

Researchers' difficulties over the past two decades in sorting out the ethical questions involved in their work make a strong case for explicit teaching about these problems in the course of professional training. The scientific community's experience in dealing with misconduct in research has demonstrated that faculty and students need a forum in which to discuss the ethical issues that may arise in a scientist's career. Ethics enters into basic questions that scientists face continuously – from their responsibilities to the human and animal subjects of their research to the social consequences of their discoveries.

Until recently, many scientists have seemed content to leave such education in ethics to the role-model format: older scientists transmitting standards to younger ones by their demeanor and through random conversations and actions. But as has been well demonstrated in clinical medicine, role models, though important, are not sufficient to educate students in the complex ethical problems of modern science.

A crucial feature of disciplines that call themselves professions is systematic reflection about the ethical traditions that govern them and their relationship with society. Such reflection is critical to fostering the public trust that sustains the professions' right of self-regulation and claims of authenticity. The consideration of the ethical dimensions of science as part of the curriculum of scientific learning and research can be tangible evidence that the scientific community warrants public trust and can serve as a major underpinning for ethical behavior in science.

Although the scientific community is developing ways to respond to unprofessional behavior, too little attention has been given to the place of education in preventing it. The time has arrived, as public and scientific concern about misconduct has demonstrated, for scientists to consider formally, through scholarship and classroom teaching, the ethical context of their work.

In 1985, prompted by an ethical conflict involving a student, and encouraged by R. W. Butcher, the dean of our graduate school of biomedical sciences, we developed a course to provide such instruction; the course has since been required of all entering graduate students in the biomedical sciences. We believed then, and believe more strongly now, that the lack of systematic teaching about the nature of scientific discovery and the scientist's life in the context of ethics leads to ambiguity about the moral aspects of gathering, interpreting, and reporting evidence; the social responsibilities of science; and the personal obligations of scientists to their colleagues, their discipline, and themselves.

The course that we designed does not enumerate standards that students must adopt or commit to memory; rather, it attempts to stimulate students' interest and to provoke them to further reading and consideration of the issues and their implications. Although honesty, integrity, truth, and professional responsibility are all key elements of the course, they are complemented by considerations of creativity, the process of discovery, and the implications of Pasteur's dictum that "in the field of experimentation, chance favors only the prepared mind."[2] The very existence of the course, and the requirement that entering graduate students in biomedical sciences attend it, demonstrates to students the commitment of the institution to examining ethical values within the scientific process.

A similar educational requirement was accepted in 1989 as part of the administrative guidelines for the National Research Service Award institutional training grant applications submitted to the Alcohol, Drug Abuse, and Mental Health Administration and the National Institutes of Health (NIH). As stated in the NIH Guide for Grants and Contracts, a program concerned with understanding the concepts of scientific integrity must be a part of any proposed research training effort.[3]

In 2000 the U.S. Public Health Service proposed a more comprehensive learning requirement for education in the responsible conduct of research, which involves a far larger range of scientific personnel that includes not only investigators but members of their research staff.[4] To share the benefits of our experience with such a program, we developed this volume. This second edition covers all the instructional areas recommended in this new policy and incorporates the latest thinking about ethical issues in the biological and health sciences.

The book is divided into twelve parts, each of which begins with an extensive essay by one of the book's authors. Each overview essay is followed by seminal readings and documents on the subject, questions to stimulate discussion, and further references. The final section provides cases on each of the book's main subjects and a discussion of how to approach case analysis.

The book attempts to do two things. First, it presents in one place a variety of readings organized according to several fundamental topics of ethics in science. Second, the introductory essays and discussion questions in each section provide a focus on aspects that we believe warrant particular consideration.

The book introduces students to the norms of ethical conduct in science as established by the profession and by legislative bodies; scientific honesty and its relationship to objectivity and self-deception; professional policies of coauthorship and plagiarism; the use of human beings and animals in research; the relationship between science, scientists, industry, and society; the ethics and process of data management, collaboration, and peer review; and the ethics of teaching and learning. The readings also provide an opportunity to discuss other issues basic to research but often not formally considered in graduate science education such as methods of scientific investigation (and scientists' difficulty thinking outside the paradigm upon which their own work is based), the creative process, and the problem of describing reality.

Many of the previously published articles reprinted here are considered classics. Some that are less well known are nonetheless personal favorites, either for their clarity, insight, or ability to spark discussion. We have reproduced these articles in as close to their original form as possible, resulting in a wide variety of reference styles and occasional editorial discrepancies across the volume. (Unfortunately, we were unable to include the figures in two articles; however, in each case the authors' respective descriptions of their data make clear what the figures were intended to illustrate.) We are thankful to the many authors and publishers who gave us permission to reprint their copyrighted works.

The three authors collectively have education and work experience in laboratory science, clinical medicine, health policy, history, and ethics and currently teach courses in the ethics of the biological and health sciences. We have used several formats in teaching this material. For some subjects we used predominantly a lecture approach, whereas other sessions were led in a Socratic style; however, time has always been reserved for group discussion, and the readings provide many issues for debate. In class we have also supplemented these readings with material from our own academic environment. For example, to consider using animals in research, the students have served as an Animal Care and Use Committee, reviewing a fictitious application on the forms used by our institution. Because many of our students have worked in a laboratory, their experiences have also been a focus for discussion. We recommend that the general material in this book be tailored similarly to the specific needs and situations of the students and institutions that will use it.

For their work on this second edition we are grateful to Janice Glover, Sheryl Hamilton, and Michael C. Rossa. Our thanks also go to Kristin Heitman and Lida Anestidou for their critical commentary on several of the essays.

As regards the contributions of Ruth Bulger to this book, her opinions and assertions are private ones and are not to be construed as official comments of, or to reflect the views of, the U.S. Department of Defense or the Uniformed Services University of the Health Sciences.

Ruth Ellen Bulger, Elizabeth Heitman, and Stanley Joel Reiser

References

1. Nash JM, Thompson D. Crisis in the labs. *Time.* August 26, 1991:44.
2. Cuny H. *Louis Pasteur: A Man and His Theories.* Evans P, trans. New York: Fawcett World Library; 1963:149.
3. *NIH Guide for Grants and Contracts.* December 22, 1989; 18;No–45.
4. U.S. Department of Health and Human Services, Office of Research Integrity. PHS Policy on Instruction in the Responsible Conduct of Research (RCR). Washington, DC:DHHS; 2000.

Introduction to the Study of Ethics in the Biological and Health Sciences

The Ethics Movement in the Biological and Health Sciences

A New Voyage of Discovery

Stanley Joel Reiser

The modern voyage to chart the ethical bases of the biological and health sciences (biohealth sciences) is an important episode in their history and also in the annals of society. Its purpose has been to identify, for scientists from different disciplines who probe human function and for the surrounding society, principles for setting the goals of this research, creating the resultant knowledge, and influencing its subsequent use. This essay traces seminal events of this journey, which began near the midpoint of the twentieth century, and seeks to identify directions the journey may take as it continues on a course into the future. This passage has occurred in four phases, in each of which biohealth scientists have altered a fundamental relationship: in the first phase with the individual research subject, in the second with society, in the third with their research procedures, and in the fourth with their institutions of learning.

Phase I 1945–1966: Fathoming the Human Subject

Revelations emerging from the Nuremberg War Crimes Trials at the end of World War II disclosed the forced induction of prisoners of war and civilians into experiments that injured and killed many. These activities were officially sanctioned and promoted by government authorities of the Nazi regime and conducted by scientists and physicians. To prevent future harm to subjects of human studies, instruct investigators about the ethical precepts needed to protect subjects, and delineate the responsibilities of investigators to carry out these goals, a set of ten principles was developed by the war crimes staff. It came to be called the Nuremberg Code.

The code focused on giving the potential subject of an experiment the opportunity to decide whether to participate. It enumerated the conditions necessary to assure the freedom and capacity of individuals to make this choice. This included the absence of a coercive environment that would hinder choice, the presence of a mental capability and adequate data about harms and benefits that would facilitate choice, and the freedom of the subject to withdraw at any time from the experiment. The code made investigators responsible for assuring the adequacy of the consent process, the scientific credibility and safety of the experiment, the qualifications of those conducting the experiment, and the ending of an experiment when the likelihood of injury or death to subjects emerged.[1]

With the code in hand, and the consequences of moral insensitivity to the possibilities of harm in human studies so starkly taught, scientists believed that major ethical problems now could be avoided or adequately handled if they occurred. As researchers entered the 1950s they were also caught up in the excitement of a period of unsurpassed growth in biomedical research. This was a time when the public accepted scientists as benevolent experts whom

3

they trusted to select the projects and determine the goals of science. Research into health and illness was a good of which the public wanted more, and they were willing to give considerable sums of money for this purpose. The National Institutes of Health (NIH) became a major scientific funder in the postwar period, its grants rising from $75 million in 1948 to $150 million in 1954.[2] Understandably, the research community wished to focus on scientific questions. Hence the 1950s produced little commentary about the ethical issues of human studies or the relation of the biohealth sciences to society.

However, in the 1950s a small group of lawyers was interested in strengthening legal protections for human subjects. They attempted to encourage research organizations in the United States to build on the ideas in the Nuremberg Code. They urged scientists to seek ways to refine scientific practices used in human studies and to develop innovative principles to guide the research. But as one of these lawyers, William Curran, who became Professor of Legal Medicine at Harvard, wrote of his efforts in the 1950s to gain attention to research ethics: "We had only very limited success in this ambitious undertaking. We were working at a time somewhat before the researchers were ready to believe such action was necessary."[3]

Attitudes changed in the 1960s. The catalysts were the discovery of particular cases in which investigators disregarded the canons of the Nuremberg Code, the burgeoning civil rights movement that heightened social sensitivity to the needs of vulnerable groups, and legislative and regulatory actions that changed the procedure of research on human subjects.

A case that drew wide attention occurred in 1963, when three physicians experimentally injected live cancer cells into twenty-two elderly and debilitated in-patients at the Jewish Chronic Disease Hospital in Brooklyn to determine whether such patients would reject such cells. Several physicians opposing this experiment and particularly concerned that the subjects never consented to participate brought the matter to the hospital's board of trustees. One of these physicians took the hospital to court to see the records of involved patients. In the complicated proceedings that followed, several of the study's investigators contended that a doctor could rightfully withhold data that patients might find threatening. This position was not upheld when the Board of Regents of the State University of New York reviewed the case. It asserted that the investigators had an experimental, not a therapeutic, relationship with subjects. Thus no basis existed for the exercise of the "usual professional judgment applicable to patient care."[4] As the story unfolded in the media, however, there was public and professional surprise and consternation that existing ethical principles of scientific research had not prevented the occurrence of such an experiment.

Federal interest in this subject had emerged a year earlier in 1962. A group of U.S. senators devoted to civil rights issues and led by New York Senator Jacob Javits added a requirement to the Food, Drug, and Cosmetic Act being amended that year. It mandated investigators of experimental drugs to obtain a formal consent from subjects in their trials. In 1965, more pressure for reform was introduced. In March of that year Harvard anesthesiologist Henry Beecher delivered a paper at a conference in which he cited cases in the published literature showing disregard of the consent process in human experiments. This speech, published in 1966 as an essay, received widespread coverage in the public media. In December 1965 The National Advisory Council to the NIH added its weight to the issue and went much further than had the food and drug legislation. It announced that guidelines would be developed requiring prior review of all research protocols on human subjects before a study could begin. A February 1966 memorandum from the U.S. Surgeon General spelled out what these guidelines would mean. Scientists now would be required to obtain an informed consent from all research subjects and provide an assessment of the possible harms and benefits of the studies they proposed. Evaluation of this material would be given to a group of peers within the investigator's institution. In a July 1966 revision these institutions were made responsible for assuring that all research funded in them by the NIH met its review requirements.[3] The panels became known as Institutional Review Boards, or IRBs.

With the IRBs in place, the private world of the individual investigator was opened not only to peers but to social others as the membership on IRBs became enlarged to include community participants who were not scientists. The IRB requirement made investigators consider and discuss explicitly with subjects ethical questions connected with their research. This discourse, involving issues of consent and the risks and benefits of medical interventions, dovetailed with and further stimulated consideration of these matters in clinical medicine. Indeed the scientists whom such regulations involved often worked in the milieu of hospitals where human subjects could be recruited from among patients. Accordingly these events influenced investigators doing basic and applied research in the clinical community more than it did those working on biologic questions in laboratories removed from patient care.

In the 1940s and 1950s social authority was used to free both the individual scientist and the research subject. The NIH increasingly freed scientists from monetary constraints to pursue their research projects; the Nuremberg Code liberated research subjects from the authority of scientists to decide their own welfare. However, in the 1960s, the introduction of the IRB diminished the scientist's authority to determine the content of research procedures used on the human subject, while it enhanced the self-determination of the subject.

Phase II 1966–1974: The Social Engagement of Scientists

While the first part of this ethics movement focused on the danger of the scientist's work to particular individuals, the second part emphasized its threat to society at large. In the context of exploring potential social threats, a searching examination was conducted concerning the respective roles of the public, government, and investigators in deciding the course of scientific work that posed a possible threat to populations. This phase began in the mid-1960s and lasted about a decade.

The proximal antecedents of this phase were calls of alarm in the early 1960s by a number of prominent intellectuals such as Lewis Mumford, Jacques Ellul, and Raymond Aron. They and others were concerned about the growing hegemony of science in determining the course of civilization. Through innovations in transportation, communication, and warfare science was altering basic patterns of life, and scientists were becoming the quintessential experts of society. As the power over the way society lived flowed to the experts upon whose scientific knowledge social change was based, anxiety arose about the ability of the laity to question their authority. Raymond Aron wondered whether democracy could function in this situation. How, he asked, could legislators, politicians, or the electorate evaluate the complex facets of social problems when the most basic knowledge about them increasingly fell into the domain of the scientific expert? He worried that democratic institutions were threatened by the emerging dominance of a scientific elite.[5]

Ironically, this problem stemmed in part from the retreat of scientists from political dialogue and not their entrance into it. Scientists, including those in the sphere of biology, generated these transforming innovations without a clear view of the changes their work produced. They largely were unprepared to discuss the social consequences of their innovations when called into public forums for this purpose. Scientists held the knowledge to create transforming social change but lacked the understanding or will to evaluate its influence on social institutions or values. They exercised power but seemed unwilling and unable to take responsibility for its effects.

The main exceptions in this period were found in the community of atomic scientists. During the late 1940s and 1950s J. Robert Oppenheimer, Leo Szilard, and other leading physicists urged scientists to participate in discussing the use of their innovations. But the example of the physicists was not widely followed in other scientific disciplines. Scientists for the most part stayed out of social controversies for several important reasons. Too much involvement would take time away from the reading, reflection, and experimental work that made them "expert" in the first place: an excessive public profile threatened their scientific status. Public discourse required oversimplification of complex issues, and too much public exposure could turn scientists into celebrities. These effects could taint their image as detached analysts. Further, their training did not prepare them intellectually or emotionally for the social and political forums of public debate. Some worried, rightly, that when they entered into social debate, they descended from the platform of the expert to the ground of the layperson.[6]

However, by the mid-1960s a small number of biologists and medical scientists began actively to embark on an involvement in social issues. They were joined by a public grown increasingly interested in, and perturbed about, the power of the biological sciences to alter human life. The trust that the public had imposed on the scientist to decide alone what research to pursue was fading. In no aspect of biology and medicine was this concern deeper than in genetics.

The modern scientific transformation of this field had occurred in 1953 when James D. Watson and Francis H. C. Crick described the structure of DNA. This development made possible dramatic advances in understanding the architecture and function of human genes. During the 1960s, particularly the latter half of the decade, discussions were held in growing numbers on the ethical, social, and medical consequences of this research. Concerns grew that a second eugenics movement would emerge as more was learned about genetic functions. Worry began to compete with exhilaration about what the knowledge might bring. One of the earliest efforts to study these issues began in 1966. A small research group at the newly created Harvard Program on Technology and Society was formed to explore the social implications of advances in the biomedical sciences. The group convened conferences that brought together scientists, humanists, and policy experts. A book describing its early work noted that the issues being addressed had "to do specifically with the social control of the new biomedical technologies. . . . They relate to how science and technology can be used to social advantage. . . . It is evident that what were once considered exclusively professional decisions are increasingly coming to be regarded as decisions that need to be made by the larger society."[7]

As the 1960s came to an end, popular books began to appear that portrayed the threatening sides of the emerging understanding of biological function. A typical one, by the journalist Gordon Rattay Taylor, was called, ominously, *The Biological Time Bomb*. The titles of its eight chapters tell its story: "Where Are Biologists Taking Us?" (a chapter describing how biological knowledge is outpacing society's ability to control it), "Is Sex Necessary?" (a view of test-tube babies), "The Modified Man" (a look at transplantation), "Is Death Necessary?" (prolonging life through hibernation and freezing), "New Minds for Old" (manipulating emotions, memory, and intelligence), "The Genetic Engineers" (the possibilities of genetic surgery and eugenics), "Can We Create Life?" (making cells and viruses), "The Future, If Any" (social discord as the aforementioned innovations mature). In this and in similar publications, analogies were made between the possible destructive force of biological discoveries and the problems caused by the knowledge of atomic energy. The book's cover included a quote from Arthur Koestler from which its title apparently was taken: "Biology is just reaching the critical point of sudden acceleration which physics reached a generation ago . . . the biological time bomb is about to explode in our face."[8]

These concerns extended into the 1970s. In 1971, ethicist Joseph Fletcher made a comment about genetic research that mirrored an emerging social fear that biological knowledge could be used to harm or control society: "Even though its medical aim were only to gain control over the basic "stuff" of our human constitution it could no doubt also be turned into an instrument of political power."[9]

It was against this background of rising anxiety that in 1971, a member of the research staff of the Cold Spring Harbor Laboratory, Robert Pollack, telephoned Stanford biochemist Paul Berg. He called to discuss his concern with Berg's research to determine if the simian virus 40 could be used to transfer a foreign gene into bacteria. Because it had been shown that this virus produced tumors in hamsters, Pollack worried about the consequences of placing it into a strain of bacteria that grew in the human intestine, such as the widely used *Escherichia coli*, the one that Berg had intended to employ. Given the possibility that the virus could cause tumors in the human population, Pollack asked whether more knowledge was needed before conducting such an experiment. After much consultation Berg decided two things: He would postpone the experiment, and he would seek to convene a conference on the hazards of using tumor viruses. The conference was held in January 1973, at Asilomar, California, with about 100 scientists attending and Berg as chair. The meeting concluded that firm evidence of hazards of laboratory viruses inducing cancer was not available but that caution should be used in work with these viruses.

Later in 1973, the ability to splice and recombine different DNAs became possible. On first learning of this possibility at a Gordon research conference in New Hampshire, several scientists became alarmed. As Donald Frederickson writes, they reacted "to this hint that biology was approaching something akin to the nuclear physicists' chilling arrival at 'critical mass.'" Maxine Singer of the NIH and Dieter Söll of Yale drafted a letter, with the backing of others attending the meeting, to the National Academy of Sciences. It asked the academy to convene a committee to study the consequences of making biological alterations such as joining DNA from animal viruses with DNA from bacteria. "In this way," they wrote, "new kinds of hybrid plasmids or viruses, with biological activity of unpredictable nature, may eventually be created."[10]

The letter, and a general societal concern that this work posed a potential threat, produced a second Asilomar Conference held in September 1974, chaired again by Paul Berg. Its explicitly announced purposes were threefold: to review progress on research on recombinant DNA molecules; to discuss whether what were called "the biohazards of the work" still required a "pause" in certain of its aspects; and to decide how to conduct this research with minimal risk to laboratory workers, the public, and plants and animals.[11]

The conferees produced a set of guidelines for recombinant DNA research. It specified that the research should proceed but that biological and physical safeguards were to be used to contain the new organisms it generated. The biological barriers were bacterial hosts that could not survive in the material environment and vectors able to grow only in specified hosts. The physical barriers were containment technologies – for instance, gloves, hoods, and filters – applied in a strategy that matched the level of containment to the risk of the experiment. However, experiments involving highly pathogenic organisms were to be deferred until more knowledge was gained. These guidelines were to be implemented by codes of practice in different countries. But until such codes were developed, scientists as individuals were to decide on how to comply. A clear statement also was made about the ethical duties of principal investigators to their staff: they were to inform the staff fully about the hazards of experiments before initiating research, assure they were properly trained in containment procedures, and monitor their health.

Like the events that led to the creation of the IRBs, Asilomar reflected a growing public need for a voice in shaping the research agenda of biological science. In this sense, as Dorothy Nelkin argues, Asilomar was a challenge to the autonomy of biological science.[12] But Asilomar also stood for the recognition by a small vanguard of biological scientists that consideration of effects of their work on society should be a factor in developing the scientific agenda. Perhaps most fundamental, concern over the social harms and benefits of biological science became appreciated more widely in the 1970s as a shared responsibility of scientists and the public. However, this phase is marked more by the public's growing interest in biological science than by scientists' concern with public issues. The large majority of scientists still were focused on performing their basic work in the laboratory.

Phase III 1975–2000 Challenges to the Process of Creating Knowledge

The third part of the ethics movement, which directed attention to the procedures within the biohealth sciences used to generate and transmit knowledge, had four distinct components. It began in 1975 with the publication of Peter Singer's book *Animal Liberation;* continued with the highly publicized events of 1981 when John Darsee, a scientist at Harvard Medical School, admitted to falsifying scientific data; kept on into mid-decade with the growth of large project grants for the biological sciences made possible by its new relation with industry, and the development of social interest in the human genome project; and concluded in 2000 when the U.S. Public Health Service proposed that required training in research integrity be given to all investigators and their staff working under its research grants. The growing density of events perceived as ethical issues by the biohealth sciences community marks this phase as one of greater openness of that community toward ethical discourse and reflection. By the end of Phase III the stage was set for the development of a collective self-consciousness among these scientists about the moral dimensions of their work and a greater understanding of why public accountability should be important to them.

In 1975, with a number of worldwide movements for human rights as background, Peter Singer published his book *Animal Liberation*. In it he disputed commonly held views about animals, such as the belief that they lack the capacity to suffer. He argued that the human claim to a right to life should be extended to animals, whom society should not cause to suffer regardless of particular characteristics (or lack of them) they might have. He urged us to "bring non-human animals within our sphere of moral concern and cease to treat their lives as expendable."[13]

This book, and the rights-conscious social environment fostered by the civil rights and medical ethics movements, were important catalysts of a re-examination of the ethical issues concerning animals in experimental work that occurred in the 1980s. Groups emerged such as the Animal Liberation Front, The International Society for Animal Rights, and the Coalition to End Animal Suffering in Experiments. By 1986, eighty bills dealing with the use of animals in research had been introduced in state legislatures around the United

States.[14] By the decade's end, federal legislation had extended to animals protections similar to those given human subjects in the mid-1960s. Institutional review boards to examine all experiments involving animals from the viewpoint of humane treatment now were required. However, the controversy over their appropriate use continued, marked by heated discussions and even violent entries by activists into laboratories to free animals being used in scientific experiments.

The second component of this phase arose at the turn of the 1980s as big business became interested in the biohealth sciences. Up to then, apart from the funding of drug research by pharmaceutical companies, key sources of revenue for the biohealth sciences were from the federal government (mainly through the NIH), private foundations, and universities. However, the possibilities to develop profitable innovations led industrial corporations to make significant investments in biohealth research. For example, in the 1980s the Massachusetts General Hospital received two major industrial grants: one of almost $50 million was from a German drug and chemical company for molecular biology research, and a second of $85 million was from a Japanese cosmetics company to study the skin. In this period, the founding of the Biogen Company by Nobel Laureate Walter Gilbert and colleagues marked another milestone – the emerging viewpoint among biohealth scientists that work in a business corporation is an appropriate extension of their lives in science. During that decade many scientists developed relationships with industry to produce commercial products. By 1984 industrial funds accounted for almost a quarter of the external support of university research in biotechnology, which included projects on genetically engineered drugs and genetically altered bacteria, cell and tissue cultures, DNA technology, monoclonal antibodies, and fermentation.[15,16]

The growing relationship between biohealth scientists and industry posed ethical issues for investigators, universities, science, and the public. With new interests in profit-making activities, would the scientific agenda of research shift from seeking basic knowledge to seeking profitable knowledge? Would openness of communication be damaged by the introduction of competition among scientists working under grants from different companies? Would industrial relationships undermine the obligations and allegiance of scientists to the universities in which they held appointments? What obligations did universities have to ensure timely dissemination of inventions developed within them that might significantly further the public's health? How could universities avoid compromising the education of students and fellows employed by faculty supervisors to work on industry-sponsored research? Studies indicated the existence of such problems.[16,17]

In addition to large grants from industry, a major effort that led government to invest, over time, several billion dollars in a single biological research project emerged in the second half of the 1980s, when proposals appeared to delineate the human genome. In 1984 Robert Sinsheimer and colleagues at the University of California at San Diego attempted to create a genome sequencing institute. "They likened the effort to the exploration of the moon, arguing it would provide insights into who we were, and serve as an integrative focus of all DNA cloning techniques," wrote R. M. Cook-Deegan.[18] The proposal failed to attract private or federal funding. But in 1984 the parallel efforts of Charles DeLise and David Smith at the U.S. Department of Energy to begin a human genome project did garner governmental and scientific support, ultimately with the NIH jointly sponsoring the project with the Department of Energy. In 1987 the NIH made an initial appropriation of $17 million, and in 1990 Congress allocated $87 million for human genome research.

The organizers of the genome program recognized the ethical implications of gaining a genetic portrait of human beings – particularly James Watson, named as head of the NIH genome office created in 1988 and then as director of the National Center for Human Genome Research initiated in 1989. As a result of this recognition, a working group was created and funds dedicated for social, ethical, and legal research as part of the project. This research brought up issues such as: How will knowledge of human propensity for genetically determined illness influence employment and insurance coverage? Will it lead to wholesale discrimination in both? What right to such information does government have? Can the confidentiality of genetic data be assured? This new project has promised to make biological scientists more sensitive to the social significance of their work. As Paul Berg put it, "Judging the ethical value of basic research prospectively and preemptively would be a considerable departure from current practice."[19]

While scientists in the 1980s debated aspects of discovery that affect society, another set of events pointed to problems within the research community itself. In 1981 John Darsee, a medical scientist working in clinical and experimental cardiology, admitted to falsifying data in one of his papers. Darsee had published 18 research papers in major biomedical journals and about 100 abstracts, book chapters, and other works. Investigations at institutions where he worked – Emory and Harvard Universities and the NIH, which funded some of his studies – revealed that his fabrication was more widespread.

What troubled many was not only that Darsee had been dishonest but that his coauthors had not detected the flaws in his work before it was published. This led to concern about whether the responsibilities of authorship are sufficiently clear to members of the scientific community. It cast doubt on what Walter W. Stewart and Ned Feder, NIH scientists at the forefront of this discussion, called "the integrity of the scientific literature." In a 1987 article in *Nature* that produced much comment and controversy, they claimed that Darsee's coauthors had not been adequately vigilant, that in some cases the contributions of coauthors were minimal and not entitling authorship. For instance, one coauthor's role had been to encourage Darsee and provide grant support.[20]

Sensitized by the Darsee case, the scientific and lay press publicized several other instances of alleged improper conduct in research during the decade. One of the most prominent of these cases involved a Nobel laureate, David Baltimore. In 1986 he was one of the authors of a published article concerning genetic influences on the immune system; the main investigator was a colleague, Thereza Imanishi-Kari of Tufts University. Baltimore's role was that of a senior advisor who reviewed the paper's data and research but did not personally participate in the laboratory work on it. Following publication of the article, Dr. Margot O'Toole, a junior researcher in molecular biology at Tufts who questioned the validity of some of its experimental data, lost her job. The ensuing controversy about the facts and meaning of these events brought the case to the NIH and to the U.S. Congress. As a result, Baltimore was called to testify before a Congressional committee about the issue, and the laboratory notebooks of the experiment were even subpoenaed by the Secret Service.[21] Responding to this case, *The New York Times* published a lead editorial headlined, "A Scientific Watergate?" The newspaper pointed out that Baltimore, who was never accused of fabrication, and several committees of scientists had investigated the affair and found no basic problems, yet a draft report by the federal investigators involved in the case did find problems. The *Times* faulted the scientific community's mechanisms for investigating such controversies.[22]

These events led, as had revelations of problems in human experiments in the 1960s, to a review of procedures of research. One of the earliest outcomes of this examination was a careful look at the duties of scientific authorship. While the subject had been discussed before, it had never received the focused attention of investigators that it did in the mid-1980s. For example, in a 1986 article Edward J. Huth, editor of the *Annals of Internal Medicine*, defined what he called "unjustifiable authorship," a situation in which authors cited in a paper lack basic involvement in its generation: that is, the gaining and analysis of the evidence, and the writing and revision of the findings.[23] Such action appeared to be a leading cause of the burgeoning number of papers cited on the vitae of scientists. Some scientists and, more emphatically, members of the public believed that this behavior, like the highly publicized cases of fraud, represented a breakdown in the fidelity of scientists to truth in the oversight and reporting of their investigations and that it thus damaged the scientific community as a whole.

But within the scientific community these discussions were received with mixed feelings. Many believed that it remained appropriate, for instance, for the persons who obtained the funds for a project to be named as authors. They pointed out that the stream of help and obligations that flows through a laboratory and touches many of its staff in the course of a study makes rigid criteria for defining authorship too difficult to devise or implement. Many preferred to determine themselves, on an ad hoc basis and with less rigidity, who should be given the credit of assistance that the title of author conveys.

These events and discussions prompted a number of private and public institutions such as Harvard University, the University of Texas Health Science Center at Houston, and the NIH, and professional societies and journals to publish corrective guidelines delineating the responsibilities of authorship.[24] They led also to two developments in 1989, which demonstrated a social and governmental interest in areas that before were the private preserve of the biological scientist: the oversight of scientific misconduct, and the teaching of students.

An announcement in the *Federal Register* of March 16, 1989, told of the establishment at the NIH of an Office of Scientific Integrity. Its task was to delineate for investigators the responsibilities of handling and reporting possible scientific misconduct, and of investigating it. The office defined such misconduct "as fabrications, falsification, plagiarism, or other practices that seriously deviate from those that are commonly accepted within the scientific community for proposing, conducting, or reporting research."[25] A parallel Office of Scientific Integrity Review was also established at this time in the Department of Health and Human Services (DHHS) under the purview of the Assistant Secretary of Health. These offices were created to carry out provisions of the 1985 Health Research Extension Act, which required all institutions receiving federal research grants to have an administrative process to examine reports of scientific fraud and to send details of serious cases to the Secretary of Health and Human Services.[26]

While some welcomed the introduction of a formal mechanism to deal with misconduct, others were concerned that because it came from government it was intimidating. An article by Bernard Davis, an emeritus professor at Harvard Medical School, titled "How Far Should Big Brother's Hand Reach?" expressed a widely held viewpoint within the scientific community. Davis was concerned that the office reached too deeply into the interstices of research and threatened its freedom. He thought that inadequate distinctions were being made between fraud and normal error and that the investigation of science by government authority could foster a repressive atmosphere that would cast a shadow over the environment of openness needed for creativity to thrive.[27]

Following this article, in December of 1989, a new administrative rule concerning teaching was placed in the NIH Guide for Contracts and Grants.[28] The rule stated that all institutions seeking National Research Service Award training grants were required to have "a program in the principles of scientific integrity" as an integral part of their efforts in researcher training. The subject matter of this program, it was suggested, could include material on conflict of interest, professional standards and codes of conduct, responsible authorship, issues of human and animal experimentation, and the recording and retention of data. The rule expressed a concern about integrity in the conduct of research and the hope that these efforts to train scientists in research ethics early in their career would be meliorative.

In the decade of the 1990s and up to the present, federal regulations concerning misconduct and teaching have continued to evolve. In 1992 the two federal offices that monitored scientific misconduct were consolidated and renamed the Office of Research Integrity (ORI), and the government established a mechanism through which scientists accused of misconduct could request a DHHS hearing on the charges against them. Of the over 1,500 allegations of misconduct handled by ORI from 1992 to 1999, some 300 were serious enough to require a formal ORI inquiry, which yielded misconduct findings in about 100 cases.[26]

Elaboration of federal policy on the teaching front also continued in this period. Reports of the National Academy of Sciences in 1992 and of the 1995 Commission on Research Integrity empaneled by DHHS reinforced the original intent of the 1989 NIH requirement while not significantly expanding it.[26] But such an expansion was recommended in 2000 by the U.S. Public Health Service (PHS). It announced a policy, which awaits action by the U.S. Congress, for an instruction program on the responsible conduct of research that would enlarge the scope of the research projects and the breadth of participants covered. The policy deals with all research conducted through PHS contracts or grants, including animal, human, and basic research as well as the research training activities to which the 1989 NIH teaching requirement had been directed. The new policy recommends that health care institutions provide ethical training for research staff not supported through the PHS and defines research staff broadly as people involved in proposing, reviewing, and reporting research. The goals of the policy are to improve the knowledge and decision-making abilities of participants to conduct research ethically, to enhance their understanding of federal policies and guidelines in the area, and to link governmental and educational institutions in an effort to elevate ethical abilities and sensibilities in the biohealth sciences. Nine core areas were identified on which to focus this education: data management, mentor and trainee responsibilities, authorship, peer review, collaboration, human subject research, animal research, research misconduct, and conflicts of interest and commitment. Implementation of this policy was projected to occur in 2002.[29]

The need for such learning was underscored during the 1990s and into the new millennium by the prominent ethical issues produced as knowledge of human biological development continued to unfold. Emblematic of these issues was the controversy surrounding research on human embryos.[30] In 1995 the U.S. Congress banned federal government funding of research in which human embryos were destroyed. However, in 2000 the Clinton Administration excluded stem cell research from the ban if no federally funded investigator had a role in obtaining the cells and thus destroying embryos. As soon as he took office, President George Bush had to decide whether or not to change the Clinton policy. The Presidents' open acknowledgment of the difficulties of this choice stimulated intense public discussion, which again demonstrated how closely science and ethics are entwined.

Embryonic stem cells, which have the capacity to develop into different cell and tissue types of the body, are thought to hold great promise in the treatment of a wide variety of diseases. But the question arose whether the moral standing of the embryo, considered by many individuals and religious traditions to have personhood from the moment of conception, should preclude this use. The embryos in question include among others those produced in laboratories through in vitro fertilization for couples seeking children and stored in freezers as unwanted extras from this process, those generated from eggs and sperm given by donors for the purpose of producing embryos for stem cell research, and the future possibility of generating embryos in laboratories specifically for therapy through the use of cloning technology. A key ethical issue is whether embryos created outside of the human body and so situated as never to have the chance to develop into people – the embryos sought for use in this research – should have the same moral weight as those developing within the body that can become people. Also ethically controversial is whether scientists should create human embryos for the sole purpose of research.

Complicating decision making on this issue is whether a credible scientific alternative to embryonic stem cells exists that would shield society from the ethical dilemmas of such embryo use. Stem cells can also be obtained from adults, but a number of scientists do not consider them as therapeutically valuable as those harvested from embryos. Should the embryo use decision be postponed until definitive scientific judgment is made on the significance of adult stem cells? Should investigation of both types of stem cells proceed simultaneously?

Such was the state of the debate when, on August 9, 2001, President Bush announced his decision: federal funds could be used to support stem cell research, but only with the cell lines from fertility clinic embryos donated before the time of this announcement.[31] He claimed that an NIH survey had identified some 60 available cell lines in laboratories around the world and that these were enough to meet current research needs. He thus sought to walk a narrow line between the parties in this debate by permitting federally funded research to go forward but limiting the further destruction of embryos to do so.

The weeks following this announcement brought a mixed reaction from the scientific community. Many scientists were relieved that some government funding remained available. Others were skeptical about the quality and readiness for use of the cell lines said to exist.[32] Some of the lines had been only recently established and were too new to evaluate for longevity. Others were held by private firms whose needs for control and profit might cause future problems. Further, most of the cell lines were grown in a mouse cell base that created an advantage and a problem. The base secreted an unknown factor that helped stem cells remain healthy but also created the risk of passing mouse viruses to human patients. This scientific feature of creating stem cell lines had not been examined in the discussion that preceded the presidential decision and appeared to take the public by surprise. The added danger it posed was a threat not only to human recipients of stem cells but to the development time of the research. Scientists now became bound to follow stringent Food and Drug Administration guidelines applied to the transplantation of animal tissue into humans. Stem cell research, with its dual effects on the work of the scientist and the welfare of society, demonstrates the crucial role that scientists should play in the public dialogue about the meaning and consequences of the advances they produce.

This phase of development uncovered ethical problems in the major procedural aspects of the work of the biohealth sciences, from its use of animal subjects to its authorship claims. Still, it seemed that many biohealth scientists and students had not yet integrated the ideas generated in the controversies of this period into the way they thought about and ran institutions. But with the series of education policies in this phase affirming that a formal examination of the ethical meanings of scientific work was important, a new pedagogic element in the development of the biohealth sciences had been introduced. The possibilities for new thinking about these issues seemed at hand.

Phase IV 2001-?: Turning Inward and Institutionalizing Ethical Discourse

The ethics movement in the biohealth sciences may now be entering a fourth phase, one that promises to enhance ethical self-awareness about research issues among scientists as education in ethics enters their institutions of learning. Evaluation of what has happened can help to determine where best to go from here. This process was started by challenges to the view that the biohealth sciences can be managed and directed essentially by the professional community of scientists. The creation of the Institutional Review Boards in 1966 in Phase I of the ethics movement, the Asilomar Conference of 1974 in Phase II, and the broad requirements for ethics education in Phase III are witness to society's efforts to join scientists in evaluating standards and setting goals. The sharing of authority with society, the voyage of the biohealth sciences from a private to a public enterprise, has been a key theme and issue of controversy in the events discussed.

The debate of the biohealth scientists among themselves and with others in society about the values that should undergird key functional activities in scientific research also has been a recurring theme that has been particularly strong in Phase III. This is mirrored in the attention given to evaluating the procedures that govern the keeping and reporting of evidence and the awarding of authorship. At the heart of the public's concern about these activities was the significance it attached to the fidelity of scientists to honestly obtain, record, evaluate, and reveal their findings and to seek to depict nature truthfully. Some members of the public thought that they could not trust scientists to use the funds given to them by society properly, or the conclusions generated by their work, if the rule of honesty seemed threatened.

While some scientists viewed this public concern as an intrusion and did not believe that significant problems existed, others became convinced that the issues were real and necessitated action. One result of this debate was the conclusion that informal attention to education in ethics is not enough. This conclusion led to the development of the 1989 and 2000 federal guidelines that advocated such education as a basic part of graduate studies and research work.

Opposition to such requirements coalesces about the view that the informal system of ethics education – observing and learning from mentors – remains adequate for the biohealth sciences. The same argument was heard during the modern medical ethics movement, a search for ethical precepts to guide practice among clinicians from different disciplines, which has run in time alongside the ethics movement in the biohealth sciences. The mentor-based argument failed to carry the day in clinical medicine because the ethical issues of patient care had grown too complex even for mentors to understand fully. Many clinicians reached the conclusion that scholars who were knowledgeable about ethics needed to join those learned in medicine in order to deal with the ethical questions of practice. A similar association between investigators and ethicists is needed now in the biohealth sciences to produce innovative educational formats and materials and to stimulate discourse on ethical issues arising in scientific work.

There are other parallels between the ethics movements in clinical medicine and in the biohealth sciences. In the medical ethics movement, the phase when medicine changed from a private calling to a public enterprise was followed by a period of self-reflection about the ethical bases of clinical practices and medicine's accountability to the public. As this self-reflection deepened, it stimulated the spread of course work and other institutional innovations in education such as ethics case rounds, which in turn caused this learning to be expressed in the policies and goals of medicine.

The question now exists whether the ethics movement in the biological sciences is evolving in this way or will continue to be driven by regulation, adopting educational interventions more as legal requirements to be met rather than ethical commitments to be honored and integrated into thoughts and actions of scientists. If this education initiative focuses scientists more on certification and less on responsibility, a great opportunity for professional enhancement of the people and institutions of the biological sciences will have been missed. I do not believe this will happen.

The movement now is entering a period in which it should, and I think will, encourage a greater sense of public accountability and self-reflection among scientists concerning the ethical parameters of actions and goals as well as institutional activities to further these developments. This activity should lead to efforts that clarify and increase the connections of the biohealth sciences with humanistic ideas and learning. It should produce more empirical and analytical research on the ethics of significant relationships in science such as those between students and teachers, researchers and funders, investigators and staff, and scientists and society. It should stir a closer examination of the institutions of the biohealth sciences – such as professional societies, research organizations, and schools – to clarify their goals and to assure that their policies do not create pressures that impede their constituents from meeting ethical responsibilities to science and society.[32] It should cause scientists to rethink the expectations and aims of their lives in science. It also should stimulate thought on how the scientific community should treat members involved in inappropriate ethical actions. No sound policy on these issues yet exists.

Conclusions

To realize the possibilities of Phase IV will require a decision by scientists to support change rather than to retain the status quo. Such a challenge is not new to science, which is perennially concerned with modification. A response to a shift in theory or technique that alters concepts and practices is continually demanded of scientists. But this situation can be difficult. Change can require new learning, disrupt research patterns, and shift institutional authority and social standing. The biohealth sciences now must consider whether a change of a kind they are not used to encountering is appropriate: to relinquish the view of science as a private professional enterprise to one that sees its activities as engaging the ideas and values of society and its institutions. Ideally, the research community will draw on its own experiences with scientific change so that it can wisely face these novel issues.

Some may find it tempting, comforting, and perhaps safer to argue that things should be left as they are. However, experiences from the medical ethics movement provide a perspective and encouragement for change. Like scientists now, clinicians felt highly uncomfortable when ethical issues arose in the 1960s concerning medical decisions such as whether to withdraw life support measures or perform abortions. Many doctors believed such decisions were personal matters and not proper issues to consider with experts outside the field of medicine or with the public, both of whom lacked the doctor's experience and knowledge. Gradually, physicians recognized that the significant ways in which society is affected by medicine required collaboration with it in discussing and defining medical problems and goals. Physicians further saw that the new ethical questions raised by advances in their own technology and in their new social relationships demanded a different experience, which they did not have. This was an expert experience in the analysis of ethical questions; in the organization and financing of health care services; and in defining the needs, values, and preferences of social institutions with which they now collaborated. As medicine has accommodated these experts into its fabric, it has emerged stronger and more able to deal with the new reality that its innovations in part created. This experience and outcome for medicine, difficult but salutary, offers the biohealth sciences an important reassurance as it charts its future course.

If the community of biohealth scientists comes to agree that change is appropriate and beneficial, then the educational efforts advocated by the NIH and the PHS can be shaped to give students and faculty the capacity to meet prospective problems. The subjects of such an education span matters from the ethical aspects of the relationships of scientists with colleagues in the work of research to the scientist's ethical obligations to society and the enterprise of science itself. Because ethics is the study of the right-making and wrong-making characteristics of action, significant features of this education involve discerning which ethical values can best serve as yardsticks to determine whether actions contemplated or taken in the biohealth sciences are right or wrong and learning how best to resolve ethical dilemmas.

Some examples of ethical values particularly relevant to the biohealth sciences are truthfulness, trustworthiness, stewardship, autonomy, and the avoidance of harm. Maintaining truthfulness as a characteristic of action is essential for scientists themselves and the public to remain open to ideas and conclusions presented by investigators and for the triumph of objectivity over bias and self-interest in science. Trust in the intentions, reliability, and honor of colleagues is necessary for the confidence it provides investigators to participate in the relationships essential for the interdependent enterprise that science is. Assuming a responsibility for safeguarding the beings, resources, and institutions used and influenced by science, embodied in the concept of stewardship, is relevant to issues that bear on how scientists should deal with the effects of their discoveries. Autonomy, or the ability to be free and self-governing, is a value that in science encourages inquiry and the creation of novel ideas. The value of avoiding harm to others is also important to an enterprise like science, which forges knowledge that produces significant power.

Ethical dilemmas arise when uncertainty exists about which ethical values are most cogent to the problem at hand, or when the relevant values are recognized but found to be in conflict with one another – for example, when pursuit of one value requires the others to be minimized or disregarded and participants must decide on the appropriate weights to give the conflicting values. In these situations, ethical analysis has as its aim delineating the balances and compromises that will produce for participants the best available choice under the given circumstances.[33]

Formal courses on the ethical dimensions of the biohealth sciences and discussions of the ethical aspects of scientific cases are the basic structures within which this education should take place. The two are complementary for ethical learning. Courses provide students with the methodological and analytical capabilities needed for ethical inquiry. Cases provide the material to which this rational approach can be applied. While the development of courses is familiar to the scientific community, the concept and formatting of case discussions generally are not.

A key aspect of the development of clinical medicine has been to record the experiences of patient care as cases. These cases provide data not only to advance knowledge but also to inform instruction.[34,35] In the medical ethics movement, ethics case discussions have been a valuable means to learn precisely what ethical problems exist in the care of patients through discussion to decide on a course of action and through record keeping to preserve important experiences otherwise lost to learning. Such case discussions that reflect the daily experiences of work and thinking in the scientific community could serve its research, education, and policy needs equally well.

This next phase of development in the biohealth sciences will produce new discoveries, but some will be of a different sort than those to which biohealth scientists are accustomed. Until this time biological scientists have single-mindedly explored the environment of nature. They must now turn their attention to the environment of their profession and focus their vision inward, on themselves.

References

1. Nuremberg Code. In: Trials of War Criminals Before the Nuremberg Military Tribunals Under Control Council Law. No. 10, Vol. 2. Washington, DC: U.S. Government Printing Office; 1949:181–182.
2. Reiser SJ. Human experimentation and the convergence of medical research and patient care. *Annals of the American Academy of Political and Social Sciences.* 1978; 8–18.
3. Curran WJ. Current legal issues in clinical investigation with particular attention to the balance between the rights of the individual and the needs of society. In: *Psychopharmacology: A Review of Progress, 1957–1967.* Washington, DC: U.S. Public Health Service; 1968:337–343. Publication no. 1836.
4. Katz J. *Experimentation with Human Beings.* New York: Russell Sage Foundation; 1972:9–65.
5. Aron R. The education of the citizen in industrial society. *Daedalus.* 1962; Spring: 253–258.
6. Reiser SJ. The public and the expert in biomedical controversies. In: *Biomedical Politics.* Washington, DC: National Academy Press; 1991:325–331.
7. Mendelsohn E, Swazey JP, Taviss I, eds. *Human Aspects of Biomedical Innovations.* Cambridge: Harvard University Press; 1971.
8. Taylor GR. *The Biological Time Bomb.* New York: The Wood Publishing Co; 1968.
9. Fletcher J. Ethical aspects of genetic controls: designed genetic changes in man. *N Engl J Med.* 1971;285:776–783.
10. Frederickson DS. Asilomar and recombinant DNA: The end of the beginning. In: *Biomedical Politics.* Washington, DC: National Academy Press; 1991:258–298.
11. Berg P. Baltimore D, Brenner S, Robin III R, and Singer MF. Asilomar Conference on recombinant DNA molecules. *Science.* 1975;188:791–794.
12. Nelkin D. Commentary. In: *Biomedical Politics.* Washington, DC: National Academy Press; 1991:299–301.
13. Singer P. *Animal Liberation: A New Ethics for Our Treatment of Animals.* New York: Discus; 1977.
14. Bulger RE. Use of animals in experimental research: a scientist's perspective. *The Anatomical Record.* 1987;210:215–220.
15. Blumenthal D, Gluck M, Louis KS, Wise D. Industrial support of university research in biotechnology. *Science.* 1986;231:242–246.

16. Blumenthal D, Gluck M, Louis KS, Stoto MA, Wise D. University-industry research relationships in biotechnology: implications for the university. *Science.* 1986;232:1361–1366.

17. Association of Academic Health Centers. *Conflicts of Interest in Academic Health Centers.* Washington, DC: Association of Academic Health Centers; 1990.

18. Cook-Deegan RM. The Human Genome Project: The formation of federal policies in the United States, 1986–1990. In: *Biomedical Politics.* Washington, DC: National Academy Press; 1991:99–168.

19. Berg P. Commentary. In: *Biomedical Politics.* Washington, DC: National Academy Press; 1991:171.

20. Stewart WW, Feder N. The integrity of the scientific literature. *Nature,* 1987;325:207–214.

21. Hilts PS. Hero in exposing science hoax paid dearly. *New York Times.* March 22, 1991; A1, B6.

22. A Scientific Watergate? *New York Times.* March 26, 1991; A14.

23. Huth EJ. Irresponsible authorship and wasteful publication. *Ann Intern Med.* 1986;104:257–259.

24. International Committee of Medical Editors. Guidelines on authorship. *BMJ.* 1985;291:722.

25. Hollum JV, Hadley SW. OSI: Why, what, and how. *ASM News.* 1990;56:647–651.

26. U.S. Department of Health and Human Services. *HHS Fact Sheet: Promoting Integrity in Research.* Rockville, MD: DHHS; October 22, 1999.

27. Davis BD. How far should Big Brother's hand reach? *ASM News.* 1990;56:643–646.

28. National Institutes of Health Guide, Requirement for Programs on the Responsible Conduct of Research in National Research Service Award Institutional Training Grants. Vol. 19. No. 30. August 17, 1990; 1.

29. Office of Research Integrity, U.S. Department of Health and Human Services. *PHS Policy on Instruction in the Responsible Conduct of Research.* Rockville, MD: DHHS; December 1, 2000.

30. Guernin LM. Morals and primordials. *Science.* 2001;2921:1659–1660.

31. Bush GW. Address on U.S. financing of embryonic stem cell research (excerpts). *New York Times.* August 10, 2001, A16.

32. Varmus H, Melton D. The stem cell compromise. *Wall Street Journal.* August 14, 2001, A14.

33. Bulger RE, Reiser SJ, eds. *Integrity in Health Care Institutions: Humane Environments for Teaching, Inquiry, and Healing.* Iowa City: University of Iowa Press; 1990.

34. Beauchamp TL, Childress JF. *Principles of Biomedical Ethics,* 5th ed. New York: Oxford University Press; 2001.

35. Reiser SJ. The clinical record in medicine, Part 1: Learning from cases. *Annals of Internal Medicine.* 1991;114:902–907.

36. Reiser SJ. Administrative case rounds: institutional policies and leaders cast in a different light. *JAMA.* 1991;266:2127–2128.

The Roots of Honor and Integrity in Science

The Roots of Honor and Integrity in Science

Historical Themes in the Practical Ethics of Research

Elizabeth Heitman

The essence of science is the pursuit, generation, and transmission of knowledge. The practical demands of these activities define an inherently moral social contract among researchers in which honesty, objectivity, and mutual trust are the standards of integrity and professional honor. Every scientist depends on the validity of others' work, whether as the foundation for new questions or as the conceptual framework in which new explanations are tested. Moreover, while individuals may conduct research, no single researcher can master every aspect of any issue – especially as multidisciplinary approaches become more common. Thus, the ethics of scientific research are based in practices designed to foster the growth of knowledge while reinforcing the bonds of the scientific community.

Much of the attention that has been paid to the ethics of life sciences research since the 1980s has focused on reports of misconduct and the threat of governmental intervention into the research process. Discussion of the ethics of scientific research in the 1980s and 1990s often illustrated unethical activities without providing more than a set of basic rules for accepted behavior against which to judge them.[1] Today, scientists, ethicists, and governmental agencies are all working to articulate the broader scope of research ethics and the demands of the responsible conduct of research.[2] It appears likely that the responsible conduct of research will itself grow into a multidisciplinary specialty field in much the same way that bioethics evolved in the 1970s and 1980s. Nonetheless, even as the responsible conduct of research emerges as an area of special expertise, it is essential for scientists and ethicists alike to recognize the ethical values and practical safeguards that have been intrinsic to modern science since its earliest stages.

Looking for the historical roots of ethical values in research presupposes a clear understanding of what is meant by *ethics*. Much of the governmental attention to the responsible conduct of research has addressed ethics in terms of the identified professional norms and practice standards of science. For example, the federal Office of Research Integrity (ORI) defines integrity in research as "adherence to rules, regulations, guidelines, and commonly accepted professional codes or norms."[3] While it is clearly important to understand and follow available guidelines and stated rules and norms, it is one of the ironies of history that clear ethical standards are usually not articulated until *after* ethical controversy demonstrates a need for them. As Stanley Reiser noted in the preceding section, efforts to promote education and research in research integrity have typically resulted from scandals over research misconduct and debates about the scope and severity of wrongdoing. Ideally, current attention to the responsible conduct of research will not only identify standards in areas where misconduct has occurred but also consider disputed areas of practice in which achieving consensus might prevent harmful controversy.

Among ethicists, the term *ethics* is most widely understood as a branch of philosophy or theology that systematically considers the bases for judging right and wrong. Ethics addresses both the responsibilities and obligations that individuals have to each other and the characteristics and behaviors that individuals and groups should adopt in order to live well together. Thus, ethics typically involves analysis of the values, choices, and actions of a community as well as its individual members. Many courses in applied ethics begin with an introduction to prominent theories and analytic methods of philosophical ethics and examine practical moral questions in light of these theories and frameworks. Courses and textbooks in professional ethics often complement this approach with consideration of the ethical basis of the concept of profession and the content of the codes of ethics that many professional groups have adopted.

Life sciences researchers cannot claim a distinct historic tradition of professionalism nor an explicit code of ethics as the basis of a contemporary moral framework for research except to the extent that physician researchers can look to the ethical traditions of medicine for guidance. However, there are other means of recognizing a group's code of behavior apart from what has been written down. The linguistic origins of both the terms *ethics* and *morals* reflect the traditional view that ethics is an extension of a group's *customs* or *mores*, the regular practices, activities, and collective rituals that give structure and purpose to the daily lives of its members. An *ethos* is generally made up of the principles that shape those customs. Like its customs, a group's ethics reflects its sense of communal identity, its aspirations, and its fears. Historians, social scientists, and ethicists are now beginning to analyze the ethical tradition that has developed from the regularized practices of scientific research and the customs of the scientific community.

The Scientific Method and the Community of Science

Historians of science can easily point to significant changes in the self-definition of the life sciences since they blossomed in the 1700s. Prior to the 1800s, life scientists understood their work as the description of nature, its processes, and its purposes. The important achievements of this era included vast collections of specimens and the generation of catalogues that both described and classified life forms and other natural phenomena as parts of an intricate and elegant created universe. Close and repeated examination of diverse natural phenomena and detailed record keeping were the essence of good science. Careful observation and discernment were considered to be the pinnacle of scientific technique.

Individual scientists built their reputations on the scope, detail, and careful documentation of their observations and the extent to which their interpretations of the natural world could be seen as rational deductions from observed facts. Natural scientists in this period were particularly concerned *not* to impose themselves on their work. Rather, they believed that their responsibility was to report what they saw as dispassionate recorders of fact and to offer purely rational interpretations of those observations. The unifying assumption behind the life sciences was that an intelligent Creator had imposed order on the universe – an order that scientists could understand and describe. This presupposition did not result from scientific observation but rather from the predominantly Christian religious beliefs of the society of which early life scientists were a part.

By the beginning of the nineteenth century, the relatively passive approach to the life sciences gave way to new efforts to understand nature's complexity through experimentation.

Inspired by the success of experimental methods in chemistry and physics, life scientists in the 1800s increasingly sought to understand the mechanisms and principles of nature by manipulating and testing them. However, the development of experimental methods posed new challenges to scientists' discernment and reason. Intervention in natural processes carried an increased risk that subjectivity and unseen factors could affect the experimentalist's observations of nature and subsequent conclusions, contaminating the essential truths of science with human bias.

Thus, in the early modern era the early life sciences adopted a rudimentary scientific method, based in researchers' foundational commitment to objectivity and truthful description. Experimental science required them not only to be truthful in their observations but also meticulous and self-critical in developing and validating their experimental procedures. In the second half of the 1800s, researchers increasingly focused on standardizing the process of experimentation, including how the experiment was devised and carried out, how the results were tested, how these outcomes compared with what was expected, and what constituted adequate proof to support the researcher's hypothesis. As in chemistry and physics, the reproducibility of individual experiments, most particularly their reproducibility by *other* researchers, became a hallmark of good science. The traditional dependence on individual scientists' discernment and objectivity evolved into reliance on the group's critical assessment, and the need for collegial interaction created a skeptical, self-correcting community.

The contemporary scientific method is both an individualized and a communal process. It requires not only that the researcher identify and test a clear hypothesis based on careful observation and rational analysis but also that this work be subjected to further testing and verification by peers. It is the responsibility of the community to challenge the theoretical underpinnings, methodology, findings, and conclusions of any research before accepting it as legitimate. Today's scientific community is said to work as an "invisible boot," kicking out invalid or inadequate work. Bentley Glass, in the first essay in this section, outlines the social contract that supports the scientific community in this role. Glass observes that, because everyone is capable of error, scientists must approach their own research critically and that of others with an open mind. Because all scientists must rely on their colleagues to verify, interpret, and expand upon their work, researchers must report their findings openly. For Glass, collegial interaction, including competition among researchers, ideally should enhance the integrity of science.

The Goal of Objectivity and the Fear of Self-Deception

This social contract also reflects the difficulty of achieving its underlying vision of scientific integrity. As a communal practice, the scientific method speaks not only to the scientific community's commitment to the goals of objectivity and the truthful depiction of nature but also to its fear of the threat that error and self-deception pose to every scientific undertaking. The scientific method is intended to limit the risks of error and self-deception by institutionalizing skepticism and self-criticism through such procedural safeguards as the use of control groups, blinding, statistical analysis, and peer review. It challenges researchers to prove that a hypothesis must be true by testing it exhaustively to eliminate other options and then subjecting their work to the scrutiny and replication of others not involved in original investigation. As sociologist of science Robert Merton has described it, the scientific method provides an unrivaled form of "rigorous policing."[4]

Researchers throughout history have had good reason to be concerned about the dangers of self-deception. Scientists' uncritical acceptance of irrational conclusions in the face of overwhelming conflicting evidence, as well as the occasional collective delusion of large numbers of researchers, has been a recurrent source of embarrassment to the scientific community. In *Betrayers of the Truth*, a far-reaching analysis of misconduct in science, journalists William Broad and Nicholas Wade portray researchers' gullibility and openness to deception as a much more serious threat to the integrity of science than overt fraud could ever be. Their chapter "Self-Deception and Gullibility," included later in this section, traces many of the more famous historical cases of self-deception among scientists, including cases in which self-deception devastated professional reputations and careers.

Broad and Wade conclude in part that even the most rigorous application of the scientific method may not prevent researchers from drawing unreasonable conclusions or accepting illogical assertions as the truth. Throughout history, an assortment of biases and contextual influences has shaped researchers' work and interpretation of their findings. Researchers' belief in their own objectivity as scientists appears to make them particularly susceptible to self-delusion as well as to deceit by others. Through the discussion of historical cases, Broad and Wade illustrate that the most insidious influences on researchers' objectivity are eagerness to make an important discovery and enthusiasm for a specific hypothesis. They conclude that "even the most rigorous training in objective observation is a feeble defense against the desire to obtain a particular result."[5]

Sources of Self-Deception and Threats to the Integrity of Research

Many of the forces that led prominent researchers into self-deception in the past are still very much a feature of twenty-first century science. While it may not be possible to eliminate the threat that they pose, understanding the factors that may predispose scientists to self-deception can help individual investigators recognize and minimize their effects as well as assist the scientific community in guarding against them in the future.

Experimenter Expectancy

As illustrated by Broad and Wade, one of the greatest obstacles to objectivity in research is the human tendency to take pride in one's work. The joy of discovery may be easily transformed into a desire to discover something of note – especially when a researcher's work appears to be promising or receives public acclaim. Young scientists are often warned not to fall in love with their hypotheses because dedication to a single answer may blind even the most skilled researcher to the shortcomings of an approach or technique. Personal, institutional, and even national pride have been common features in cases of expectancy bias in which inaccurate observations and false conclusions appeared to support the hopes and prejudices of the researchers and their communities.

Expectancy bias may also take more systemic forms. As philosopher of science Thomas Kuhn described in his classic work *The Structure of Scientific Revolutions*,[6] the range of "acceptable" questions, answers, and interpretations of data is established by traditional paradigms that define the explanatory frameworks in which legitimate science may operate. Such paradigms and the specific beliefs that support them often dictate how new findings should be viewed and whether new ideas are received as creative variations of established work or as pseudoscience that fails to meet the theoretical or methodological standards of the field.

Methodological Conceptions

Like Kuhn, sociologist Bernard Barber has observed that scientists are often resistant to novelty and that the research community's claim to open-mindedness is limited by a number of substantive concepts and methodological preconceptions.[7] Citing the initial rejection of Mendelian genetics and the germ theory of disease as prime examples of this resistance, Barber maintains that researchers may reject important discoveries or even fail to recognize obvious new insights because they are committed to theories and conceptual frameworks in which such discoveries do not make sense. Moreover, even when researchers do recognize the potential of new discoveries, they may also consciously shape their work to conform to prevailing conceptual and methodological standards – especially in order to have their work published in mainstream journals. Because publication is essential to the development of any line of research, questions and findings that would not be publishable are often ignored or neglected.

Similarly, scientists' reliance on established models in the interpretation of their work may lead them to reject new ideas and experimental findings that cannot be expressed in terms of a model that they recognize. Barber's example of biologists' initial resistance to the introduction of mathematical models in the early 1900s provides a particularly ironic example of methodological bias in light of the vital role that statistical significance now plays in validating biomedical research. Whereas biological scientists at the turn of the century harbored "anti-mathematical preconceptions," the work of today's life science researchers often reflects the assumption that statistical analysis is essential to scientific investigation.

Like other methodological presuppositions, the assumption that counting, measurement, and other mathematical processes are inherently objective may itself introduce bias into a researcher's analysis or disguise biases already at work. As a human enterprise, mathematics is not value free. Numbers have powerful symbolic value in every culture.[8] Even in direct measurement, mathematical systems may be subject to human biases. Certain numbers' association with bad luck and death, good luck and prosperity, or completeness and balance may affect researchers' observations and calculations in subtle ways. Moreover, even how something is measured may be affected by cultural attitudes toward numbers or mathematical systems. U.S. scientists' ambivalence toward the metric system and cultural resistance to its widespread adoption in the United States may lead to confusion and error in many endeavors. The catastrophic effects of such error in scientific projects was publicly emphasized in September 1999, when NASA engineers mixed English and metric units in their calculation of the Mars Climate Orbiter's trajectory into Martian orbit, sending the probe crashing into the planet.

Statisticians themselves are also quick to point out the possible abuses of statistical methods and mathematical tests by individuals and groups who seek to legitimate questionable research. John C. Bailar III, whose essay on statistics and deception in science is included in Section III, identifies eight common ways in which statistics can be misused to give deceptive conclusions.[9] The American Statistical Association's *Ethical Guidelines for Statistical Practice* directs statisticians to "guard against the possibility that a predisposition by investigators or data providers might predetermine the analytic result." The guidelines offer a comprehensive series of professional standards for statistical practice that are intended to limit methodological biases.[10]

Religious and Political Views

In the premodern world, when science was clearly in the service of religion, the fundamental premises, models, and questions of natural science in the West were indelibly shaped by the Judeo–Christian worldview of nature as a creation of a rational, all-powerful God. When natural science moved away from its religious foundations in the 1800s, the scope of the questions that researchers began to address grew tremendously. The fundamental premises and models were somewhat slower to change, however, for the entire conceptual framework of the West was shaped by deep, often unconscious, Christian religious convictions. Yet, Barber notes that historically it has not been the religious forces external to science that have posed the greatest resistance to scientific discovery but rather the religious beliefs and presuppositions of scientists themselves.

Darwin's theory of evolution has undoubtedly generated more scientific debate and resistance than any development in the life sciences. The scientific community, and later most mainline Christian traditions, ultimately came to respect Darwin's observations and accept his conclusions. Moreover, in the 1960s and 1970s, many religious scholars concluded that apparently contradictory statements of religious truth and scientific truth could coexist because religion and science address different dimensions of knowledge. However, since the 1980s, there has been a resurgence of resistance to the theory of evolution among conservative Christian scientists.[11] Their efforts to restore the concept of an intelligent Creator to the conceptual framework of natural science has met with mixed results in the academic world but is increasingly well received by the lay public. While public sentiment has few immediate consequences for research, it can be quite influential in shaping public science policy and, more important, how science education defines legitimate science. The full effects of the growing support for the intelligent design theory may not be evident until members of the current generation of school children enter college and consider careers in the life sciences.

Barber's observations about the effects of religious belief on scientific inquiry also hold true for the effects of politics. When science serves the state, the state's views of meaningful research may shape both the research agenda and definition of good science. The corruption of German medical research by Nazi racism is a horrifying example of how political motives can completely overwhelm scientific objectivity and intellectual freedom.[12] Researchers may also be rewarded or punished for their personal allegiance and commitments to particular political regimes. In the post–World War II United States, government officials sought to identify scientists with any affiliation with the Communist party in order to exclude them from funded research opportunities. In contrast, during that same period, researchers in many Communist countries were expected to be members of the Communist party as a function of their importance to society. Irrespective of how Communist beliefs themselves might shape the conduct and outcome of specific studies, the perceived trustworthiness of scientists and the value of their research were clearly affected by political considerations.

Professional Standing, Affiliation, and Specialization

Barber's final sources of resistance to objective scientific discovery relate to the researcher's own position in the scientific community, both in terms of academic credentials and seniority, as well as specialization and area of expertise. Researchers' institutional affiliations (academic or commercial, general university or academic medical center, private or public institution), positions within these institutions (full professor or postdoctoral fellow), and status in scientific professional organizations have implications for the presumed quality of their research. Professional standing often confers authority on ideas and data that might be dismissed as unimportant if they came from other sources. Conversely, brilliant insights may be discounted if their author is unknown. Barber contends that Mendel's groundbreaking genetics work was ignored by leading European botanists because he was an obscure German monk whom they considered to be "an insignificant provincial."[7] Assumptions about the possibility of good research coming from nontraditional sources continue to delay the consideration of significant new findings today as well.

Barber also notes that even the valuable work of well-trained, experienced researchers from prestigious institutions may face resistance if the investigators come from specialties other than those traditionally considered to have authority over a given issue. The differences in training among researchers from different specialties may foster mistrust and anxiety about others' grasp of central concepts and thus the quality of their work. Just as nineteenth century physicians rejected Pasteur's germ theory because they discounted his understanding of disease, a true innovation may be rejected by traditionalists when an outsider approaches a familiar problem from an unfamiliar direction.

Some potential examples of this effect are evident in contemporary scientific controversies. The work of 1954 Chemistry Nobel Prize winner Linus Pauling[13] on the positive health effects of vitamin C is widely heralded by lay readers and practitioners of alternative medicine but is harshly criticized by physicians and dieticians. Similarly, life scientists from many different fields have rejected astrophysicist and cosmologist Sir Fred Hoyle's[14] work supporting the concept of *panspermia* (the seeding of ancient Earth with genetic material from space) and his argument that such human scourges as the influenza virus and the cockroach originated in outer space. While both Pauling and Hoyle have made brilliant contributions to the physical sciences, among life sciences researchers their names are often linked to pseudoscience. If their "outrageous" ideas are one day validated by mainstream research, the change will likely stem from shifts in the standard methods and questions of cancer biology, virology, and entomology rather than reconfiguration of the data.

Conclusions

The growing field of research integrity is in many ways the latest expression of a tradition that defines good science in terms of its processes as well as its products. The integrity of individual scientists and that of the scientific enterprise as a whole clearly depends on researchers' adherence to procedural rules and concern for the legitimacy of methods and data. But, as seen throughout the history of the modern life sciences, integrity also demands the scientific community's ongoing consideration of why customary practices are standard. Continual examination of its communal goals is essential to the health and growth of the scientific community – especially in times of complexity and change. Often the answers to new ethical questions have precedents in history, and a critical historical perspective can highlight the strengths and weaknesses of proposed solutions to recurrent challenges to the integrity of science.

Ideas that have been transmitted through history reinforce the bonds of the scientific community over time and provide the foundation for new growth. The readings included in this book offer signposts through the history of thought on the responsible conduct of research as well as insights into the ethical standards of science today. Readers are encouraged to examine these readings for patterns and trajectories in the practical ethical commitments of research and to consider how they shape both the past and the future integrity of the biological and health sciences.

References

1. Reiser SJ. Overlooking ethics in the search for objectivity and misconduct in science. *Acad Med.*1993;68 (Suppl.):S84–S87.
2. Macrina FL. *Scientific Integrity: An Introductory Text with Cases*, 2nd ed. Washington, DC: ASM Press; 2000.
3. Office of Research Integrity. *Research on Research Integrity*, RFA-NS-02–005. May 7, 2001.
4. Merton RK. The normative structure of science. In: NW Storer, ed. *The Sociology of Science. Theoretical and Empirical Investigations.* Chicago: University of Chicago Press; 1973.
5. Broad W, Wade N. *Betrayers of the Truth.* New York: Simon & Schuster;1982:107.
6. Kuhn T. *The Structure of Scientific Revolutions.* Chicago: University of Chicago Press; 1970.
7. Barber B. Resistance by scientists to scientific discovery. *Science.* 1961;134:596–602.
8. Schimmel A, Carl F. *The Mystery of Numbers.* New York: Oxford University Press; 1994.
9. Bailar JC III. Science, statistics, and deception. *Ann Int Med.* 1986;104:259–260.
10. American Statistical Association. *Ethical Guidelines for Statistical Practice.* Alexandria, VA: ASA, Aug. 7, 1999. Available at http://amstat.org
11. Dembski WA, Behe MH. *Intelligent Design: The Bridge Between Science & Theology.* Downers Grove, IL: InterVarsity Press;1999.
12. Lifton RJ. *The Nazi Doctors: Medical Killing and the Psychology of Genocide.* New York: Basic Books;1986.
13. Pauling L. *How to Live Longer and Feel Better.* New York: W.H. Freeman; 1986.
14. Hoyle F. *Diseases from Space.* New York: Harper & Row; 1980.

The Ethical Basis of Science

Bentley Glass

It has been said that science has no ethical basis, that it is no more than a cold, impersonal way of arriving at the objective truth about natural phenomena. This view I wish to challenge, since it is my belief that by examining critically the nature, origins, and methods of science we may logically arrive at a conclusion that science is ineluctably involved in questions of values, is inescapably committed to standards of right and wrong, and unavoidably moves in the large toward social aims.

Human values have themselves evolved. Man arose after some two billions of years of organic evolution, during which species after species originated, flourished, and fell, or occasionally became the progenitors of species that were new and better adapted, on the basis of the evolutionary scheme of values. Fitness, like it or not, in the long run meant simply the contribution of each trait and its underlying genes to survival. High mortality or sterility led to extinction; good viability and fertility enabled a gene or a trait, an individual or a species, to be perpetuated. Man's own values grew out of his evolutionary origins and his struggle against a hostile environment for survival. His loss of certain unnecessary structures, such as bodily hair once clothing was invented; the homeostatic regulation of his body temperature and blood pressure, breathing, and predominant direction of blood flow; his embryonic and fetal growth inside the mother and his prolonged dependence upon maternal lactation; the slow maturation that enabled his brain to enlarge so greatly; the keen vision so necessary to the hunter using his weapons – all of these and many other important human characteristics that contributed to the social nature of man and cemented the bonds of family and tribe arose adventitiously, were improved step by step, and endured because they promoted human survival. Our highest ethical values – the love of the mother for her child and of the man for his mate, the willingness to sacrifice one's own life for the safety of the family or tribe, and the impulse to care for the weak, the suffering, the helpless – all of these too had the same primitive beginnings.

But these ethical values are always, in the evolutionary scheme of things, relative, and never absolute. Whenever the environment becomes changed, the adaptiveness of existing traits becomes maladjusted, and the forces of natural selection lead to a realignment of the genotype, an alteration of the external features and modes of behavior, a modification of the species. What was once good is so no longer. Something else, in terms of reproductive fitness, has become better.

Finally, a crude, embryonic form of science entered the scheme of things, a method of observing and reporting accurately to other persons the movements of the stars, the planets, and the sun and moon, the behavior and migrations of the food animals, the usefulness of certain seeds for food and of certain stems for fibers, the poisonous properties of others. For generations all such practical lore was transmitted only by word of mouth, but the day came when useful knowledge could be written down and preserved inviolate from the forgetfulness and the twists of memory. These were the first simple steps in the development of science: observation, reporting, written records, communication. To such must be added the processes of human reasoning, at first mostly by analogy, so often wrong; then by improved analysis, by deduction from an established truth, or by induction of an established truth from a multitude of observations.

Seen aright, science is more than the instrument of man's increasing power and progress. It is also an instrument, the finest yet developed in the evolution of any species, for the malleable adaptation of man to his environment and the adjustment of his environment to man. If the human species is to remain successful, this instrument must be used more and more to control the nature and the rate of social and technological change, as well as to promote it. In this sense, at least, science is far more than a new sense organ for comprehending the real relations of natural phenomena and the regularities we call "laws of nature." It is also man's means of adjustment to nature, man's instrument for the creation of an ideal environment. Since it is preeminently an achievement of social man, its primary function is not simply that of appeasing the individual scientist's curiosity about his environment – on the contrary it is that of adjusting man to man, and of adjusting social groups in their entirety to nature, to both the restrictions and the resources of the human environment.

Ethics is a philosophy of morals, a moral system that defines duty and labels conduct as right or wrong, better or worse. The evolutionist is quite prepared to admit the existence of right and wrong in terms of the simple functions of biological structures and processes. The eye is for seeing, an evolutionary adaptation that enables an animal to perceive objects at a distance by means of reflected light rays. Sight conveys information about food, water, danger, companionship, mating, the whereabouts and doings of the young ones, and other vitally important matters. Should one not then say, "To see is right; not to see is wrong"? Similarly, the mind reasons as it does because in the countless ages of evolutionary development its characteristic mental processes led to successful coping with the exigencies of life. Humans whose mental processes, because of different genes, too often led them to wildly erroneous conclusions did not so often leave children to reason in similar ways. It is thus right to be guided by reason, wrong to distrust it. Does it not follow, finally, from consideration of the social role and function of science, that it is *right* to utilize science to develop and regulate human social life, adjustment to change, and rate of social transformation? Conversely, it is *wrong* – morally and ethically wrong – not to do so. We must use whatever light and whatever reason we have to chart our course into the unknown.

Those who distrust science as a guide to conduct, whether individual or social, seem to overlook its pragmatic nature, or perhaps they scorn it for that very reason. Rightly understood, science can point out to us only probabilities of varying degrees of certainty. So, of course, do our eyes and ears, and so does our reason. What science can do for us that otherwise we may be too blind or self-willed to recognize is to help us to see that what is right enough for the individual may be wrong for him as a member of a social group, such as a family; that what is right for the family may be wrong for the nation; and that what is right for the nation may be wrong for the great brotherhood of man. Nor should one stop at that point. Man as a species is a member – only one of many members – of a terrestrial community and an even greater totality of life upon earth. Ultimately, what is right for man is what is right for the entire community of life on earth. If he wrecks that community, he destroys his own livelihood. In this sense, coexistence is not only necessary but also right, and science can reveal to us the best ways to harbor our resources and to exploit our opportunities wisely.

The Subjectivity of Science

From the foregoing description of science as itself an evolutionary product and a human organ produced by natural selection, it may already be guessed that I do not adhere to the view that either the processes or the concepts of science are strictly objective. They are as objective as man knows how to make them, that is true; but man is a creature of evolution, and science is only his way of looking at nature. As long as science is a *human* activity, carried on by individual men and by groups of men, it must at bottom remain inescapably subjective.

Our sensory apparatus and the structure of the human nervous system, within which arise our sensations, grow and develop as they do from the first beginnings in the human embryo because of the particular genetic constitutions we inherit from our parents. First and foremost, we are *human* scientists, not insect scientists, nor even monkey scientists. The long past of our evolutionary history, with its countless selections and rejections of various kinds of genes and combinations of genes, has made us what we are. Try as we will, we cannot break the bonds of our subjective interpretations of the physical events of nature. We are born blind to many realities, and at best can apprehend them only by translating them by means of our instruments into something we can sense with our eyes or ears, into something we can then begin to reason about by developing abstract mental concepts about them, by making predictions on the basis of our hypotheses, and by testing our theories to see whether reality conforms to our notions.

This line of reasoning leads us to the conclusion that the objectivity of science depends wholly upon the ability of different observers to agree about their data and their processes of thought. About quantitative measurements and deductive reasoning there is usually little dispute. Qualitative experiences like color, or inductive and theoretical types of reasoning, leave great room for disagreement. Usually they can be reduced to scientific treatment only if the subjective color can by agreement be translated into some quantitative measurement such as a wavelength, only if the reasoning can be rendered quantitative by use of a calculus of probability. It nevertheless remains a basic fact of human existence that the subjectivity of the individual personality cannot be escaped. We differ in our genes, each of us possessing a genotype unique throughout all past and future human history (unless we happen to possess an identical twin). To the extent that our genes endow us with similar, though not identical, sensory capacities and nervous systems, we may make similar scientific observations, and we may agree to ignore the existence of the variables in our natures that prevent us from ever making exactly the same measurements as someone else or arriving at exactly the same conclusions. But it is perilous to forget our genetic individuality and our own uniqueness of experience. These form the basis of the ineradicable subjectivity of science. In the last analysis science is the common fund of agreement between individual interpretations of nature. What science has done is to refine and extend the methods of attaining agreement. It has not banished the place of the individual observer, experimenter, or theoretician, whose work is perhaps subjective quite as much as objective.

These considerations may seem so obvious as not to require the emphasis just given them. Yet I believe not. Somehow there has crept into our writings about the nature and methods of science a dictum that science is objective while the humanistic studies are subjective, that science stands outside the nature of man. What a profound mistake! Science is ultimately as subjective as all other human knowledge, since it resides in the mind and the senses of the unique individual person. It is constrained by the present evolutionary state of man, by the limitations of his senses and by the even more significant limitations of his powers of reason. All that can be claimed for science is that it focuses upon those primary observations about which human observers (most of them) can agree, and that it emphasizes those methods of reasoning which, from empirical results or the successful fulfillment of predictions, most often lead to mental constructs and conceptual schemes that satisfy all the requirements of the known phenomena.

Science, Integrity, and Intellectual Freedom

From a consideration that science is a human activity, inescapably subjective, and a product of biological evolution, it is possible to derive a genuine ethical basis of science. J. Bronowski, in an essay entitled "The Sense of Human Dignity" (*1*, p. 63), has sketched a treatment that serves well for a beginning. The values and duties which are the concern of ethics are social, he affirms. The duties of men hold a society together, he says; and "the problem of values arises only when men try to fit together their need to be social animals with their need to be free men." Philosophy must deal with both the social and individual aspects of value. Most philosophical systems have found this very difficult to do. Thus dialectical materialism swings far to the side of social values and leaves little scope for individual freedom. Positivism and analytic philosophy, as typified by Bertrand Russell and Wittgenstein, on the other hand, emphasize the values of the individual.

Hence, continues Bronowski, because the unit of the positivist or the analyst is one individual man, "positivists and analysts alike believe that the words *is* and *ought* belong to different worlds, so that sentences constructed with *is* usually have a verifiable meaning, but sentences constructed with *ought* never have" (*1*, p. 72).

The issue, then, is simply whether verification can indeed be assumed to be carried out by one man. Bronowski concludes, and I find it impossible to deny, that in the practice of science this supposition is sheer nonsense. Verification depends completely on the existence of records that may be consulted, of instruments that may be used, of concepts that must be understood and be properly utilized. In all these ways, knowledge is a social construct, science a collective human enterprise, and verification is no procedure of the naked, unlettered, resourceless man but an application of the collective tools of the trade and the practiced logic of science to the matter at hand. It is a fallacy to assume that one can test what is true and what is false unaided. But then it must follow that all verification, all science, depends upon communication with others and reliance upon others. Thus we come straight to the *ought* of science, for we must be able to trust the word of others. A full and true report is the hallmark of the scientist, a report as accurate and faithful as he can make it in every detail. The process of verification depends upon the ability of another scientist, of any other scientist who wishes to, to repeat a procedure and to confirm an observation.

Neither the philosophy of dialectical materialism nor that of the individualist accords with the basic nature of man and of scientific truth. The extreme social position leaves no room for the conscience of man and the exercise of intellectual freedom because the community dictates what is right and what a man *ought* to do. Yet the positivist's position is also faulty because "how a man *ought* to behave is a social question, which always involves several people; and if he accepts no evidence and no judgment except his own, he has no tools with which to frame an answer" (*1*, p. 72). Again, "All this knowledge, all our knowledge, has been built up communally; there would be no astrophysics, there would be no history, there would not even be language, if man were a solitary animal" (*1*, p. 73).

"What follows?" asks Bronowski, and answers (*1*, p. 73): "It follows that we must be able to rely on other people; we must be able to trust their word. That is, it follows that there is a principle which binds society together, because without it the individual would be helpless to tell the true from the false. This principle is truthfulness. If we accept truth as a criterion, then we have also to make it the cement to hold society together." Whence he derives the social axiom:

"We OUGHT to act in such a way that what IS true can be verified to be so."

So Bronowski. If his reasoning be accepted, and to me it seems unarguable, we must conclude that the cement of society is nothing less than the basic ethical tenet of science itself. The very possibility of verification, the assurance that one's own conclusions are not dreams, hallucinations, or delusions rests upon confirmation by others, by "competent" observers whom we trust to tell the truth.

The Scientist's Integrity

Ethics rests upon moral integrity. Science rests upon the scientist's integrity. This is so implicit in all of our science that it is rarely expressed and may be overlooked by novice or layman. Bronowski mentions examples of what happens when this basic moral commandment is violated by a scientist. Lysenko is held up to scorn throughout the world and eventually is deposed (*2*). Kammerer commits suicide (*3*). It is very interesting that both of these notorious examples, and others less well known, such as that of Tower, a quondam professor of biology at the University of Chicago, have related to attempts to "prove" or bolster the theory of the inheritance of acquired characteristics. The singular attractiveness of this theory for violators of scientific integrity is no doubt owing to its social significance, since if true it would offer a quick and easy way for man to control the direction of human evolution and would lessen the obdurate qualities of genes modifiable only by mutation in uncontrollable directions.

It is not so generally recognized by these superficial evolutionary philosophers that, if true, the inheritance of characters produced through modifications of the environment would call in question the value of all evolutionary gains, since the modified characters would themselves have no real genetic permanence and would shift and vary with every change of environment. They also do not recognize one of the most essential aspects of heredity: the protection of the genetic nature against vicissitudes. The reason why death is so necessary a part of life is that the ground must be cleared for fresh life. The reason why the genotype must remain unmodifiable by ordinary environmental causes is because the course of life for every individual involves the cumulative effects of injury, disease, and senescence. The new generation must indeed start *fresh* – that is, free from all the disabilities incurred during life by its parents and remoter ancestors. Evolution through the action of natural selection upon mutations, most of which are harmful and nonadaptive, while only a rare exemplar among them is possibly advantageous, is a process slow in the extreme. But it preserves the gains of the past, and it permits every generation to be born anew, unburdened by decrepitude, to try out its varieties of genotypes in each niche of the environment.

The loss of scientific integrity through deliberate charlatanry or deception is less common than the violation of scholarly honesty through plagiarism. The theft of another man's ideas and the claim that another's discovery is one's own may do no injury to the body of scientific knowledge, if the substance of what is stolen be true. It may even do no harm to the original discoverer, who may be dead or in no need of further credit to advance his own career. It is nevertheless a canker in the spirit of the thief and does damage to the fabric of science by rendering less trustworthy the witness of the scientist.

Plagiarism shades into unacknowledged borrowing. Which of us in fact can render exactly the sources of all his ideas? Psychologists have now amply demonstrated the ease with which self-deception enters into the forgetfulness of borrowed benefits. The wintry wind of man's ingratitude blows only on the donor of benefits forgot. Around the self-deluded recipient blow only the mildest, gentlest zephyrs of spring. The newer patterns of scientific publication and support of research have multiplied a thousandfold the opportunities for the scientist's self-deception. Editors of scientific journals today customarily rely upon referees for opinions regarding the merit of manuscripts submitted for publication. The enormous expansion of scientific activity and the development of hundreds of new specialities have made this referee system necessary. The best referee is of course some other scientist who is working closely on the same scientific problems but is not associated with the author in the actual work – in other words, a competitor, since we must not forget that scientists are people who must earn a living, and since compensation and repute follow productivity and publication. Natural selection is at work among scientists, too! What is most alarming about the workings of the referee system is not the occasional overt lapse of honesty on the part of some referee who suppresses prompt publication of a rival's work while he harvests the fruit by quickly repeating it – perhaps even extending it – and rushing into publication with his own account. What is far more dangerous, I believe, because it is far more insidious and widespread, is the inevitable subconscious germination in the mind of any referee of the ideas he has obtained from the unpublished work of another person. If we are frank with ourselves, none of us can really state where most of the seminal ideas that lead us to a particular theory or line of investigation have been derived. Darwin frankly acknowledged the ideas of Malthus, which led him to the Theory of Natural Selection; but although he was one of the most honest of men, and one who was deeply troubled when Alfred Russel Wallace sent him in 1858 the brief paper setting forth his own parallel derivation of Darwin's theory, Darwin nevertheless never made the slightest acknowledgment of the idea of natural selection which he had surely read in the work of Edward Blyth in 1835 and 1837 (*4*). We may guess that Darwin's reasoning at the time went rather as follows:

Blyth's conception is that natural selection leads to a restriction of hereditary variation in populations. Through elimination of the more variable specimens in a species, nature keeps the species true to type and prevents it from becoming maladapted to its environment. Blyth's Natural Selection is not an evolutionary force at all, but instead is a force for maintenance of the status quo.

Yet it is very hard to understand why, when the full significance of the action of natural selection dawned upon Darwin, he did not reexamine the ideas of Edward Blyth. It should have been perfectly evident to him that the very same force that would eliminate variation and maintain the status quo of the species in a stationary environment would operate quite differently in a changing environment. Will we then ever know the extent to which Darwin was really indebted to Blyth, or how the ideas he probably rejected as invalid actually prepared the way for his reception of Malthus's thoughts in 1838?

The conscientious referee of unpublished scientific manuscripts is similarly a gleaner in the harvest fields of others. The only possible way to avoid taking an unfair advantage would be to refuse to referee any manuscripts that might conceivably have a relationship to one's own research work. The consequences for editors left with piles of unevaluated manuscripts might become desperate, were there not, as I believe, a reasonable solution in the possibility that the role of referee could be limited to scientists who have ceased to do active experimental work themselves. What with the increasing life span and the large number of retired but mentally vigorous older scientists, the supply of competent referees would perhaps be sufficient. To be sure, the criticism may be raised that the older scientific men cannot properly evaluate the significance and merit of really revolutionary new ideas and lines of work. Neither, for the most part, can the young! A combination of older referees in the field and younger ones knowledgeable but not working in the same speciality might solve this difficulty.

What has been said about referees applies with even greater force to the scientists who sit on panels that judge the merit of research proposals made to government agencies or to foundations. The amount of confidential information directly applicable to a man's own line of work acquired in this way in the course of several years staggers the imagination. The most conscientious man in the world cannot forget all this, although he too easily forgets when and where a particular idea came to him. This information consists not only of reports of what has been done in the recent past but of what is still unpublished. It includes also the plans and protocols of work still to be performed, the truly germinal ideas that may occupy a scientist for years to come. After serving for some years on such panels I have reached the conclusion that this form of exposure is most unwise. One simply cannot any longer distinguish between what one properly knows, on the basis of published scientific information, and what one has gleaned from privileged documents. The end of this road is self-deception on the one hand, or conscious deception on the other, since in time scientists who must make research proposals learn that it is better not to reveal what they really intend to do, or to set down in plain language their choicest formulations of experimental planning, but instead write up as the program of their future work what they have in fact already performed. Again, the integrity of science is seriously compromised.

Science and Intellectual Freedom

The first commandment in the ethical basis of science is complete truthfulness, and the second is like unto it:

Thou shalt neither covet thy neighbor's ideas nor steal his experiments.

The third is somewhat different. It requires fearlessness in the defense of intellectual freedom, for science cannot prosper where there is constraint upon daring thinking, where society dictates what experiments may be conducted, or where the statement of one's conclusions may lead to loss of livelihood, imprisonment, or even death.

This is a hard ethic to live by. It brought Giordano Bruno to the stake in 1600. The recantation of Galileo was an easier way; the timidity of Descartes and Leibniz, who left unpublished their more daring scientific thoughts, was understandably human but even less in the interest of science or, ultimately, of the society that felt itself threatened. Whether in the conflict of science with religion, or with political doctrine (as in Nazi Germany), or with social dogma (as in the Marxist countries), scientists must be willing to withstand attack and vilification, ostracism and punishment, or science will wither away and society itself, in the end, be the loser.

From the beginning the inveterate foe of scientific inquiry has been authority – the authority of tradition, of religion, or of the state – since science can accept no dogma within the sphere of its investigations. No doors must be barred to its inquiries, except by reason of its own limitations. It is the essence of the scientific mind not only to be curious but likewise to be skeptical and critical – to maintain suspended judgment until the facts are in, to be willing always, in the light of fresh knowledge, to change one's conclusions. Not even the "laws" of science are irrevocable decrees. They are mere summaries of observed phenomena, ever subject to revision. These laws and concepts remain testable and challengeable. Science is thus wholly dependent upon freedom – freedom of inquiry and freedom of opinion.

But what is the value of science to man, that it should merit freedom? There are those, indeed, who say that science has value only in serving our material wants. To quote one of them: "Science is a social phenomenon, and like every other social phenomenon is limited by the injury or benefit it confers on the community. . . . The idea of free and unfettered science . . . is absurd." Those were the words of Adolf Hitler, as reported by Hermann Rauschning (*5*). In Soviet states a similar view is held officially; and in the Western democracies, likewise, not a few scientists as well as laymen have upheld a similar opinion. The British biologist John R. Baker has pointed out that this view shades through others, such as the admission that scientists work best if they enjoy their work, and the supposition that science has value in broadening the outlook and purging the mind of pettiness, to the view that a positive and primary value of science lies in its creative aspect "as an end in itself, like music, art, and literature"(*6*). "Science aims at knowledge, not utility," says Albert Szent-Györgyi (*7*), and Alexander von Humboldt wrote in his masterpiece, *Cosmos*, that "other interests, besides the material wants of life, occupy the minds of men" (*8*).

It is readily demonstrated that the social usefulness of the conclusions of science can rarely be predicted when the work is planned or even after the basic discoveries have been made. John R. Baker, in his book *Science and the Planned State*, has cited numerous examples that show the impracticability of too narrowly planned a program of scientific research. The sphere of investigation must be determined by the investigator's choice rather than by compulsion – by perception of a problem to be solved rather than by a dogma to be accepted blindly. Science must be free to question and investigate any matter within the scope of its methods and to hold and state whatever conclusions are reached on the basis of the evidence – or it will perish. But science is represented only by the individual scientists. These persons must acknowledge the moral imperative to defend the freedom of science at any cost to themselves. Every Darwin needs a Thomas Henry Huxley. Every Lysenko demands his martyred Vavilov, his hundreds of displaced geneticists before he is finally deposed. Modern science, from its very beginnings near the end of the 16th century, became immediately concerned with a major political issue, the freedom of the scientist to pursue the truth wherever it might lead him, even though that conclusion might be highly disturbing to settled religious beliefs or social conventions and practice. The pyre of Bruno and the ordeal of Galileo led directly in spirit to the attacks on Charles Darwin 250 years later and to latter-day instances of the social suppression of scientific findings. The distortion of genetics by racists in Nazi Germany finds a counterpart in the United States. Mendelian genetics in the U.S.S.R. and the nutritive qualities of oleomargarine in Wisconsin share a similar fate. The third commandment then reads:

Thou shalt defend the freedom of scientific investigation and the freedom of publication of scientific opinion with thy life, if need be.

Science and Communication

Inasmuch as science is intrinsically a social activity and not a solitary pleasure, another primary aspect of the ethics of science is the communication to the world at large, and to other scientists in particular, of what one observes and what one concludes. Both the international scope of scientific activity and the cumulative nature of scientific knowledge lay upon the individual scientist an overwhelming debt to his colleagues and his forerunners. The least he can do in return, unless he is an ingrate, is freely to make his own contributions a part of the swelling flood of scientific information available to all the world.

There are at least five distinct obligations his indebtedness places upon each scientist. The first of these is the obligation to publish his methods and his results so clearly and in such detail that another may confirm and extend his work. The pettiness and jealousy that lead some scientists, in their effort to stay ahead of the ruck, to withhold some significant step of procedure or some result essential to full understanding of the stated conclusions have no place in the realm of science. In other instances it is sheer laziness or procrastination that is at fault. Whatever the only-too-human reason, science suffers.

A second obligation that is far more frequently neglected is the obligation to see that one's contributions are properly abstracted and indexed, and thus made readily available to workers everywhere. Many scientists ignore this obligation completely. Yet, as the sheer volume of scientific publication passes a half-million and soon a million articles a year, it is obviously insufficient to add one's own leaflet to the mountains of paper cramming the scientific libraries of the world. The need to have scientific findings abstracted and indexed has been fully recognized by such international bodies as the International Council of Scientific Unions: its Abstracting Board has urged every author to prepare an abstract in concise, informative style, to be printed at the head of each scientific paper; and the editors of most scientific journals have now made this a requirement for acceptance and publication of a paper. Nevertheless, few authors prepare their abstracts without a reminder, and few heed the requirements for a concise, informative summary that will permit proper indexing of the major items treated in the paper.

A third obligation is that of writing critical reviews, which will be true syntheses of the knowledge accumulating in some field. I firmly believe that there is no scientific activity today more necessary and at the same time less frequently well done than this one. I have said elsewhere (9):

To be sure, the scientist seeks for facts – or better, he starts with observations. . . . But I would say that the real scientist, if not the scholar in general, is no quarryman, but is precisely and exactly a builder – a builder of facts and observations into conceptual schemes and intellectual models that attempt to present the realities of nature. It is the defect and very imperfection of the scientist that so often he fails to build a coherent and beautiful structure of his work . . .

The creativity of scientific writing lies precisely here. The task of the writer of a critical review and synthesis . . . is not only indispensable to scientific advance – it surely constitutes the essence of the scientific endeavor to be no mere quarryman but in some measure a creator of truth and understanding. The aesthetic element that makes scientist akin to poet and artist is expressed primarily in this broader activity.

The critical nature of the critical review grows from our constant forgetfulness of all this. The young scientist is taught carefully and methodically to be a quarryman or a bricklayer. He learns to use his tools well but not to enlarge his perspective, develop his critical powers, or enhance his skill in communication. The older scientist is too often overwhelmed by detail, or forced by the competition of the professional game to stick to the processes of "original research" and "training." The vastness of the scientific literature makes the search for general comprehension and perception of new relationships and possibilities every day more arduous. The editor of the critical review journal finds every year a growing reluctance on the part of the best qualified scientists to devote the necessary time and energy to this task. Often it falls by default to the journeyman of modest talent, a compiler rather than critic and creator, who enriches the scientific literature with a fresh molehill in which later compilers may burrow.

All this need not be so, but it will remain so without a deeper sense of the obligation of the scientist to synthesize and present his broadest understanding of his own field of knowledge. Tomorrow's science stands on the shoulders of those who have done so, no less than on the shoulders of the great discoverers.

A fourth obligation is communication to the general public of the great new revelations of science, the important advances, the noble syntheses of scientific knowledge. There have always been a few eminent scientists who did not scorn to do this: Thomas Henry Huxley, John Tyndall, and Louis Pasteur set the pattern in the 19th century, and in our own time there have indeed been many who followed their precedent. Yet there seems to be a growing tendency to turn this obligation over to professional science writers who, however good, should not replace the direct, personal, and authoritative appeal of the scientist to the general public. As our culture and civilization become day by day more completely based on scientific discovery and technological application, as human exploration becomes ever more restricted to the endless frontiers of science, every citizen must know whereby he lives and whereupon he leans. A democracy rests secure only upon a basis of enlightened citizens who have imbibed the spirit of science and who comprehend its nature as well as its fruits. In fulfilling the requirement of our age for the public understanding of science the scientist must shirk no duty.

A final obligation in the total purview of scientific communication is the obligation to transmit the best and fullest of our scientific knowledge to each succeeding generation. It is well said that genetic transmission of human characteristics and powers is now far overshadowed by cultural inheritance. The transmission of knowledge is the role of the teacher, and the obligation of the scientist to teach is his last and highest obligation to the society that gives him opportunity to achieve his goals.

To every scientist – to some sooner, to some only late – there comes the realization that one lifetime is too short and that other hands and other minds must carry on and complete the work. Only a few scientists are therefore content to limit their entire energies to exploration and discovery. Research is one end, but the other must be the training of the new generation of scientists, the transmission of knowledge and skill, of insight and wisdom. The latter task is no less necessary, no less worthy. From the beginnings of human history, the exponentially accelerating growth of human power . . . has required each generation to instruct and inform the next.

This is the challenge that faces every teacher of a science as he steps into the classroom or guides the early efforts of an individual student. Here, in this sea of fresh faces – here, amidst the stumblings and fumblings – may be the Newton or Einstein, the Mendel or Darwin of tomorrow. For few – so very few – men are self-taught. The teacher cannot supply the potentialities of his students, but he is needed to see that the potentialities will unfold, and unfold fully. His is not only the task of passing on the great tradition of the past, with its skills and accumulated knowledge; he must also provide breadth and perspective, self-criticism and judgment, in order that a well-balanced scientist may grow to full stature and continue the search.

Of all the resources of a nation, its greatest are its boys and girls, its young men and women. Like other material resources, these can be squandered or dissipated. They are potential greatness, but they are only potentialities. Science creates knowledge and knowledge generates power, but knowledge resides only in the minds of men who first must learn and be taught, and power is tyranny unless it be guided by insight and wisdom, justice and mercy. The greatest of men have been teachers, and the teacher is greatest among men (*10*).

The Social and Ethical Responsibilities of Scientists

The scientist escapes lightly – instead of ten commandments only four: to cherish complete truthfulness; to avoid self-aggrandizement at the expense of one's fellow-scientist; fearlessly to defend the freedom of scientific inquiry and opinion; and fully to communicate one's findings through primary publication, synthesis, and instruction. Out of these grow the social and ethical responsibilities of scientists that in the past 20 years have begun to loom ever larger in our ken.

These may be considered under the three heads of proclamation of benefits, warning of risks, and discussion of quandaries. The first of these, the advertisement of the benefits of science, seems to be sufficiently promoted in these days when science is so well supported by government and private agencies and when grants are justified on the basis of social benefits. Every bit of pure research is heralded as a step in the conquest of nuclear or thermonuclear power, space exploration, elimination of cancer and heart disease, or similar dramatic accomplishments. The ethical problem here is merely that of keeping a check-rein on the imagination and of maintaining truthfulness. But the truth itself is so staggering that it is quite enough to bemuse the public.

Since 1945 more and more scientists have become engaged in warning of the great risks to the very future of man of certain scientific developments. First the atomic bomb and then the hydrogen bomb brought swift realization of the possibility of the destruction of all civilization and even the extinction of all human life were a nuclear war to break out. The atomic scientists, conscience-stricken, united to secure civilian control of nuclear energy. Albert Einstein and Bertrand Russell issued an appeal to scientists to warn the world of the tragic consequences of overoptimism and of an unbridled arms race. Joined by a dozen notable scientists, they initiated the "Pugwash" Conferences on Science and World Affairs in 1957. In these conferences scientists of East and West sat down together to talk, in objective scientific terms, of the military and political problems of the world and their resolution. It was not that the scientists at all felt themselves to be more highly qualified than diplomats and statesmen, economists or lawyers, to find solutions of the most difficult and delicate problems of international relations. They acted on two grounds only: that they understood the desperate nature of the situation about which the world must be warned in time; and that they hoped discussions by persons accustomed to argue in objective, scientific terms might pave the way for better understanding and more fruitful negotiation on the part of officials. In the ensuing discussions of the effects of fallout from nuclear weapons tests on persons now living and on the generations yet unborn, scientists played a very important role. In no small measure, I believe, historians of the future will recognize how great a part was played by the scientists in bringing about the partial nuclear weapons test ban. Scientists are now deeply involved in politics, and naturally enough often on both sides of the argument, for although they may agree upon the basic scientific facts which are relevant to the issue, there are rarely enough established facts to clinch the argument and there is always room for differences of opinion in interpreting the facts. In these matters the ethic of the matter requires the scientist to state his opinion on matters of social concern, but at the same time to distinguish clearly between what he states to be fact and what opinion he holds. Moreover, his opinion about matters within his technical sphere of competence is an "informed" opinion; his opinion about other matters, even other scientific matters, is that of a layman. He must in all honesty make clear to the public in what capacity he speaks.

Nuclear war is only one of the dire misfortunes that are poised above the head of modern man. The unrestricted and appalling rate of population increase in most countries of the world, if projected just a few decades into the future, staggers the imagination with its consequences. Effective control of the birth rate is the only conceivable answer to effective reduction by modern health measures of the death rate. This is the world problem second in importance at the present time, and must engage the conscience of the scientist.

The problem of the future is the ethical problem of the control of man over his own biological evolution. The powers of evolution now rest in his hands. The geneticist can define the means and prognosticate the future with some accuracy. Yet here we enter the third great arena of ethical discussion, passing beyond the benefits of science and the certain risks to the nebulous realm of quandaries. Man must choose goals, and a choice of goals involves us in weighing values – even whole systems of values. The scientist cannot make the choice of goals for his people, and neither can he measure and weight values with accuracy and objectivity. There is nonetheless an important duty he must perform, because he and he alone may see clearly enough the nature of the alternative choices, including laissez faire, which is no less a choice than any other. It is the social duty and function of the scientist in this arena of discussion to inform and to demand of the people, and of their leaders too, a discussion and consideration of all those impending problems that grow out of scientific discovery and the amplification of human power. Science is no longer – can never be again – the ivory tower of the recluse, the refuge of the asocial man. Science has found its social basis and has eagerly grasped for social support, and it has thereby acquired social responsibilities and a realization of its own fundamental ethical principles. The scientist is a man, through his science doing good and evil to other men, and receiving from them blame and praise, recrimination and money. Science is not only to know, it is to do, and in the doing it has found its soul.

References

1. J. Bronowski, *Science and Human Values* (Messner, New York, 1956).
2. B. Glass, "Dialectical materialism and scientific research," *Quart. Rev. Biol.* 23, 333–337 (1948); D. I. Greenberg, "Lysenko: Soviet science writes finis to geneticist's domination of nation's biological research," *Science* 147, 716–717 (1965).
3. R. B. Goldschmidt, "Research and politics," *Science* 109, 219–227 (1949).
4. L. C. Eiseley, "Charles Darwin, Edward Blyth, and the Theory of Natural Selection," *Proc. Amer. Phil. Soc.*, 103, 94–158 (1959).

5. H. Rauschning, *Hitler Speaks: A Series of Political Conversations with Adolf Hitler on His Real Aims* (Butterworths, London, 1939), pp. 220–221.

6. J. R. Baker, *Science and the Planned State* (Macmillan, New York, 1945).

7. A. Szent-Györgi, *World Digest* 55, 50 (1943).

8. A. von Humboldt, *Cosmos: A Sketch of a Physical Description of the Universe*. E. C. Otté, transl. (Bohn, London, 1849).

9. B. Glass, "The critical state of the critical review article," *Quart. Rev. Biol.* 39, 182–185 (1964).

10. ———. "The scientist and the science teacher," *Amer. Assoc. Univ. Professors Bull.* 50, 267–268 (1964).

Self-Deception and Gullibility

William Broad and Nicholas Wade

In 1669 the distinguished English physicist Robert Hooke made a wonderful discovery. He obtained the long-sought proof of Copernicus' heliocentric theory of the solar system by demonstrating stellar parallax – a perceived difference in position of a star due to the earth's motion around the sun. One of the first to use a telescope for this purpose, Hooke observed the star Gamma Draconis and soon reported to the Royal Society that he had found what he was looking for: the star had a parallax of almost thirty seconds of arc. Here at last was impeccable experimental proof of the Copernican theory.

This heartening triumph of empirical science was only momentarily dashed when the Frenchman Jean Picard announced he had observed the star Alpha Lyrae by the same method but had failed to find any parallax at all. A few years later England's first Astronomer Royal, the brilliant observer John Flamsteed, reported that the Pole Star had a parallax of at least forty seconds.

Hooke and Flamsteed, outstanding scientists of their day, are leading lights in the history of science. But they fell victim to an effect that to this day has continued to trap many lesser scientists in its treacherous coils. It is the phenomenon of experimenter expectancy, or seeing what you want to see. There is indeed a stellar parallax, but because of the vast distance of all stars from earth, the parallax is extremely small – about one second of arc. It cannot be detected by the relatively crude telescopes used by Hooke and Flamsteed.[1]

Self-deception is a problem of pervasive importance in science. The most rigorous training in objective observation is often a feeble defense against the desire to obtain a particular result. Time and again, an experimenter's expectation of what he will see has shaped the data he recorded, to the detriment of the truth. This unconscious shaping of results can come about in numerous subtle ways. Nor is it a phenomenon that affects only individuals. Sometimes a whole community of researchers falls prey to a common delusion, as in the extraordinary case of the French physicists and N-rays, or – some would add – American psychologists and ape sign language.

Expectancy leads to self-deception, and self-deception leads to the propensity to be deceived by others. The great scientific hoaxes, such as the Beringer case and the Piltdown man discussed in this chapter, demonstrate the extremes of gullibility to which some scientists may be led by their desire to believe. Indeed, professional magicians claim that scientists, because of their confidence in their own objectivity, are easier to deceive than other people.

Self-deception and outright fraud differ in volition – one is unwitting, the other deliberate. Yet it is perhaps more accurate to think of them as two extremes of a spectrum, the center of which is occupied by a range of actions in which the experimenter's motives are ambiguous, even to himself. Many measurements that scientists take in the laboratory admit judgment factors to enter in. An experimenter may delay a little in pressing a stopwatch, perhaps to compensate for some extraneous factor. He can tell himself he is rejecting for technical reasons a result that gives the "wrong" answer; after a number of such rejections, the proportion of "right" answers in the acceptable experiments may acquire a statistical significance that previously was lacking. Naturally it is only the "acceptable" experiments that get published. In effect, the experimenter has selected his data to prove his point, in a way that is in part a deliberate manipulation but which also falls short of conscious fraud.

The "double-blind" experiment – in which neither doctor nor patients know who is receiving a test drug and who a placebo – has become standard practice in clinical research because of the powerful effects of the doctor's expectancy, to say nothing of the patients'. But the habit of "blinding" the experimenter has not become as universal in science as perhaps it should. A dramatic demonstration of experimenter expectancy has been provided in a series of studies by Harvard psychologist Robert Rosenthal. In one of his experiments he gave psychology students two groups of rats to study. The "maze-bright" group of rats, the students were told, had been specially bred for its intelligence in running mazes. The "maze-dull" group were genetically stupid rats. The students were told to test the maze-running abilities of the two groups. Sure enough, they found that the maze-bright rats did significantly better than the maze-dull rats. In fact there was no difference between the maze-bright and maze-dull animals: all were the standard strain of laboratory rats. The difference lay only in the students' expectancies of each group. Yet the students translated this difference in their expectancies into the data they reported.[2]

Perhaps some of the students consciously invented data to accord with the results they thought they should be getting. With others, the manipulation was unconscious and much more subtle. Just how it was done is rather hard to explain. Perhaps the students handled more gently the rats they expected to perform better, and the treatment enhanced the rats' performance. Perhaps in timing the run through the maze the students would unconsciously press the button on the stopwatch a fraction too early for the maze-bright rats and a fraction too late for the maze-dull animals. Whatever the exact mechanism, the researchers' expectations had shaped the result of the experiment without their knowledge.

The phenomenon is not just a pitfall for laboratory scientists. Consider the situation of a teacher administering IQ tests to a class. If he has prior expectations about the children's intelligence, are these likely to shape the results he gets? The answer is yes, they do. In an experiment similar to that performed on the psychology students, Rosenthal told teachers at an elementary school that he had identified certain children with a test that predicted academic blooming. Unknown to the teachers, the test was just a standard IQ test, and the children identified as "bloomers" were chosen at random. At the end of the school year, the children were retested, by the teachers this time, with the same test. In the first grade, those who had been identified to the teachers as academic bloomers gained fifteen IQ points more than did the other children. The "bloomers" in the second grade gained ten points more than the controls. Teachers' expectancies made no or little difference in the upper grades. In the lower grades, comments Rosenthal, "the children have not yet acquired those reputations that become so difficult to change in the later grades and which give teachers in subsequent grades the expectancies for the pupil's performance. With every successive grade it would be more difficult to change the child's reputation."[3]

A particularly fertile ground for scientific self-deception lies in the field of animal-to-man communication. Time and again, the researcher's expectation has been projected onto the animal and reflected back to the researcher without his recognizing the source. The most famous case of this sort is that of Clever Hans, a remarkable horse that could apparently add and substract and even solve problems that were presented to it. He has acquired immortality because his equine spirit returns from time to time to haunt the laboratories of experimental psychologists, announcing its presence with ghostly laughter that its victims are almost always the last to hear.

Hans's trainer, a retired German schoolteacher named Wilhelm Von Osten, sincerely believed that he had taught Hans the ability to count. The horse would tap out numbers with his hoof, stopping when he had reached the right answer. He would count not just for his master but for others as well. The phenomenon was investigated by a psychologist, Oskar Pfungst, who discovered that Von Osten and others were unconsciously cuing the equine prodigy. As the horse reached the number of hoof taps corresponding to the correct answer, Von Osten would involuntarily jerk his head. Perceiving this unconscious cue, Hans would stop tapping. Pfungst found that the horse could detect head movements as slight as one-fifth of a millimeter. Pfungst himself played the part of the horse and found that twenty-three out of twenty-five questioners unwittingly cued him when to stop tapping.

Pfungst's celebrated investigation of the Clever Hans phenomenon was published in English in 1911, but his definitive account did not prevent others from falling into the same trap as Von Osten. Man's age-old desire to communicate with other species could not so easily be suppressed. By 1937 there were more than seventy "thinking" animals, including cats and dogs as well as horses. In the 1950's the fashion turned to dolphins. Then came an altogether new twist in the dialogue between man and animals. The early attempts to teach speech to chimpanzees had faltered because of the animals' extreme physical difficulty in forming human sounds. Much greater progress was made when Allen and Beatrice Gardner of the University of Nevada taught American Sign Language to their chimpanzee Washoe.

Washoe and her imitators readily acquired large vocabularies of the sing language and, even more significantly, would string the signs together in what appeared to be sentences. Particularly evocative was the apes' reported use of the signs in apposite novel combinations. Washoe was said to have spontaneously made the signs for "drink" and "fruit" on seeing a watermelon. Gorilla Koko reportedly described a zebra as a "white tiger." By the 1970's the signing apes had become a flourishing subfield of psychological research.

Then came a serious crisis in the form of an ape named Nim Chimpsky, in honor of the well-known linguist Noam Chomsky. Nim's trainer, psychologist Herbert Terrace, found he learned signs just like the other chimps and started using them in strings. But were the strings of signs proper sentences or just a routine that the crafty ape had learned would induce some appropriate action in its human entourage? Certain features in Nim's linguistic development threw Terrace into a crisis of doubt. Unlike children of his age, Nim suddenly plateaued in his rate of acquisition of new vocabulary. Unlike children, he rarely initiated conversation. He would string signs together, but his sentences were lacking in syntactic rigor: Nim's longest recorded utterance was the sixteen-sign declarative pronouncement, "Give orange me give cat orange me eat orange give me eat orange give me you."

Terrace was eventually forced to decide that Chimpsky, and indeed the other pointing pongids, were not using the signs in a way characteristic of true language. Rather, they were probably making monkeys out of their teachers by imitating or Clever Hansing them. Nim's linguistic behavior was more like that of a highly intelligent, trained dog than of the human children he so much resembled in other ways.

The critics began to move in on the field. "We find the ape 'language' researchers replete with personalities who believe themselves to be acting according to the most exalted motivations and sophisticated manners, but in reality have involved themselves in the most rudimentary circus-like performances," wrote Jean Umiker-Sebeok and Thomas Sebeok.[4] At a conference in 1980, Sebeok was even more forthright: "In my opinion, the alleged language experiments with apes divide into three groups: one, outright fraud; two, self-deception; three, those conducted by Terrace. The largest class by far is the middle one."[5] The battle is not yet over, but the momentum at present lies with the critics. Should they prove correct, the whole field of ape language research will slide rapidly into disrepute, and the ghost of Clever Hans will once again enjoy the last laugh.

Researchers' propensity for self-delusion is particularly strong when other species enter the scene as vehicles for human imaginings and projections. But scientists are capable of deluding themselves without any help from other species. The most remarkable known case of a collective self-deception is one that affected the community of French physicists in the early 1900's. In 1903 the distinguished French physicist René Blondlot announced he had discovered a new kind of rays, which he named N-rays, after the University of Nancy, where he worked.

In the course of trying to polarize X-rays, discovered by Röntgen eight years earlier, Blondlot found evidence of a new kind of emanation from the X-ray source. It made itself apparent by increasing the brightness of an electric spark jumping between a pair of pointed wires. The increase in brightness had to be judged by eye, a notoriously subjective method of detection. But that seemed to matter little in view of the fact that other physicists were soon able to repeat and extend Blondlot's findings.

A colleague at the University of Nancy discovered that N-rays were emitted not just by X-ray sources but also by the nervous system of the human body. A Sorbonne physicist noticed that N-rays emanated from Broca's area, the part of the brain that governs speech, while a person was talking. N-rays were discovered in gases, magnetic fields, and chemicals. Soon the pursuit of N-rays had become a minor industry among French scientists. Leading French physicists commended Blondlot for his discovery. The French Academy of Sciences bestowed its valuable Leconte prize on him in 1904. The effects of N-rays "were observed by at least forty people and analyzed in some 300 papers by 100 scientists and medical doctors between 1903 and 1906," notes an historian of the episode.[6]

N-rays do not exist. The researchers who reported seeing them were the victims of self-deception. What was the reason for this collective delusion? An important clue may be found in the reaction to an article written in 1904 by the American physicist R. W. Wood. During a visit to Blondlot's laboratory, Wood correctly divined that something peculiar was happening. At one point Blondlot darkened the laboratory to demonstrate an experiment in which N-rays were separated into different wavelengths after passing through a prism. Wood surreptitiously removed the prism before the experiment began, but even with the centerpiece of his apparatus sitting in his visitor's pocket, Blondlot obtained the expected results. Wood wrote a devastating account of his visit in an English scientific journal. Science is supposed to transcend national boundaries, but Wood's critique did not. Scientists outside France immediately lost interest in N-rays, but French scientists continued for several years to support Blondlot.

"The most astonishing facet of the episode," notes the French scientist Jean Rostand, "is the extraordinarily great number of people who were taken in. These people were not pseudo-scientists, charlatans, dreamers, or mystifiers; far from it, they were true men of science, disinterested, honorable, used to laboratory procedure, people with level heads and sound common sense. This is borne out by their subsequent achievements as Professors, Consultants and Lecturers. Jean Bacquerel, Gilbert Ballet, André Broca, Zimmern, Bordier – all of them have made their contribution to science."[7]

The reason why the best French physicists of their day continued to support Blondlot after Wood's critique was perhaps the same as the reason for which they uncritically accepted Blondlot's findings in the first place. It all had to do with a sentiment that is supposed to be wholly foreign to science: national pride. By 1900 the French had come to feel that their international reputation in science was on the decline, particularly with respect to the Germans. The discovery of N-rays came just at the right time to soothe the self-doubts of the rigid French scientific hierarchy. Hence the Academy of Sciences, faced after the Wood exposé with almost unanimous criticism from abroad and strong skepticism at home, chose nonetheless to rally round Blondlot rather than ascertain the truth. The members of the academy's Leconte prize committee, which included the Nancy-born Henri Poincaré, chose Blondlot over the other leading candidate, Pierre Curie, who had shared the Nobel prize the year before.

Most historians and scientists who have written about the N-ray affair describe it as pathological, irrational, or otherwise deviant. One historian who is not part of this consensus is Mary Jo Nye. To seek an understanding of the episode, she chose to examine "not the structure of Blondlot's psyche, but rather the structure of Blondlot's scientific community, its organization, aims and aspirations around 1900." Her conclusion, in brief, is that the episode arose from at most an exaggeration of the usual patterns of behavior among scientific communities. The N-ray affair, she says, "was not 'pathological,' much less 'irrational' or 'pseudo-scientific.' The scientists involved in the investigations and debate were influenced in a normal, if sometimes exaggerated, way by traditional reductionist scientific aims, by personal competitive drives, and by institutional, regional, and national loyalties."[8]

That a whole community of scientists can be led astray by nonrational factors is a phenomenon that bears some pondering. To dismiss it as "pathological" is merely to affix a label. In fact the N-ray affair displays in extreme form several themes endemic to the scientific process. One is the unreliability of human observers. The fact is that all human observers, however well trained, have a strong tendency to see what they expect to see. Even when subjectively assessed qualities such as the brightness of a spark are replaced by instruments such as counters or print-outs, observer effects still enter in. Careful studies of how people read measuring devices has brought to light the "digit preference phenomenon" in which certain numbers are unconsciously preferred over others.[9]

Theoretical expectation is one factor that may distort a scientist's observation. The desire for fame and recognition may prevent such distortions from being corrected. In the case of N-rays, a nexus of personal, regional, and national ties combined to carry French physicists far away from the ideal modes of scientific inquiry, and not only that, but to persist in gross error for long after it had been publicly pointed out.

Do scientists take adequate steps to protect themselves from experimental pitfalls of this nature? "Blinded" studies, in which the researcher recording the data does not know what the answer is supposed to be, are a useful precaution but are not sufficient to rule out self-deception. So pervasive are the coils of self-deception in the biological sciences that a foolproof methodology is hard to devise. Theodore X. Barber compiled a manual of pitfalls in experimental research with human subjects, which he concluded with the following poignant postscript: "Before this text was mailed to the publisher, it was read critically by nine young researchers or graduate students. After completing the text, three of the readers felt that, since there were so many problems in experimental research, it may be wiser to forsake experimentation in general (and laboratory experiments in particular) and to limit our knowledge-seeking attempts to other methods, for example, to naturalistic field studies or to participant observation."[10]

The bedrock of science is observation and experiment, the empirical procedures that make it different from other kinds of knowledge. Yet observation turns out to be most fallible when it is most needed: when an experimenter's objectivity falters. Take the case of the eighteenth-century savant Johann Jacob Scheuchzer, who set out to find evidence that mankind at the time of Noah had been caught up in a terrible flood. Find it he did, and Scheuchzer hailed the skeletal remains of his flood man as *Homo diluvii testis*. Examination years later showed the fossil to be a giant amphibian, long ago extinct.

Twentieth-century science has not escaped the danger to which Scheuchzer fell victim. When the American astronomer Adriaan van Maanen announced in 1916 that he had observed rotations in spiral nebulae, the result was accepted because it confirmed a prevailing belief that the nebulae were nearby objects. Later work by Edwin Hubble, van Maanen's colleague at the Mount Wilson Observatory, showed that, to the contrary, the spiral nebulae are galaxies at an immense distance from our own, and that they do not rotate in the manner described by van Maanen. What made van Maanen's eyes deceive him?

The standard explanation, promulgated in such publications as the *Dictionary of Scientific Biography,* is that "the changes he was attempting to measure were at the very limits of precision of his equipment and techniques."[11] But random error of the sort suggested cannot explain the fact that van Maanen over the course of a decade reported many nebulae to be rotating in the same direction (unwinding rather than winding up). The subjectivity of scientific observers has prompted a historian of the van Maanen affair, Norriss Hetherington, to comment that "today science holds the position of queen of the intellectual disciplines. . . . The decline of the dominance of theology followed from historical studies that revealed the human nature and thus the human status of theology. Historical and sociological studies that begin to investigate a possible human element of science similarly threaten to topple the current queen."[12]

Self-deception is so potent a human capability that scientists, supposedly trained to be the most objective of observers, are in fact peculiarly vulnerable to deliberate deception by others. The reason may be that their training in the importance of objectivity leads them to ignore, belittle, or suppress in themselves the very nonrational factors that the hoaxster relies on. The triumph of preconceived ideas over common sense has seldom been more complete than in the case of Dr. Johann Bartholomew Adam Beringer.

A physician and learned dilettante of eighteenth-century Germany, Beringer taught at the University of Würzburg and was adviser and chief physician to the prince-bishop. Not content with his status as a mere healer and academician, he threw himself into the study of "things dug from the earth," and began a collection of natural rarities such as figured stones, as fossils were then called. The collection assumed a remarkable character in 1725, when three Würzburg youths brought him the first of a series of extraordinary stones they had dug up from nearby Mount Eivelstadt.[13]

This new series of figured stones was a treasure trove of insects, frogs, toads, birds, scorpions, snails, and other creatures. As the youths brought further objects of their excavations to the eager Beringer, the subject matter of the fossils became distinctly unusual. "Here were leaves, flowers, plants, and whole herbs, some with and some without roots and flowers," wrote Beringer in book of 1726 describing the amazing discovery. "Here were clear depictions of the sun and moon, of stars, and of comets with their fiery tails. And lastly, as the supreme prodigy commanding the reverent admiration of myself and of my fellow examiners, were magnificent tablets engraved in Latin, Arabic, and Hebrew characters with the ineffable name of Jehovah."

Shortly after the publication of his book, historical accounts relate, Beringer discovered on Mount Eivelstadt the most unusual fossil of all, one that carried his own name.

An official inquiry was held, at Beringer's request, to discover who was responsible for perpetrating the hoax. One of the young diggers turned out to be in the employ of two of Beringer's rivals, J. Ignatz Roderick, professor of geography, algebra, and analysis at the University of Würzburg, and the Honorable Georg von Eckhart, privy councillor and librarian to the court and to the university. Their motive had been to make Beringer a laughingstock because "he was so arrogant."

What also emerged at the inquiry was that the hoaxsters, apparently fearful that things might go too far, had tried to open Beringer's eyes to the prank before the publication of his book. They started a rumor that the stones were fakes, and when that didn't work they had him told directly. Beringer could not be persuaded that the whole thing was a massive piece of fakery; he went ahead and published his book.

Even within Beringer's lifetime, the legend of the "lying stones" began to gain momentum. By 1804, James Parkinson in his book *Organic Remains of a Former World* mentioned the debacle and drew out a lesson: "It plainly demonstrates, that learning may not be sufficient to prevent an unsuspecting man, from becoming the dupe of excessive credulity. It is worthy of being mentioned, on another account: the quantity of censure and ridicule, to which its author was exposed, served, not only to render his contemporaries less liable to imposition; but also more cautious in indulging in unsupported hypotheses."[14]

Parkinson was not the only observer to comment on the salutary effect of hoaxes in promoting skepticism. In 1830, in his book *Reflections on the Decline of Science in England*, Charles Babbage remarked: "The only excuse which has been made for them is when they have been practised on scientific academies which had reached the period of dotage." By way of example he noted how the editors of a French encyclopedia had credulously copied the description of a fictitious animal that a certain Gioeni claimed to have discovered in Sicily and had named after himself, *Gioenia sicula*.[15]

When hoaxes go awry, it is often for want of occasion, not of gullibility on the part of the intended victims, as in the case of the Orgueil meteorite, a shower of stones that fell near the village of Orgueil, France, on the night of May 14, 1864. A few weeks earlier, Louis Pasteur had started a furious debate in France by delivering the famous lecture before the French Academy in which he derided the long-standing theory of spontaneous generation, which held that life-forms can develop from inanimate matter. Noticing that the material of the Orgueil meteorite became pasty when exposed to water, a hoaxter molded some seeds and particles of coal into a sample of the meteorite and waited for them to be discovered by Pasteur's opponents. The hoaxter's motive was presumably to let them adduce the seeds as evidence for life spontaneously generating in outer space, whereupon he would pull the rug out from under them by announcing the hoax.

What went wrong with the scheme was that the doctored fragment was never examined during the debate. Though other pieces of the meteorite were intensively studied at the time, the hoaxster's carefully prepared fragment lay unexamined in a glass display jar at the Musée d'Histoire at Montauban, France, for ninety-eight years. When its turn at last came, in 1964, the incentive for belief had disappeared, and the forgery was immediately recognized as such.[16]

Had the fragment been studied at the time, the hoax would doubtless have been successful. When the conditions are right, there is no limit to human gullibility, as was proved by the remarkable incident of the Piltdown man.

British national pride in the early years of the twentieth century suffered from a matter of serious disquiet. The Empire was at its height, the serenity of the Victorian era was still aglow, and to educated Englishmen it was almost self-evident that England had once been the cradle, as it was now the governess, of world civilization. How then to explain that striking evidence of early man – not just skeletal remains but Paleolithic cave paintings and tools as well – was coming to light in France and Germany but not in Britain? The dilemma was exacerbated in 1907 with the discovery near Heidelberg, Germany, of a massive, early human jawbone. It seemed depressing proof that the first man had been a German.

The discovery of the Piltdown man was made by Charles Dawson, a lawyer who maintained a quiet practice in the south of England and dabbled in geology. A tireless amateur collector of fossils, Dawson noticed a promising-looking gravel pit on Piltdown Common, near Lewes in Sussex. He asked a laborer digging there to bring him any flints he might find. Several years later, in 1908, the laborer brought him a fragment of bone that Dawson recognized as part of a thick human skull. Over the next three years further bits of the skull appeared.

In 1912 Dawson wrote to his old friend Arthur Smith Woodward, a world authority on fossil fishes at the geology department of the British Museum of Natural History, saying he had something that would top the German fossil found at Heidelberg. Woodward made several visits with Dawson to the Piltdown gravel pit. On one of these expeditions, Dawson's digging tool struck at the bottom of the pit and out flew part of a lower jaw. Close examination led Woodward and Dawson to believe that it belonged to the skull they had already reconstructed.

In great excitement, Smith Woodward took everything back to the British Museum, where he put the jaw and cranium together, filling in missing parts with modeling clay and his imagination. The result was truly remarkable. The assembled skull became the "dawn man" of Piltdown. Kept secret until December 1912, it was unveiled before a full house at the Geological Society in London, where it created a sensation. Some skeptics suggested that the human skull and apelike jaw did not belong together; others pointed out that two characteristically abraded molar teeth were not enough to prove the jaw was human. But these objections were ignored, and the find was accepted as a great and genuine discovery.[17]

The talk in clubs and pubs could note with satisfaction the new proof that the earliest man was indeed British. The Piltdown skull was also of scientific interest because it seemed to be the "missing link," the transitional form between ape and man that was postulated by Darwin's still controversial theory of evolution. Subsequent excavations at the gravel pit were not disappointing. A whole series of new fossils emerged. The clinching evidence came from a pit a few miles away – the discovery a few years later of a second Piltdown man.

Yet some were troubled by the Piltdown finds, among them a young zoologist at the British Museum, Martin A. C. Hinton. After a visit to the site in 1913, Hinton concluded that the whole thing was a hoax. He decided to smoke out the tricksters by planting clearly fraudulent fossils and watching the reactions. He took an ape tooth from the collection at the museum and filed it down to match the model canine tooth that Smith Woodward had fashioned out of clay. Hinton had the obvious forgery placed in the pit by an accomplice and sat back to wait for it to be discovered and the entire Piltdown collection to be exposed.

The tooth was discovered, but nothing else went right with Hinton's plan. All involved with the "discovery" seemed delighted and soon notified the nation about the new find. Hinton was astonished that his scientific colleagues could be taken in by so transparent a fake, and he suffered that additional mortification of seeing Charles Dawson, whom he suspected to be the culprit, acquiring kudos for his handiwork. He decided to try again, only this time with something so outrageous that the whole country would laugh the discoverers to scorn.

In a box in the British Museum he found a leg bone from an extinct species of elephant. He proceeded to carve it into an extremely appropriate tool for the earliest Englishman – a Pleistocene cricket bat. He took the bat to Piltdown, buried it, and waited for the laughter.

It was a long wait. When the bat was unearthed, Smith Woodward was delighted. He pronounced it a supremely important example of the work of Paleolithic man, for nothing like it had ever been found before. Smith Woodward and Dawson published a detailed, serious description of the artifact in a professional journal but stopped short of calling it an actual cricket bat.[18] Hinton was astonished that none of the scientists thought of trying to whittle a bit of bone, fossil or fresh, with a flint edge. If they had, they would have discovered it was impossible to imitate the cuts on the cricket bat. "The acceptance of this rubbish completely defeated the hoaxsters," notes a historian of the Piltdown episode.[19] "They just gave up, and abandoned all attempts to expose the whole business and get it demolished in laughter and ridicule." Perhaps Hinton and friends should have considered planting a bone on which the name Smith Woodward had been carved.

Piltdown man retained its scientific luster until the mid-1920's and the discovery of humanlike fossils in Africa. These indicated a very different pattern of human evolution to that suggested by the Piltdown skull. Instead of a human cranium with an apelike jaw, the African fossils were just the reverse – they had humanlike jaws with apelike skulls. Piltdown became first an anomaly, then an embarrassment. It slipped from sight until modern techniques of dating showed in the early 1950's that the skull and its famous jaw were fakes: an ape jaw, with filed-down molars, and a human skull had each been suitably stained to give the appearance of great age.

Circumstantial evidence pointed to the skull's discoverer, Dawson, as the culprit. But many have doubted that he could have been the instigator; although he was best placed to salt the gravel pit, he probably lacked access to the necessary fossil collections as well as the scientific expertise to assemble fossils of the right age for the Piltdown gravel. Indeed, the real mystery is not who did it but how a whole generation of scientists could have been taken in by so transparent a prank. The fakery was not expert. The tools were poorly carved and the teeth crudely filed. "The evidences of artificial abrasion immediately sprang to the eye. Indeed so obvious did they seem it may well be asked – how was it that they had escaped notice before," remarked anthropologist Le Gros Clark.[20]

The question is one that the victims always ask in retrospect yet seldom learn to anticipate. A group of scientists particularly plagued by tricksters and charlatans are parapsychologists, researchers who apply the scientific method to the study of telepathy, extrasensory perception, and other paranormal phenomena. Because parapsychology is widely regarded as a fringe subject not properly part of science, its practitioners have striven to be more than usually rigorous in following correct scientific methodology.

The founder of parapsychology, J. B. Rhine, made great strides in putting the discipline on a firm scientific footing. As a mark of its growing scientific acceptability, the Parapsychological Association in 1971 was admitted to the American Association for the Advancement of Science. The field seemed to be making solid headway toward the goal of scientific acceptability. Noting this progress with satisfaction, Rhine in 1974 commented on the decline of fraudulent investigators: "As time has passed our progress has aided us in avoiding the admission of such risky personnel even for a short term. As a result, the last twenty years have seen little of this cruder type of chicanery. Best of all, we have reached a stage at which we can actually look for and to a degree choose the people we want in the field." Rhine also warned against the danger of relying on automatic data recording as a means of avoiding the pitfalls of subjective measurement: "Apparatus can sometimes also be used as a screen to conceal the trickery it was intended to prevent," he noted.[21]

Less than three months after his article had appeared, Rhine's Institute for Parapsychology in Durham, North Carolina, was rocked by a scandal that involved Walter J. Levy, a brilliant young protégé whom Rhine had planned to designate his successor as director of the institute.

Levy had developed a highly successful experiment for demonstrating psychic ability in rats: through psychokinetic powers, the animals could apparently influence an electric generator to activate electrodes implanted in the pleasure centers of the brain. For more than a year the experiment had given positive results, and Rhine urged Levy to have it repeated in other labs. The work, however, quickly took a turn for the worse; results fell back to the chance level.

At this point one of the junior experimenters noticed that Levy was paying more than usual attention to the equipment. He and others decided to check out their suspicions by observing their senior colleague from a concealed position. They saw Levy manipulating the experimental apparatus so as to make it yield positive results. To Rhine's credit, he published an article recounting the whole episode.[22] "Right from the start the necessity of trusting the experimenter's personal accuracy or honesty must be avoided as far as possible," he concluded.

Most parapsychologists have training in a conventional scientific discipline, and they bring their scientific training to bear on the study of the paranormal. The competence with which the study is conducted is probably a measure of that training. But if so, scientists have not shown themselves to be highly successful in dealing with the unexpected problems of the occult world. Their subjects, those who claim occult powers, have invariably followed one of two patterns when put under systematic observation: either their powers "fade" or they are exposed as tricksters. That background might lead parapsychologists to approach new claimants with a certain degree of skepticism. But when the Israeli mentalist Uri Geller toured the United States demonstrating his psychic powers, the parapsychologists gave an enormous boost to his claims by confirming them in the laboratory.

Harold Puthoff and Russell Targ, two laser physicists at the Stanford Research Institute, wrote a scientific article corroborating Geller's ability to guess the number on a die concealed in a metal box. The article was accepted and published by *Nature*, a leading scientific journal.[23] Other scientists, such as the English physicist John Taylor of London University, endorsed Geller's psychic abilities. It fell to a professional magician, not a scientist or a parapsychologist, to explain to the public what was behind the Geller phenomenon. James Randi, of Rumson, New Jersey, showed audiences that he could duplicate all Geller's feats, but by simple conjury. "Any magician will tell you that scientists are the easiest persons in the world to fool," says mathematical columnist Martin Gardner.[24] Geller, note two students of deception, "prefers scientists as witnesses and will not perform before expert magicians, and for good reason. Scientists, by the very nature of their intellectual and social training, are among the easiest persons for a conjuror to deceive. . . . "[25]

For an extreme example of gullibility among some of America's best physicists and engineers, consider the remarkable case of the Shroud of Turin Research Project, a group of scientists devoted to studying a relic that believers say is the true burial cloth of Christ. Members of the group work at the Los Alamos National Laboratory, where America's nuclear weapons are designed, and at other military research centers. "The great majority of them are, or until recently were, engaged in the design, manufacture, or testing of weapons, from simple explosives to atomic bombs to high-energy 'killer' lasers," notes an admiring article.[26]

In their spare time the scientists study the Shroud of Turin with the most modern scientific instruments. Through careful not to say it is genuine, they say they cannot prove it is a fake, leaving the strong impression that it is the real thing. They add that there are features of the shroud that cannot be explained by modern technology; its image, of a full-length crucified man, was not painted, they say, because there is no sign of pigment. It is a reverse image, like a photographic negative, and encodes three-dimensional information. From what they tell reporters, they seem to favor a short intense burst of light, presumably from inside the body, as the cause of the image.

But consider some brief facts about the Shroud of Turin: (i) it first came to light in about 1350, at a time when medieval Europe was swamped with purported Holy Land relics of all kinds; (ii) the bishop of Troyes, France, in whose diocese it first appeard, "discovered the fraud and how the said cloth had been cunningly painted, the truth being attested by the artist who had painted it," according to a letter written to the Pope in 1389 by one of the bishop's successors; (iii) traces of two medieval pigments have been discovered in particles lifted off the shroud.[27] The negative image with its three-dimensional encoded information is simply the result of an artist trying to paint an image as it might be expected to register on a cloth covering a dead body. He put in shading to indicate the body's contours, and used so dilute a pigment that even modern tests mostly fail to reveal it. How did a group of the nation's elite bomb designers get so far along the road of persuading themselves (and numerous reporters) that they had a miracle on their hands?

"In entering upon any scientific pursuit," said the nineteenth-century astronomer John Herschel, "one of the student's first endeavours ought to be to prepare his mind for the reception of truth, by dismissing, or at least loosening, his hold on all such crude and hastily adopted notions respecting the objects and relations he is about to examine, as may tend to embarrass or mislead him." Good advice but hard to follow, as the long and continuing history of self-deception and gullibility in science repeatedly shows.

The frequency of scientific self-deception and hoaxes takes on special significance when it is remembered that the skeptical frame of mind is supposedly an essential part of the scientist's approach to the world. The scientific method is widely assumed to be a powerful and self-correcting device for understanding the world as it is and making sense of nature. What is the scientific method, and what are the flaws that make this adamantine armor so strangely vulnerable to the unexpected?

Notes

1. It is interesting to note that historians espousing the conventional ideology of science have tried to save appearances by assuming that Hooke and Flamsteed were observing another phenomenon known as stellar aberration, which they innocently mistook for the stellar parallax. This explanation will not wash. Stellar aberration is an apparent displacement similar to which a raindrop seen from a moving car seems to fall slantwise instead of straight down. It was discovered in 1725 by James Bradley in the very course of trying to repeat Hooke's observation of the stellar parallax. Bradley himself specifically stated that Hooke's data could not be measurements of stellar aberration. Hooke's observations were "really very far from being either exact or agreeable to the phenomena," Bradley reported. "It seems that Hooke found what he expected to find," notes Norriss Hetherington of the University of California, Berkeley, in an account of this episode ("Questions About the Purported Objectivity of Science," unpublished MS).
2. Robert Rosenthal, *Experimenter Effects in Behavioral Research* (Appleton–Century–Crofts, New York, 1966), pp. 158–179.
3. *Ibid.*, pp. 411–413.
4. Jean Umiker-Sebeok and Thomas A. Sebeok, "Clever Hans and Smart Simians," *Anthropos*, 76, 89–166, 1981.
5. Nicholas Wade, "Does Man Alone Have Language? Apes Reply in Riddles, and a Horse Says Neigh," *Science*, 208, 1349–1351, 1980.
6. Mary Jo Nye, "N-rays: An Episode in the History and Psychology of Science," *Historical Studies in the Physical Sciences*, 11:1, 125–156, 1980.
7. Jean Rostand, *Error and Deception in Science* (Basic Books, New York, 1960), p. 28.
8. Nye, op. cit., p. 155.
9. Rosenthal, op. cit., pp. 3–26.
10. Theodore Xenophon Barber, *Pitfalls in Human Research* (Pergamon Press, New York, 1973), p. 88.
11. Richard Berendzen and Carol Shamieh, "Maanen, Adriann van," *Dictionary of Scientific Biography* (Charles Scribner's Sons, New York, 1973), pp. 582–583.
12. Norriss S. Hetherington, "Questions about the Purported Objectivity of Science," unpublished MS.
13. Melvin E. Jahn and Daniel J. Woolf, *The Lying Stones of Dr. Johann Bartholomew Adam Beringer* (University of California Press, Berkeley, 1963).
14. Ibid.
15. Charles Babbage, *Reflections on the Decline of Science in England* (Augustus M. Kelley, New York, 1970).
16. Edward Anders *et al.*, "Contaminated Meteorite," *Science*, 146, 1157–1161, 1964.
17. J. S. Weiner, *The Piltdown Forgery* (Oxford University Press, London, 1955).
18. Charles Dawson and Arthur Smith Woodward, "On a Bone Implement from Piltdown," *Quarterly Journal of the Geological Society*, 71, 144–149, 1915.
19. L. Harrison Matthews, "Piltdown Man: The Missing Links," *New Scientist*, a ten-part series, beginning April 30, 1981, pp. 280–282.
20. Quoted in Stephen J. Gould, *The Panda's Thumb* (W. W. Norton, New York, 1980), p. 112.

21. J. B. Rhine, "Security versus Deception in Parapsychology," *Journal of Parapsychology*, 38, 99–121, 1974.
22. J. B. Rhine, "A New Case of Experimenter Unreliability," *Journal of Parapsychology*, 38, 215–225, 1974.
23. Russell Targ and Harold Puthoff, "Information Transmission under Conditions of Sensory Shielding," *Nature*, 251, 602–607, 1974.
24. Martin Gardner, "Magic and Paraphysics," *Technology Review*, June 1976, pp. 43–51.
25. Umiker-Sebeok and Sebeok, *op. cit.*
26. Cullen Murphy, "Shreds of Evidence," *Harper's*, November 1981, pp. 42–65.
27. Walter C. McCrone, "Microscopical Study of the Turin 'Shroud,' " *The Microscope*, 29, 1, 1981.

Questions for Discussions

1. Why are honesty and openness essential to the practical goals of science as well as its ethical goals?
2. How does peer review guard against self-deception and subjective interpretation of data? How can peer review fall prey to these same forces?
3. What is "pseudoscience?" What practices or fields might be considered pseudo-sciences? What distinguishes them from "true" sciences? How have these distinctions changed through history?

Recommended Supplemental Reading

Barber B. Resistance by scientists to scientific discovery. *Science.* 1961;134:596–602.
Broad W, Wade N. *Betrayers of the Truth.* New York: Simon & Schuester; 1982.
Bronowski J. *Science and Human Values*, New York: Messner; 1956.
Callahan JC. Professions, institutions, and moral risk. In DE Wueste, ed. *Professional Ethics and Social Responsibility.* Totowa, NJ: Rowman and Littlefield; 1994:243–270.
Kohn A. *False Prophets: Fraud and Error in Science and Medicine.* Oxford: Basil Blackwell; 1986.
Medawar P. *The Limits of Science.* New York: Oxford University Press, 1984.

The Responsible Conduct of Research

The Responsible Conduct of Biological and Health Research

Ruth Ellen Bulger

During this time of rapid change in the environment of science, sensitivity to and understanding of the relevant issues of responsible conduct in science are important to both scientists and university administrators. Knowing the accepted scientific norms in situations in which norms have been defined as well as how to understand complex situations for which norms have not been defined or generally accepted by the majority of scientists are both aspects to be considered.

There are many reasons why understanding these principles is essential to all scientists. Louis Pasteur said, "In the field of experimentation, chance favors only the prepared mind." Teaching principles of scientific integrity is one way to prepare the mind for ethically problematic situations that scientists may encounter in their careers. There are many ways to teach concepts of responsible conduct of research. The most common is for an experienced scientist to teach a novice by example in the laboratory. All scientists working with others, but particularly those serving as mentors for students, are teaching by example in their laboratory endeavors.

Reading about and having discussions of real cases, newspaper articles, or other pertinent materials about ethical quandaries in science can be done alone or with the mentor as situations arise. Similar discussions can occur in small group sessions in the classroom in which students are interacting with each other and with an instructor. These discussions are particularly helpful in the gray areas of science in which one particular answer may not be the only answer or clearly the best. Certain types of material that scientists need to know but which are not intuitively or rationally apparent, such as the content of local, state, or federal regulations, also can be taught in a lecture situation or by selected readings. Because ethical quandaries abound, the best approach would be a combination of these methods.

There are many goals in teaching scientific responsibility. The instruction should serve to stimulate the scientist's sensitivity to and interest in ethical issues relating to his or her work. If education about the responsible conduct of science is required by an institution, it says that the institution finds this to be an important subject to which the scientists and students need to be exposed. Such classes should open lines of communication about the expected norms of behavior and why they exist – especially between those who are early in the learning process and more experienced scientists. Formal, prescribed educational programs can communicate to students and other scientists the standards and regulations in areas such as intellectual property, conflict of interest, authorship, or data management for which general agreement about standards has been reached. Discussing these issues with others should strengthen the sense of moral obligation and personal responsibility in the scientists as well as help them recognize ethical problems related to their research practices in the gray areas in which one must weigh many factors to choose the most acceptable course. Discussions of ethically difficult situations can help students understand and use various methods for ethical decision making related to scientific issues.

In dealing with complex issues of scientific responsibility, the environment in which scientists work has many potentially perverse incentives that must be overcome. For example, the environment is competitive for obtaining grant funds to support research, good academic positions, and subsequent promotions. To succeed, it is important to publish an adequate number of high-quality papers in a relatively short time. Yet there are conflicts among the various roles required of each scientist: doing the science well, producing quality articles, becoming a respected expert in one's area of research, teaching others not only in the scientist's research area but in other fields of knowledge, and providing services to one's institution. All are expected of a faculty member. In addition, scientists have the usual responsibilities to their families and loved ones that must also be met.

Values in Science

The customary way to teach the responsible conduct of science has been to examine the *spheres of scientific activity* such as data management, authorship policy, or conflicts of interest. The teaching quickly becomes an abbreviated discussion of what the accepted standards are, if in fact they have been delineated, and what the various local, state, and federal regulations are that the scientists must follow. It is no wonder that holding the interest of students and other scientists during an ethics course can sometimes be difficult. However, knowing research regulations is essential to doing science in a responsible manner, and thus this book has information dealing with these spheres of scientific activity.

However, what is really important to scientists are the values that underlie these various rules or standards. Why have scientists decided to act in a certain way? It is the system of underlying values that also must be understood. This is clearly seen if we consider the important ethical issues involved with the inclusion of human volunteers in biomedical studies. Studies involving human participants have clearly been key to improving the health status of the population.

Values that must be respected when research involves humans were clearly enunciated in the Belmont Report,[1] a six-page masterpiece written in 1979 as a summary of the deliberations of the National Commission for the Protection of Human Subjects of Biomedical and Behavioral Research. The National Commission had written about a dozen longer documents on various aspects of including human volunteers in research and then summarized what the commissioners felt to be the most important principles in the Belmont Report.

The National Commission identified three basic ethical principles on which the ethical inclusion of human volunteers must be based: *respect for persons*, *beneficence* (and non-maleficence), and *justice*. Investigators doing research with humans as subjects consider these three principles even today, for they continue to serve as an analytical framework for proposing and conducting ethical research studies involving human volunteers. For example, if individuals are to be treated with *respect as autonomous agents* when they are being asked to participate in a research study, it becomes essential that they have adequate, understandable information on all aspects of the study in language they can understand. In addition, individuals need to enter the research voluntarily, knowing that they can withdraw from the study whenever they choose without losing any of their rights.

Therefore, because this text aims to describe and examine the essential values underlying the rules and regulations of biomedical research, it must first address the *values* that control scientists' behavior in other areas besides the inclusion of human volunteers in research. Clear underlying principles have not been enunciated for some areas of basic biomedical research in a way that provides an analytical framework analogous to that for human investigation articulated in the Belmont Report.[1] Bulger reviewed the pertinent earlier work and then attempted to group these underlying values into four basic areas for principles of responsible conduct of science: the *honesty of scientists*, *respect for others*, *scholarly competence*, and *stewardship of resources*.[2] Although these categories as defined contain overlapping issues, they provide one way of thinking about the values of scientists in general and of biomedical scientists in particular.

Honesty of Scientists

Honesty, truthfulness, objectivity, and integrity are premier values held by scientists in how they observe, record, and interpret everything that they do. Because all information passes through the mind of the scientist, objectivity is something that the scientist must constantly strive to obtain. A variety of experimental methods are used by scientists to safeguard objectivity. Scientists use serially repeated experiments or experiments in which they have been "blinded" to which data are coming from the experimental subjects and which are from the control subjects. Researchers use concurrent control experiments to rule out confounding factors and often use multiple independent observers. Then they subject their data to appropriate statistical analysis to ensure that the data are significant. In addition, to strive for objectivity, scientists should examine their intellectual biases and limit their conflicts of interest based on financial or intellectual considerations.

Honesty, moreover, involves being complete in publishing the methods and results so that experiments can be repeated by others. This principle of honesty also provides guidance for the accurate quotation of the work and ideas of others.

Respect for Others

The term *others* in this context groups the way scientists respect human volunteers and animal subjects in research studies as well as their colleagues and environment. One of the principles of the Belmont Report is respecting the autonomy of individuals. Similarly, using animals in research studies entails a commitment to their humane care and treatment. In 1959, Russell and Burch[3] proposed three Rs as principles to guide the use of animals in research: refinement of the experiments, reduction in the use of animals, and replacement of living animals with alternative techniques. The principles of the inclusion of human subjects in research and the humane care and use of animals are so crucial to biomedical practices that each topic will be considered as separate chapters in this book.

How do scientists show *respect for the environment*? One way would be to avoid unnecessary duplication of experiments by conducting a complete literature review of the previous work done by others before initiating an experiment. This principle of respect for the environment implies a commitment to decrease waste of all types. Recycling paper and other substances, reclaiming certain expensive chemicals when feasible, and sharing infrequently used chemicals should become part of routine laboratory practice. Proper and safe disposal of excess chemicals, microbiological agents, and other wastes according to accepted safety procedures is essential.

We demonstrate our *respect for colleagues* in sharing knowledge and resources with them and in the proper attribution of their words and ideas to them. If information and resources are shared among scientists, society can benefit more rapidly in reaching the goal of better health outcomes for all of the population. *Respect for student colleagues* is demonstrated by being considerate of their needs and in not taking advantage of their status to encroach on their time or ideas for the adviser's personal advantage. Helping students build an area of their own expertise, not just using them to fulfill one's own research agenda, is an essential component for proper mentorship.

An additional area in which one demonstrates respect for colleagues (including students and laboratory technicians) is in maintaining the shared laboratory as a safe working environment. If I had a dime for every time I had to remove a coffee cup from a sink used to dispose of noxious chemicals, I would be rich. Eating, drinking, or storage of food in a laboratory can be a dangerous activity. Careful preparation and labeling of chemical solutions is another way of protecting those colleagues working in the same laboratory. Dangerous microbiologic agents, chemicals, or radioactive agents require knowledge of and commitment to appropriate procedures for their use and disposal and in the cleanup of any spills. Written instructions and education on the dangers involved with handling chemicals used in the laboratory must be readily available to all laboratory personnel.

Showing respect for colleagues, both faculty and students, can be a complex area because of the many barriers to collegiality that seem to exist in academia.[4] Tensions sometimes develop over issues such as salary differentials, time available for research, availability of institutional resources, or the amount of teaching time required from an individual faculty member. The number of tasks and the pace of life in a highly competitive academic environment place additional stresses on establishing collegial relationships. Yet, treating colleagues with respect is essential to responsible working relationships.

Scholarly Competence

Responsible conduct of science requires *competence* in obtaining and transmitting information. To demonstrate scholarly competence in *obtaining knowledge*, the scientist must undertake experiments that use valid, up-to-date procedures that collect sufficient data and that are conducted in such a way that the results derived are useful to the scientific community. Scholarly competence in *transmitting* scientific knowledge requires that the study results be published so others can benefit from their dissemination. There are other critical issues in transmitting information such as the ability to communicate information to other scientists, to students, and to society, the treatment of trainees and students with justice and caring, and the stimulation of creativity in students.

Stewardship of Resources

The great majority of medical and health-related scientific research being accomplished is paid for by the public, through grants from the NIH, other government agencies, voluntary foundations, or by the price that the public pays for products that have been developed by industry. Therefore, the scientist has an obligation to be a good steward of these resources. How to discharge this obligation is an issue on which scientists do not agree. Most scientists believe that they have an obligation to do science responsibly. Other possible ways to express stewardship are to choose an important research topic that should provide information useful to society, to ensure that the information gained from the research is published promptly for others to use, to avoid undue repetition of experiments done by others, or to identify ethical quandaries and work with one's institution or scientific society to help resolve such ethical issues that may arise from scientific developments.

How Does Science Advance?

Thomas Kuhn, in his 1962 book (republished in 1970) *The Structure of Scientific Revolutions*, points out that the kind of science that most scientists do for the vast majority of their careers is what he calls "normal science."[5] In doing normal science, a gap in knowledge is identified. To try to fill that gap, a hypothesis is designed that, if correct, would explain the perceived situation. The hypothesis is tested by doing experiments, analyzing the results, and seeing whether what appears to be the interpretation of the results fits the hypothesis. If the results support the hypothesis, they might lead to further hypotheses or to a broader theory. However, if the results do not support the hypothesis, the hypothesis must be reconceptualized and then retested.

A good hypothesis would be simple but broad, be internally consistent as well as consistent with what is already known, be able to unify the disparate observations seen previously, and be testable experimentally with results that would lead to further research ideas to be tested.

According to Kuhn, as scientists continue to test hypotheses, anomalies and discrepancies occur with the expectations and predictions of the prevailing theories. These anomalies frequently occur when newer experimental methods or refined instruments are developed and used. New measurements can lead to results that do not agree with currently held views. Kuhn points out that, as these discrepancies occur, theories of so-called normal science lose their power to suppress the breakthroughs, and a paradigm change occurs. That happens when someone recognizes the group of anomalies as a new set, and this recognition leads to a conceptual breakthrough or a paradigm switch. Yet Kuhn stressed how difficult it can be for a new concept to be assimilated.

However, Jasanoff points out that there is no one abstract scientific method that guides all kinds of research.[6] Because so many different methods are used, there are situations in which defining appropriate standards is difficult and still controversial among scientists. This is reminiscent of the *New Yorker* cartoon showing two individuals in jail in which one says to the other, "I thought I was well within the community standard for misconduct." Jasanoff believes that there is less agreement about what constitutes acceptable norms of scientific behavior than most people assume and that this lack of clarity and resulting criticism of the integrity of scientists needs to be recast in a new style of prospectively creating acceptable research practices. She believes that confronting and dismantling structural barriers to collegiality in research, such as the "winner-take-all" philosophy, will be necessary for improving the environment for scientists and obtaining the confidence of the public in the scientific endeavor.

If clear guidelines for scientific behavior do not now exist, are they needed? Scientists join a profession. Society has entrusted internal oversight and self-correction mechanisms to this profession as part of the responsibilities of membership. As infractions of the professions' norms occur and are reported by the media to the public, public confidence is shaken.

In modern society, there are no longer well-developed, shared religious and political values as existed in previous times. In addition, the value-laden nature of scientific endeavors was not as widely recognized as it is now. When there is a loss in public confidence in scientists, the government continues to develop regulations in an attempt to ensure that scientists behave ethically. For example, institutions receiving public research funding are required to have written policies about how to react when charges of misconduct are leveled at any member of their community.

To sustain public trust in the research enterprise and in the interest of achieving uniformity in federal policies, a notification of final federal policy on research misconduct was published by the Executive Office of the President in the *Federal Register* in December 2000.[7] This policy establishes the scope of the federal government's interest in the accuracy and reliability of research records and processes. It consists of guidelines for the response of federal agencies and research institutions to allegations of research misconduct and a new definition of research misconduct. Before the newly suggested definition of misconduct is accepted, each agency must officially move to accept the definition.

Because of the importance of these new definitions, they are quoted here even before any government agency has accepted them officially. "Research misconduct is defined as fabrication, falsification, or plagiarism in proposing, performing, or reviewing research or in reporting research results." . . . "Research, as used herein, includes all basic, applied, and demonstration research in all fields of science, engineering, and mathematics. This includes, but is not limited to, research in economics, education, linguistics, medicine, psychology, social sciences, statistics, and research involving human subjects or animals." All misconduct must be avoided in science because "advances in science, engineering, and all fields of research depend on the reliability of the research record, as do the benefits associated with them in areas such as health and national security."[7] Although this policy applies to research done by or funded by the government, or both, most institutional misconduct policies include all research performed at researchers' institutions regardless of funding sources. The misconduct policy applies to all research but does not supersede regulations concerning unethical treatment of human research subjects, mistreatment of laboratory animals, or other types of misconduct (e.g., financial mismanagement, vandalism, sexual harassment).

The definition continues,

Fabrication is making up of data or results and recording or reporting them. Falsification is manipulating research materials, equipment, or processes, or changing or omitting data or results such that the research is not accurately represented in the research record. The research record of data or results that embody the facts resulting from scientific inquiry includes, but is not limited to, research proposals, laboratory records, both physical and electronic, progress reports, abstracts, theses, oral presentation, internal reports, and journal articles.

Plagiarism is the appropriation of another person's ideas, processes, results, or words without giving appropriate credit. The new definition retains the concept from previous definitions that research misconduct does not include honest error or differences of opinion.[7]

In addition, on November 28, 2000, the Department of Health and Human Services published a notice of rule making in the *Federal Register* that would require universities to provide due process protections for so-called whistle blowers, that is, those who have brought charges of scientific misconduct against others.[8] If implemented, the regulation, which protects persons who make good-faith allegations or who experience retaliation as the result of being whistle blowers, would pertain to any organization that applied for or received grants or contracts from the Public Health Service (http://www.access.gpolgov/su_doce/aces/aces 140.html).

The Institutional Role

Classic studies like *Asylums* by Erving Goffman[9] or the studies on Nazi doctors by Robert J. Lifton[10] serve as stark reminders that the institutions in which we work can have detrimental effects on individuals under their purview. When considering the role of the university in providing ethical leadership for its community, Harold Shapiro, head of the National Bioethics Advisory Board and president of Princeton University, has reminded us that, "In the final analysis it is a society that is full of hope rather than fear, full of trust rather than alienation, full of knowledge rather than ignorance, full of confidence rather than helplessness, that will survive and progress. It is to these issues, therefore, that the nation and the university must address themselves."[11]

Conclusion

Because science moves ever forward, building on the work of previous scientists, it is important to decide on and then articulate a shared understanding of what is entailed by the responsible conduct of science. Science has only partly achieved this goal of a shared understanding, and much remains for individuals and their scientific societies to accomplish to delineate appropriate shared standards more clearly.

References

1. The Belmont Report: ethical principles and guidelines for the protection of human subjects. In: *Institutional Review Guidebook*. Bethesda, MD: National Institutes of Health; 1993. Available at: http://ohrp.osophs.dhhs.gov/human subjects/guidance/belmont.htm.
2. Bulger RE. Toward a statement of the principles underlying responsible conduct in biomedical research. *Acad Med.* 1974;68:102–107.
3. Russell WMS, Burch RL. *The Principles of Humane Experimental Technique.* Springfield, IL: Charles C. Thomas; 1959.
4. Bulger RJ, Bulger RE. Obstacles to collegiality in the academic health center. *Bull NY Acad Med.* 1992;68:303–307.
5. Kuhn TS. *The Structure of Scientific Revolutions*, 2nd Ed. Chicago, IL: University of Chicago Press; 1970.
6. Jasanoff S. Innovation and integrity in biomedical research. *Acad Med.* 1993;68(suppl. 3): S91–S95.
7. Executive Office of the President. Notification of final federal policy on research misconduct, 65 *Federal Register* 76260–76264 (2000).
8. Notice of rule making: standards for the protection of research misconduct whistleblowers, 65 *Federal Register* 70830–70841 (2000).
9. Goffman E. *Asylums: Essays on the Social Situation of Mental Patients and Other Inmates.* New York: Anchor Books; 1990.
10. Lifton RJ. *The Nazi Doctors: Medical Killing and the Psychology of Genocide.* New York: Basic Books; 1986.
11. Shapiro H. The research university. In: *The Bridge* Vol. 22. Washington, DC: National Academy Press; 1992.

The Pathogenesis of Fraud in Medical Science

Robert G. Petersdorf

Recently I had a disquieting experience. A young faculty member about to be appointed in a clinical department was discovered to have submitted several papers containing fraudulent data to several reputable journals. Up to this shocking discovery he had not been suspected of malfeasance. In fact, he was considered somewhat of a "child prodigy." He had done superbly in medical school and was excellently trained; during his fellowship he wrote over 30 papers. When he was proposed for his initial faculty appointment, he had authored in excess of 100 papers.

In assembling the proposal for this man's academic appointment, a senior member of the department reviewed some of these publications. The data of several control groups were the same in several papers: normally, different experiments should have different controls. The senior faculty member consulted with the coauthors. They had never seen the papers. Technicians in the laboratory could not recall the experiments. The data books could not be found. No purchase orders for the animals used in the experiments could be found. The grants to which the work had been credited had not contained enough money to purchase the animals used in the work that was published. When the young investigator was confronted with these doubts, he denied all the allegations but was unable to marshal proof that the allegations were false. His letter of resignation from the faculty followed shortly thereafter.

One might think that the episode ends here. Although a full investigation has corroborated the fraud in some papers, others need to be reviewed. The investigation will need to be continued: to protect the coauthors; to salvage the reputations of the research fellows who worked with the culpable investigator (but who can give them back the years of fellowship?); and to protect the granting agencies.

The "Premed Syndrome"

How have we gotten into this sorry mess? Believe it or not, it probably began with the "pre-med syndrome," painfully familiar to many in medical education. It begins with fierce competition in college, excessive emphasis on grades, and the rise of students who become 22-hour-a-day study machines. The syndrome was analyzed in detail in the May 1985 issue of *The Washington Monthly* (1). Some quotes from this article are instructive.

A recent study of 400 medical students by doctors at two Chicago medical schools revealed that 88% of the subjects had cheated at least once while they were pre-meds. The researchers found widespread cynicism among their subjects as demonstrated by frequent agreement with statements such as "people have to cheat in this dog-eat-dog world."

From *Annals of Internal Medicine*, 1986, 104, pp. 252–254. Reproduced by permission.

The majority of students continued to cheat in medical school:

The most disturbing finding was that there was a continuum from cheating in college to cheating in medical school in didactic areas to cheating in clerkships and patient care. Cheating in medical school may be a predictor to cheating in practice.

The culture in which we train our young promotes cheating:

From crib notes in organic chemistry to Medicare fraud and fudged results in medical research, the connection may be there.

The Large Size of Science

A second factor in the pathogenesis of scientific fraud is the very size of science itself. Despite some recent erosion of research budgets, they are much greater in absolute terms than ever before. The department of medicine that I chaired for 15 years, from 1964 to 1979, serves as an example (2). During this 15-year period the research budget quintupled while the teaching load only tripled. This increase in the research enterprise was accompanied by an increase in the size of graduate training programs. The number of housestaff tripled, the number of graduate students and postdoctoral fellows increased markedly, and the number of clinical fellows increased most of all.

In fellowship training groups in internal medicine, as many as 18 fellows in a group is not unusual. Despite claims that more than 50% of these clinical fellows go into academic medicine – claims that I have never believed even in the days of training grants – I have real doubts as to whether we need so many persons in advanced training, either for the academy or for practice. In fact, there is now good evidence that we do not need them for practice, where there is a surfeit of almost all types of specialists and subspecialists (3). The penchant for procreation among directors of clinical programs and among trainers of basic scientists knows no bounds; they feel that they have a right to generate the intellectual progeny of the future, whether that progeny becomes an overpopulation or not.

What are the consequences of big science? First, there is the inability to say grace over the large research groups that now exist. Thus these groups have an intermediate layer of junior faculty, many of whom are relatively inexperienced in training people and supervising research. It also results in group projects. There are not enough good ideas to go around to keep the excessive number of trainees busy. As a consequence, group projects abound with the inevitable result, the multiauthored paper. Characteristic of the multiauthored paper is that it is often not completely reviewed, and usually not in detail by every author. A few decades ago the department chair read every paper emanating from his department. This is clearly no longer possible, but now even division heads do not read the papers, as some in whose divisions fraud has occurred now ruefully admit.

Competition

A third factor in the pathogenesis of fraud is competition itself – not necessarily the competition to be first in press but, more often, the competition for grants. The progressive funding of grants with higher priorities does not connote that the science is necessarily better. It only means that competition for the research dollar is greater. Getting new grants or successful renewals requires productivity, and productivity, in turn, requires training of new people who can then publish more papers.

There is also competition for position, and our system of academic promotions is the prime example. Promotions committees count and weigh papers but do not read them. The reported research is usually narrow in scope, and the promotions committees quite often are unable to understand the nature of the work. It is much easier, therefore, for them to judge quantity not quality. Unfortunately, it is also far easier to judge quantity or quality of research than excellence in teaching and excellence in clinical care.

Academic personnel policies such as tenure exacerbate competition. Tenure appointments are guarded with jealousy and are made with a sense of false elitism, and tenure is often based on faulty criteria. Competition among young faculty for the scarce tenured slot returns the faculty to the days of the "pre-med syndrome." Tenure as a personnel policy in medical schools assures only a small fraction of the faculty member's income (4). The good do not need it and the mediocre use it as a shield. Tenure tends to perpetuate mediocrity.

Some academicians contend that the intense competition, both professional and economic, in science makes an occasional instance of research fraud inevitable. I do not share this fatalistic attitude. I believe firmly that the committed scientist cannot alter the truth. But even if some research fraud is inevitable, it is probably preventable, if not by the sponsoring institution, then by the principal investigator himself.

In this era of big science, principal investigators must be more careful in screening their associates. All too often younger investigators are invited to join a laboratory because the funds are available to support them or because they provide an extra pair of hands to do the work. Principal investigators must learn to contain the size of their laboratories. I have from time to time seen the size of a laboratory equated with the quality of work emanating from it. In science, as in all else, big is sometimes beautiful, but often it is not.

Original research data need to be checked at several levels; graduate students, postdoctoral fellows, and junior and senior faculty members must check and cross-check the raw data and not just the computer printouts, graphs, or figures that are often an intermediate product of research. Although data books may clutter the laboratory, they must be retained so that in case of doubt they will be available for review. Multiauthored papers require input and checking by all persons named as authors and not just the senior author. Heads of divisions, departments, institutes, and schools should be sufficiently familiar with the laboratories under their administrative purview so that they will be able to launch an investigation of alleged fraud when such an investigation is needed.

Conclusions

Medical science today is too competitive, too big, too entrepreneurial, and too much bent on winning. Gone is the threadbare gentility when science depended on philanthropy for its support and was carried out by a solo investigator with perhaps one fellow and one technician (5). That era is gone if for no other reason than our science today is technically so sophisticated. But while science may be less genteel, less threadbare, and less fun, none of these is an excuse for fraud or lesser abuses. Those who have chosen science for a career have, in a sense, taken an oath to discover and disseminate the truth, much as physicians have sworn the Oath of Hippocrates. Beyond these individual commitments, the institutions in which science is performed – the medical schools, research institutes, and universities – need to create an environment in which truth prevails. They must have mechanism (6) in place to ferret out untruths and to set their house in order, when untruths are discovered.

References

1. Barrett PM. The premed machine. *The Washington Monthly* 1985;May:41–51.
2. Petersdorf RG. The evolution of departments of medicine. *N Engl J Med.* 1980;**303**:489–96.
3. Petersdorf RG. Is the establishment defensible? *N Engl J Med.* 1983;**309**:1053–7.
4. Petersdorf RG. The case against tenure in medical schools. *JAMA.* 1984;**251**:920–4.
5. Petersdorf RG. Academic medicine: No longer threadbare or genteel. *N Engl J Med.* 1981;**304**: 841–3.
6. Petersdorf RG. Preventing and investigating fraud in research [Editorial]. *J Med Educ.* 1982;**57**:880–1.

Science, Statistics, and Deception

John C. Bailar III

In science, lying is condemned, even by some of its few practitioners. Deliberate or careless deception short of lying, however, seems to be universally accepted and sometimes even promoted as a part of the culture of science. I do not suggest that scientists as a group are careless, venal, or otherwise depraved: they may even be above the human average in developing and adhering to detailed, albeit tacit, standards of professional conduct. Those who are clearly violators are drummed out of our ranks, loudly and publicly. But what about less clearcut deception?

My thesis is that our professional norms are incomplete and that several kinds of widely accepted practices (Table 1) should also be widely recognized as potentially deceptive and harmful. Some of these practices also have much value, but at times they are inappropriate and improper and, to the extent that they are deceptive, unethical.

The scientific method is fundamentally concerned with the processes of inference, generally from data that are necessarily inaccurate to some degree, incomplete, drawn from small samples, or not quite appropriate for a specific task. Inference – that is, drawing conclusions or making deductions from imperfect data – provides most of the excitement and intellectual ferment of science. Scientific rewards are probably more closely related to valid inferences established than to such related activities as imaginative hypotheses formulated, elegant experiments designed and conducted, or new methods developed. The rewards for publishing a first-class inference can include income, position and power, professional status, and the respect of colleagues. Such rewards may sometimes count for more than self-respect and the joy of discovery. We must therefore be attentive to scientific norms and activities that may distort the processes of inference.

An example of a deceptive practice is the statistical testing (such as the calculating of p values) of *post hoc* hypotheses. It is widely recognized that t-tests, chi-square tests, and other statistical tests provide a basis for probability statements only when the hypothesis is fully developed before the data are examined in any way. If even the briefest glance at a study's results moves the investigator to consider a hypothesis not formulated before the study was started, that glance destroys the probability value of the evidence at hand. Certainly, careful and unstructured review of data for unexpected clues is a critical part of science. Such review can be an immensely fruitful source of ideas for new, before-the-fact hypotheses that can be tested in the correct way with other new or existing data, and sometimes findings may be so striking that independent confirmation by a proper statistical test is superfluous. Statistical "tests" are also used sometimes in nonprobability ways as rough measures of the size of an effect rather than to test hypotheses. (An example is the column of p values

From *Annals of Internal Medicine*, 1986, 104, pp. 259–260. Reprinted by permission.

Table 1. *Some Practices that Distort Scientific Inferences*

Failure to deal honestly with readers about nonrandom error (bias)
Post hoc hypotheses
Multiple comparisons and data dredging
Inappropriate statistical tests and other statistical procedures
Fragmentation of reports
Low statistical power
Suppressing, trimming, or "adjusting" data; or undisclosed repetition of "unsatisfactory"
   experiments
Selective reporting of findings

that sometimes accompanies a table comparing the pretreatment characteristics of patient groups in a randomized clinical trial.) When either the test itself or the reporting of the test is motivated by the data, a probability statement such as "$p < 0.05$" is deceptive and hence damaging to inference.

Other potential problems are the selective reporting of findings and the reporting of a single study in multiple fragments. These practices can obscure critical aspects of an investigation, so that readers will misjudge the evidential value of the data presented. Such reporting may be deceptive, whether deliberately or accidentally. On the other hand, these practices sometimes have positive value that should be preserved. For example, they can facilitate the tasks of both the investigator and the user when a demand for a monolithic analysis might seriously delay or frustrate the progress of both.

"Negative" conclusions of low statistical power – that is, reporting that no effect was found when there was little chance of detecting the effect – can also distort inference, especially when investigators do not report on statistical power. The concept of power is formally defined in terms of the random variability of results that is inherent in a specific combination of data structure, sample size, statistical models, and analytic method; but I believe that the concept should be substantially broadened to include the likelihood that a particular effect would be detected and reported if it were present to some specified degree. Such an analysis rarely accompanies "negative" findings, and readers may be left with an unjustified sense that an effect not demonstrated is an effect not present. Again, however, there are counterarguments: a report with low power may be better than no report (and no power), or meta-analysis (1) of several low-power reports may come to stronger conclusions than any one of them alone. Reporting negative studies of low power can create ethical problems, but those problems may be largely mitigated if the low power is accurately and clearly reported as well. Too many scientists resist the objective reporting of this kind of weakness in their work, and pressure for "strong" results may be greatest during the formative years of graduate training and career entry. Thus we may be training new scientists in unethical methods.

Despite the occasionally useful roles of these and other practices listed in Table 1, each can seriously distort the processes of inference and should therefore be an object of concern. Where the practices have legitimate applications, they should, of course, be used; but even then they should be fully and explicitly disclosed by the investigator, justified in some detail, and accepted with caution by readers. A combination of restraint in their overall use, limiting their use to clearly appropriate situations, providing full disclosure and justification, and maintaining the readers' skepticism will help to diminish the frequency and severity of ethical problems. Full disclosure here means more than a few words buried in the fine print of a Methods section; it means not just that the author send a message, but that the author also work to ensure that the message is received and correctly interpreted by readers. There are parallels here to the evolving requirements for informed consent by experimental subjects.

Pressures to publish can be great and may account for many of the abuses suggested by Table 1. I fear that even the constrained use of these potentially damaging practices will leave attractive loopholes for an army of ambitious practitioners of science, each feeling great pressure to publish, who will rush in to explain why his or her situation is different, why full disclosure is inappropriate, and so forth. I am convinced that science, scientists, and society as a whole would benefit from substantially broader concepts, ultimately based on the need to protect the processes of inference, about ethical standards and violations in science.

Reference

1. Louis TA, Fineberg HV, Mosteller F. Findings for public health from meta-analysis. *Annu Rev Public Health*. 1985;6:1–20.

Innovation and Integrity in Biomedical Research

Sheila Jasanoff

Science's reputation for purity has suffered two major setbacks in the past ten years. First, we learned to question the capability of scientists to regulate themselves. Promising young researchers at some of the nations' premier academic institutions were shown to have falsified and fabricated data, and senior colleagues had taken years in some cases to discover their misconduct. Second, while policymakers and university administrators were still reeling from these revelations, we learned that burgeoning entanglements between universities and industry were creating additional incentives for misconduct in research. Cutting methodological corners, misrepresenting results, evading peer review – these and other questionable practices seemed to flow unchecked from a generation of scientists who had acquired multimillion-dollar stakes in the commercial successes of their own inventions. Ethical standards of scientific inquiry seemed to be under assault on many fronts. Organizations responsible for the support of science understandably turned their attention to investigating and remedying the problem.

More than a decade of national preoccupation with scientific integrity has bred in some respects a surprising complacency among regulators (and perhaps also scientists) about ensuring the quality of biomedical research. Conventional wisdom holds that the standards of accepted behavior are not problematic; they should be familiar to all scientists worth their salt, in universities, in industry, or in government. Policy accordingly has been directed toward making individuals and institutions comply better with the supposedly well-known rules of the scientific game. Policymakers have scrambled to find the right mix of incentives, penalties, and institutional supports for attaining this desired end point.

My aim in this article is to shift our attention from compliance to the definition of the standards themselves and to suggest that there is in fact less agreement about acceptable norms of behavior than is commonly supposed among policy critics of science. I argue further that this lack of clarity is in part a consequence of the fragmentation of research communities at the forefront of science. Standards for scientific work, as we now know, vary across time, across disciplines, and across institutions. There is no abstract, universal "scientific method" that guides practice in all situations. Data-reporting techniques that were right for Gregor Mendel would not necessarily pass muster with geneticists in the late twentieth century, who must look for guidance to contemporary practices within their own communities.

The notion of scientific community, however, has become increasingly ambiguous as science itself has diversified and grown more complex. Scientific specialties are at once

From *Academic Medicine*, 1993; 68: S91–S95. Reprinted by permission.

more narrowly subdivided and more fluid in relation to each other than at previous times in history. As a result, practitioners in closely related fields may disagree even on such basic methodological issues as the use of controls.[1] The newer and more loosely organized the field, the less likely it is that its members will belong to clearly defined peer groups adhering to precisely the same standards of practice. In some areas of clinical and experimental science – for example, studies of animal or human exposure to toxic substances – it has taken years for common practices to develop and be standardized. Moreover, what comes to be regarded as normatively acceptable behavior in science is not always controlled by scientists alone; standards can be driven by societal pressures originating outside science, as in the cases of regulations on human experimentation, guidelines for recombinant DNA research, and rules governing the ethical use of animals.

In many areas of modern bio-medical science, innovative work is done to please multiple audiences – Congress, regulators, university administrators, funding agencies, Wall Street, the press, and the public – each imposing its own demands and standards on the conduct of research. Furthermore, the researchers themselves are not necessarily organized in well-demarcated communities from which they can learn authoritative rules of practice – and to which they can be answerable in turn for deviations from the common code. Yet, in misconduct cases, the scientific community is asked to act as if this heterogeneity did not exist and as if the applicable norms should have been discernible in advance.

The incentive structure of science is another factor that stands in the way of achieving workable standards of integrity at the frontiers of biomedical research. Embedded in a competitive society, science is subject to deep-seated conflicts between individualistic and communal values. The success of a laboratory or start-up firm may depend on dedicated teamwork by technicians, students, and other support staff, but recognition and rewards flow disproportionately to the senior scientists at the top of the pyramid. As we shall see, these pressures erode the collegiality that is a prerequisite for shared standards of behavior; the practices developed by scientific competitors in the race to innovate run an especially high risk of subsequently being labeled deviant.

Past Experience and Present Malaise

Since Henry K. Beecher[2] published his controversial exposé on human experimentation in 1966, U.S. biomedical researchers have known that their enterprise is neither so altruistic nor so disinterested as might be expected from followers of the Hippocratic tradition. Yet, although examples such as the deliberate failure to treat syphilis-infected patients or the injection of live cancer cells into healthy patients aroused universal revulsion, a widespread response in the medical community was to dismiss Beecher's examples as isolated aberrations from ethically correct behavior. A similar reaction greeted the publication in *Nature* of the now famous attack by Stewart and Feder on the integrity of the scientific literature.[3] The article analyzed a corpus of work coauthored by a single researcher, Dr. John Darsee, who had been discovered fabricating data at Harvard Medical School. The piece could therefore be seen as an extended case study of a particular deviant individual rather than as a generalized critique of science, and many in the scientific community chose to read Stewart and Feder's charges in this relatively comforting light. Others, however, wondered whether Darsee would have flourished as long or as dramatically in an environment that was genuinely committed to upholding integrity.

As new disclosures followed, explanations for scientific dishonesty crystallized into the aptly named "rotten apple" and "rotten system" theories.[4] The former attributed instances of fraud to flaws in the individual researcher's character, while the latter held that the entire environment for research was culpable for the misbehavior of individuals. Proponents of the "rotten apple" theory focused on the uncontrolled ambitions and weak moral instincts of guilty scientists such as John Darsee. The less sanguine "rotten system" theorists asserted that fraud was only to be expected in a work environment characterized by lax supervision from above, competitive relations among colleagues of the same rank, and emphasis on quantity over quality in the reporting of results. Critics of the research system saw the reported instances of fraud as just "the tip of the iceberg" and speculated that misconduct was much more prevalent than these small numbers appeared to suggest. Disagreements between the two schools thus focused on the questions of how big the problem was and who should be blamed for it. Participants in the debate tacitly assumed that there was little or no contest as to what kinds of conduct were actually worthy of blame.

Throughout the 1980s, however, there were episodes that hinted at a deeper level of complexity. Thus, the prolonged investigation of David Baltimore's laboratory at MIT's Whitehead Institute raised questions about whether fraud could always be clearly distinguished from error in scientific work. This potentially troublesome issue lost its centrality when congressional investigators produced seemingly irrefutable proof that Thereza Imanishi-Kari, Baltimore's accused coworker, had fabricated some of the data that she had claimed as authentic. Attempts by federal agencies to define scientific misconduct led to more serious disagreements about the boundary between acceptable and unacceptable behavior. Scientists took particular issue with the decision by the Public Health Service and the National Science Foundation to include in their definitions not just the relatively uncontested categories of fabrication, falsification, and plagiarism but also the catch-all category of "other serious deviations from accepted research practices.[5,6] Many found this formulation unacceptably vague and feared that it would allow federal enforcers to sweep legitimate instances of scientific innovation into the domain of misconduct.

A number of recent controversies about scientific integrity suggest that the scientific community's concerns about the definition of "accepted practices" were not entirely unfounded. Although incidents of plagiarism, data fabrication, and falsification continue to be reported, some highly publicized and consequential instances of questionable conduct appear to fall within the category of serious deviations from accepted practice. Yet, the borderline between deviant and nondeviant behavior has proved difficult to draw even in seemingly straightforward cases of plagiarism. When does a review article, for example, cross the boundary between responsible summary and unacceptable appropriation of the words or ideas of other authors? In cases involving more complex charges of improper research or reporting, scientists from different institutional perspectives have come to quite different conclusions about what constitutes misconduct. Indeed, the heterogeneity of the institutions that claim to set standards for science is an important factor in explaining the conflicting assessments that surfaced in the cases described below.

In the spring of 1992, a rift developed between the NIH's Office of Scientific Integrity (OSI) and a panel of independent researchers investigating the conduct of Dr. Robert Gallo, codiscoverer of the AIDS virus.[7] In particular, the outside panel criticized the OSI's decision to blame only Mikulas Popovic, Gallo's junior coauthor, for four instances of misconduct in their joint 1984 article announcing the discovery. NIH director Bernadine Healy defended her agency's exoneration of Gallo, but Congress and the press appeared inclined to accept the advisory panel's contrary judgment. It took another half-year for the newly created Office of Research Integrity in the Department of Health and Human Services to sort through the impasse and to conclude that Gallo himself had been guilty of false reporting in the AIDS article. These investigators also found Gallo substantially responsible for the instances of misconduct previously attributed to Popovic alone. In the course of the investigation, however, some charges against Gallo and Popovic were deemed not to constitute misconduct, such as the authors' failure to give credit for the cell line in which the AIDS virus was eventually grown. This protracted episode illustrated both how institutional factors influenced the assessment of a noted scientist's behavior and how troublesome it was to decide whether particular statements and practices constituted carelessness, error, or blameworthy scientific conduct.

In October 1992, U.S. Army officials notified Congress that they were investigating Lt. Col. Robert Redfield, one of their leading AIDS researchers and a noted advocate of vaccine therapy, for making a possibly misleading report of clinical trial data at a public meeting.[8] As the investigation unfolded, debate centered on the method chosen by Redfield to detect increases or decreases in the amounts of viral material in patients' blood cells. A statistician from a private research foundation disagreed with one of Redfield's statistical techniques, observing that it was biologically unmotivated and therefore arbitrary. Some of Redfield's own colleagues were troubled by his failure to consult them before presenting his analysis to a wider audience. At the same time, others familiar with the investigation speculated that the issue would never have arisen but for the charged political climate surrounding a $20-million appropriation by Congress for the army to test a particular AIDS vaccine. Rivalry between the army and the other services was also cited as a factor precipitating the investigation. This case pointed to the possibility that variations in scientific practice that would normally pass as innocent, though ill considered, might be reclassified as "misconduct" under less friendly political circumstances.

In January 1993, a small drug company named Centocor, Inc. announced that it was withdrawing its extremely promising antisepsis drug Centotoxin from the European countries where it had already been marketed.[9] Once projected to save many thousands of lives each year, the drug had turned out in clinical studies to be of doubtful usefulness; the death rate in one group of patients treated with the drug was higher than that in an untreated group. An inquiry into the incident showed that Centocor had pushed ahead with early clinical tests based on a promising scientific idea and positive early experiments, although other scientists had held back because they had been unable to replicate the key animal tests. An advisory committee of the Food and Drug Administration (FDA) certified Centocor's approach as legitimate, but then it emerged that, in violation of FDA rules, the company had changed its standards for determining success during its first clinical study of the drug. The FDA thereupon demanded a second study, which resulted in the problematic survival rates. Possible defects in Centocor's market-driven approach to drug testing thus came to light only when the company was required to comply with the FDA's more cautious, risk-averse rules of practice.

In each of these three cases – Gallo, Redfield, Centocor – we sense that something more than the "rotten apple" or the "rotten system" theory is needed to explain the investigator's apparent failure to conform to socially acceptable norms of scientific inquiry. To begin with, neither theory satisfactorily explains why the existence of improper behavior was itself a contested issue in these cases. Why did it take three years of federal investigation, with contradictory findings in between, to reach a consensus that Gallo as well as Popovic was guilty of misconduct? Why did Redfield's conduct become the object of investigation in the first place, and did his faulty methodology represent a moral failing or poor scientific judgment? How was it possible for Centocor to market its product in ten European countries and win initial approval from the FDA's scientific advisers if its approach to clinical trials was fundamentally flawed in ways that should have been apparent to responsible scientific reviewers? One must conclude from examples like these that the messiness of actual scientific practice resists easy partitioning into the black-and-white judgments that are called for in misconduct investigations.

A second and related point is that in each case a variety of institutions were engaged in the process of determining whether scientific integrity had been violated. This multifaceted engagement was most dramatically visible in the Gallo investigation, where Gallo himself, his supporters and colleagues, his French competitors, and the independent scientific community, as well as Congress, the Department of Health and Human Services, the NIH, and the investigative press, all asserted a right to speak to the question of misconduct. More limited kinds of interinstitutional negotiation took place in the Redfield and Centocor cases as well: for example, behind-the-scenes conflicts among the armed services in the former and the partly public disagreements among the FDA, its advisers, and the drug company in the latter. Debated in mixed scientific and political, private and public communities, the issue of integrity clearly involved considerably more than the application of well-understood criteria of accepted practice to instances of questioned conduct.

Third, there are common elements in these stories that are frequently underemphasized in conventional explanations for scientific misconduct. Intellectual commitment is one such factor, one that is almost always in play when one looks at innovative research. At least in the Redfield and Centocor cases, and arguably also in the case of Gallo, the investigators were driven by a belief that the natural world would behave in certain ways; and their publications, presentations, and studies were designed to reinforce these beliefs – at times with pronounced disregard for competing or contradictory opinions from their peers. In each case, moreover, scientific research was conducted in the knowledge that success might bring very substantial rewards in money as well as recognition. This knowledge led to a perceptible narrowing of the researchers' formal and informal relationships within the scientific community, as reflected in decisions to deny credit or exclude potential coauthors (in the Gallo case), to bypass possibly critical coworkers (in the Redfield example), and to ignore scientists whose results did not confirm one's own expectations (in the Centocor example). In each case, too, the questionable practices occurred in an atmosphere of haste, with the investigators' desire for priority apparently taking precedence over science's traditional bent toward caution. In all, the circumstances were far better calculated to promote individualized and idiosyncratic behavior than to make scientists adhere to consistent, communally endorsed, and critically tested standards of research practice.

Rebuilding Scientific Community

Setting aside the relatively uncontroversial questions of falsification, fabrication, and plagiarism, the exercise of determining the acceptability of innovative research practices turns out to be unexpectedly complex. The examples cited above suggest that in fast-track areas of science there may not in fact be any a priori standards for distinguishing deviant from normal behavior. Standards may come into being only after work is challenged, through a laborious, sometimes contested, multi-institutional process of negotiation, whose end point is to find the accused scientist guilty or not guilty of misconduct. That standards are thus retroactively determined does not, of course, make them any the less credible as statements of a communal viewpoint. Indeed, in science as in democratic politics, the fact that blame is apportioned through a long and deliberative process makes the final judgment perhaps all the more compelling.

Here, however, we confront a paradox. How can we expect scientists to conform to codes of accepted research practice if they cannot be sure until after a complex inquiry whether their conduct will be deemed innocent, careless, unwise, uncollegial, or absolutely unacceptable? Put more provocatively, how should Robert Gallo have known in 1984 that the article he wrote with Popovic constituted scientific misconduct if it took more than three years of investigation for his adversaries to come to that conclusion, and if an intermediate report even exonerated him of wrongdoing?

The most promising way out of the paradox may be to recast the problem of scientific integrity as one of prospectively creating acceptable research practices rather than retrospectively finding and applying them. Recognizing that rules of acceptability arise from the actual doing of science, our aim should be to encourage those forms of scientific practice that are most likely to resist charges of deviance. Scientists cannot in principle be constrained by standards in areas of science where the rules of acceptable behavior are still evolving, but they can be asked to carry out their work in ways that will not court widespread censure by other members of the community. Arguably the most effective way of accomplishing that is to build a stronger sense of science as a collaborative activity among those engaged in innovative research. Criticism, cooperation, and data sharing, for example, have proved to be reliable techniques for assuring the communal acceptability of scientific practices. They may well offer researchers the surest guarantee against charges of misconduct.

To achieve conditions that foster integrity, however, will require more than the teaching of research ethics to graduate students or the education of senior scientists in better methods of mentoring. The entire culture of science will need to confront and, where necessary, dismantle the structural barriers to collegiality in research. Integrity, as we have seen, is most secure when it is grounded in a strong communal tradition of research practice. Acceptance by others, the ultimate indicator of honesty, demands that scientists submit their work to testing and criticism by peers. The rewards for discovery in science are oblivious to claims of community, however, and go almost entirely to the heroic individual or team that produces the new result. The major institutions of science are structured accordingly. Thus, journal editors compete intensely to capture pathbreaking articles, thereby reinforcing the image of science as a place of tight races and photo finishes. Patents, under U.S. law, are bestowed on the first to discover a new process or invent a new product. Prizes go to the first to publish a brilliant and unexpected finding. Science, as is often noted, is a winner-take-all game, with no glory or comfort for the also-ran.

Would a more collaborative science, with better distributed rewards and fewer incentives for speeding, produce as many dazzling results? Would progress in research or industry be seriously slowed if science became a more mannerly and collegial enterprise? As always, the burden of proof rests on those who would change the status quo. Nonetheless, with the public image of science hanging in the balance, the time may be ripe for taking up the challenge.

References

1. Jasanoff, Sheila. The Fifth Branch: Science Advisers as Policymakers. Cambridge, Massachusetts: Harvard University Press, 1993.
2. Beecher, H. K. Ethics and Clinical Research. *N. Engl. J. Med.* **274**(1966): 1354–1368.
3. Stewart, W. W., and Feder, N. The Integrity of the Scientific Literature. *Nature* **325**(1987): 207–214.
4. Engler, Robert L., Covell, James W., Friedman, Paul J., Kitcher, Philip S., and Peters, Richard M. Misrepresentation and Responsibility in Medical Research. *N. Engl. J. Med.* **317**(1987): 1383–1389.
5. Abelson, Philip H. Integrity of the Research Process. *Science* **256**(1992): 1257.
6. National Academy of Sciences. *Responsible Science: Ensuring the Integrity of the Research Process.* Washington, D.C.: National Academy Press, 1992.
7. Palca, Joseph. 'Verdicts' Are in on the Gallo Probe. *Science* **256**(1992): 735–737.
8. Cohen, John. Army Investigates Researcher's Report of Clinical Trial Data. *Science* **258**(1992): 883–884.
9. Kolata, Gina. Halted at Market's Door: How a $1 Billion Drug Failed. *New York Times,* February 12, 1993, p. A1.

Preventing Scientific Misconduct

Douglas L. Weed

When a case of serious scientific misconduct comes to light, reactions from scientists, legislators, journal editors, and the press are often swift and impassioned, reflecting the importance of a problem that strikes at the heart of the scientific enterprise. Science, after all, is a search for the truth. Misconduct, especially in the form of falsification or fabrication, is its antithesis. Biomedical science seems especially vulnerable to the serious consequences forecast by those involved in the extended discussion: Congressional oversight could become a reality, public trust could fray, and perhaps most ominous of all, patients could be harmed. Few authors agree on the frequency of scientific misconduct, owing to differing definitions and difficulties in measurement. Estimates vary widely. Nevertheless, nearly everyone agrees that preventing scientific misconduct is a worthy goal. How best to achieve that goal is not so clear. The purpose of this paper is to develop a framework for the prevention of scientific misconduct based on models familiar to public health professionals, to discuss some problems that emerge from such an analysis, and to propose tentative solutions to those problems. I begin with two questions: What is scientific misconduct, and how much of it exists?

The Nature and Extent of Scientific Misconduct

Two definitions of scientific misconduct, one from the National Science Foundation and the other from the Department of Health and Human Services, emerged in the early 1990s.[1] In both, scientific misconduct was defined as fabrication, falsification, plagiarism, or any other serious deviation from accepted scientific practices in proposing, conducting, or reporting research. A debate ensured over the inclusion of the words "other serious deviation." Proponents argued that this broad term permitted scientific communities to define what constituted ethical conduct and appropriate practices specific to their branches of science.[2,3] Opponents argued that the term was too broad.[4] Although its inclusion appeared to allow sanctions against scientists who undertook innovative, ground-breaking science – which could be construed as a "serious deviation from accepted practice" – no such cases were known.[5] Recently, a federally appointed commission recast the definition in terms of a principle with examples.[6] The commission's report stated that "research misconduct is [a] serious violation of the fundamental principle that scientists be truthful and fair in the conduct of research and the dissemination of research results." It said that unethical conduct includes misappropriation (plagiarism or breaches of confidentiality), interference,

From *American Journal of Public Health*. 1998;88:125–129. Reproduced by permission.

misrepresentation (falsification or fabrication), obstruction of investigations of misconduct, and noncompliance with research regulations.

Not everyone agrees with the commission's expansion of the definition of misconduct.[7] Some believe such a broad definition could increase the number of investigations because it includes any type of behavior judged to be untruthful or unfair.[8] On the other hand, some authors have for years insisted that misconduct should be very broadly defined to include behaviors not only beyond falsification, fabrication, and plagiarism, but also beyond the categories included in the expanded definition introduced by the commission.[9-11] Deceptive scientific practices, such as the misrepresentation of research results, are the most commonly cited behaviors. Failure to explain weaknesses in data, selective reporting of results, failure to publish a study with negative results, and reporting as "negative" a study with low power are a few examples of this less serious form of misconduct.[9,10] Practices of irresponsible authorship and wasteful (i.e., repetitive) publication have also been designated misconduct.[11]

It is important to distinguish between error and misconduct. Science makes progress because error exists, in measurement and in interpretation of evidence. But these are unintentional errors. Misconduct involves intentional misrepresentation or misappropriation. To put the relationship of error to misconduct in perspective, it may be helpful to consider scientists' conduct to range across a continuum. At one end are serious forms of misconduct, followed by deceptive reporting practices and then, toward the middle, what might best be called sloppiness. At the other end of the continuum lies appropriate scientific and professional conduct, including unintentional error.

Estimating the occurrence of scientific misconduct is not made easier by conceptualizing such a continuum. The many published opinions on the topic are polarized between the belief that scientific misconduct is a rare event[12] and the belief that it is rampant.[13] A recent *Lancet* editorial claims that the prevalence of fraud alone in research studies is between 0.1% and 0.4%, although no source for this estimate is provided.[14]

Three types of empirical estimation studies of scientific misconduct have been undertaken. In the first, written records (e.g., published papers and employment applications) were examined for accuracy (see references 15 through 17). Sekas and Hutson for example, recently found that 30% of applicants for a gastroenterology fellowship who claimed prior publications fabricated either the article or the journal cited.[16] A slightly higher percentage misrepresented their research experience. Lower but significant rates of misrepresentation were found in applications to emergency medicine residency programs, with the number of misrepresentations increasing with the number of citations.[17]

In the second type of study, questionnaires were used to assess respondents' knowledge of misconduct among academic colleagues.[18,19] Swazey et al., for example, estimated that 9% of 2600 students and faculty from several university departments had "direct knowledge" of faculty members who had plagiarized.[20] When the definition of misconduct was expanded from fabrication, falsification, and plagiarism to include a long list of questionable practices such as honorary authorship, sexual harassment, misuse of research funds, and safety violations, the percentage of those who had observed or had direct evidence of these practices increased to 44% of students and 50% of faculty.

The third type of study reported the results of routing data auditing of investigational drug programs.[21,22] Shapiro and Charrow found that the percentage of serious deficiencies had diminished between 1985 and 1988 from 12% to 7% in the work of nearly 2000 investigators.[22] The occurrence of scientific misconduct can also be tracked through the records of cases investigated by the Office of Research Integrity of the US Public Health Service and other investigational bodies.

Although quantitative assessments will help answer the question of how much misconduct exists, it is an unfortunate fact that big effects may arise from small numbers. A single well-publicized case of serious misconduct, such as the recent case of fabrication in a large government-sponsored cancer treatment trial,[23,24] can do considerable damage to institutions, to scientists' reputations, and to the public's already precipitously balanced perception of science. Therefore, scientific misconduct must not be ignored or trivialized, regardless of its prevalence.[25]

A Framework for Prevention

Preventing scientific misconduct is a widely recognized goal.[1,26–30] Attainment of this goal may require that we consider misconduct a professional affliction amenable to both primary and secondary prevention efforts. The implications of such an analysis have not been carefully examined.

Primary Prevention of Scientific Misconduct

Primary prevention is typically conceived as identifying and removing causes of events and as identifying factors whose presence (rather than absence) actively reduces the occurrence of those events. Frequently proposed causes of scientific misconduct fall into two categories overlapping those mentioned above, and in some cases overlapping each other. There are causes *external* to the individual scientist, such as publication pressure,[18,31–34] competition,[35,36] the large scale of science (reducing opportunities for effective mentoring),[34,35] and mentors setting bad examples.[36] There are also *internal* causes, such as personal financial gain,[28,29] ego or vanity,[28–30] and psychiatric illness.[13,28]

Psychiatric illness readily fits the traditional conception of primary prevention. "Remove" it by effective psychiatric treatment and some cases of scientific misconduct, specifically those involving mentally impaired yet employable scientists, could be prevented. How much misconduct is attributable to mental disease is an open and important question. Any answer must consider the possibility that those accused of misconduct may run (perhaps instinctively) to a psychiatrist, claiming illness and thereby avoiding responsibility for what may best be described as a character flaw rather than an uncontrollable personality disorder.

The most frequently posited causes of misconduct are publication pressure and competition. However, it is not clear how reducing – much less eliminating – these factors would reduce scientific misconduct without also reducing some of that which makes science the rigorous and productive enterprise it has become. Perhaps it is a matter of degree. Indeed, to reduce publication pressure, suggested interventions typically involve emphasizing quality over quantity in academic appointments and promotions as well as eliminating honorary authorship.[34] Although these are reasonable proposals, they may have little impact on the publication pressure inherent in science.

Another proposed external cause of scientific misconduct – ineffective mentoring owing to the large scale of science – reflects the idea that having too few senior scientist mentors relative to the number of junior scientists reduces the ability to monitor the (mis)behavior of those mentored. Nor can good examples be set if there are too few mentors. In either case, recommendations to increase opportunities for mentoring by increasing the ratio of senior to junior scientists seem reasonable, assuming resources are available. Nevertheless, providing more mentors and providing good mentors may not be equivalent. Indeed, bad mentoring (a proposed external cause of scientific misconduct) and the proposed internal causes of personal financial gain and vanity – which Kassirer combined into one "fame and fortune viper"[29] – together reveal an implicit claim regarding the etiology of scientific misconduct: that many scientists, because of ignorance or by design, are seriously unskilled in ethics, if not morally bankrupt. Indeed, descriptions of some cases make it reasonable to wonder if scientific misconduct is a product of basic flaws in the characters of scientists. To what extent, then, can ethics training shore up what has eroded or was never planted: a coherent and useful professional scientific ethic?

An often-cited approach to teaching ethics within the context of scientific misconduct involves codes of responsible conduct, that is, rules or guidelines for good (appropriate) scientific and professional practice.[1,28] Yet there are some fundamental problems with teaching ethics as a set of rules just as it would be seriously deficient to teach science as a set of rules for the laboratory or for the computer. In any professional scientific practice there are thousands of decisions not covered in the rules. In addition, there is the issue (at least in ethics) of what kind of individual follows rules in the first place. Ethics, like science, has its theories and methodologies beyond the rules that help to interpret the rules and to guide practice where the rules are missing.[37,38] Which of these theories and methods will prove most helpful as a foundation for preventing scientific misconduct is an important question, given the prominent theoretical plurality in contemporary bioethics.

It is beyond the scope of this paper to fully discuss the role of moral theory in ethics education. Nevertheless, one such theory – the theory of virtue ethics or character ethics – may be necessary in any account of the ethics of scientific misconduct and so deserves attention.[25] The virtues are traits of character habitually exhibited and important for attaining the goods internal to a practice.[39] By many accounts, the good internal to the practice of science is the truth; science is a search for the "really real" of the world. Fabrication and falsification, or misappropriation and misrepresentation, are direct affronts to this search, as are deceptive scientific practices. While there are many virtues to consider,[40] those of honesty, self-effacement, and excellence seem best suited to helping scientists stay on their appointed path. Put another way, scientists should develop and habitually exhibit honesty rather than dishonesty, and they should put the interests of the profession and of society (especially those of research subjects) before their personal interests, whether financial gain or fame or both. Scientists should habitually exhibit excellence rather than sloppiness. These virtues provide a moral foundation for preventing not only serious forms of misconduct (e.g., fabrication and falsification) but also the lesser offenses (e.g., misrepresentation of research results) that Bailar[9] and others have argued are part of the continuum of misconduct.

An obvious concern regarding virtue ethics as one pillar of ethics education is how to go about developing character traits within individual scientists. Pellegrino argues that virtue ethics, like all moral theories, can be taught from the literature and from case studies illustrating its dimensions, although the most efficacious approach may be to learn by example – by observing, emulating, and reflecting upon the virtuous behavior of a respected mentor.[25,40] Clearly, such mentors must not only possess the requisite virtues but also habitually display them in their everyday scientific practice. Judging from recent cases of serious misconduct, remedial ethics education for some senior scientists may be necessary. There is no guarantee, of course, that learning the virtuous scientific life from a virtuous mentor will lead to right actions or the right motivations for actions. Nevertheless, if the virtues of honesty, self-effacement, and excellence could be instilled in scientists during their training, three of the seven causes of scientific misconduct – mentors' setting bad examples, personal financial gain, and ego or vanity – could potentially be modified.

Problems Emerging within a Framework of Primary Prevention

Three problems deserve scrutiny. First, on what evidentiary and inferential bases have the proposed causes of scientific misconduct been judged? Second, how much scientific misconduct can be attributed to these causes, and how much misconduct remains unexplained? Finally, how can we determine whether suggested preventive interventions, inasmuch as they relate directly to purported causes of scientific misconduct, are effective in reducing the occurrence of misconduct, however broadly defined? These are closely related questions in the public health model. Attribution requires a decision regarding causality. Thus, to attribute cases of misconduct to a particular factor is to assume implicitly that the factor is (or can reasonably be judged to be) causal. In turn, an answer to the intervention question may help answer the question regarding cause. One of the best tests of a causal hypothesis is to remove the cause and observe the effect of the preventive intervention. But to observe preventive effects, surveillance systems must be in place to track the occurrence of misconduct before and after the intervention. In addition, primary preventive interventions in public health are rarely attempted without a reasonable body of evidence supporting the underlying causal hypothesis. The evidence supporting proposed causes of scientific misconduct is extraordinarily weak; it consists solely of expert opinion, an evidentiary category almost always fraught with opposing views. For example, Pellegrino states that "fraud is not the product of deranged or unhinged minds,"[25] while the Royal College of Physicians report states that "a . . . cause of scientific misconduct is psychiatric illness," with an accompanying note that "there [are] no data on [this issue]."[28]

Perhaps it is time to formally study the determinants of scientific misconduct.[41] This task will require behavioral and social science methodologies if scientific misconduct represents, for the most part, deliberate and conscious acts on the part of its perpetrators. Its causes, therefore, are more "historical" than "natural," according to Collingwood's classic categorization of causation.[42] A difficult aspect of such a study will be to tease out the effects of the most commonly cited causes, publication pressure and competition, because they are analogous to universal environmental factors; nearly everyone in science is exposed to them.[43] Furthermore, they are not independent of one another. Nevertheless, it makes sense to undertake surveys of professional groups regarding their knowledge, attitudes, and beliefs about misconduct in science; to obtain better empirical estimates of prevalence and incidence rates of misconduct; and to conduct case-control studies in which case subjects are those who have committed misconduct. Problems of case ascertainment, recall and other forms of information bais, and confounding should be expected.

Secondary Prevention of Scientific Misconduct

In the classic public health model, secondary prevention involves early detection of disease events coupled with effective treatment. For the secondary prevention of scientific misconduct, early detection involves increasing opportunities for discovering instances of misconduct, and "treatment" refers to procedures for investigating cases as well as the sanctions delivered to those responsible for the misconduct.

Auditing is the most obvious strategy for finding instances of scientific misconduct, although less drastic measures have been suggested: periodic review of scientific records, publications, and workloads.[18,22,28] Increasing the ratio of senior to junior scientists, discussed previously, is also a form of secondary prevention, inasmuch as one role for the mentor is to monitor the behavior of junior colleagues. These approaches to early detection require the concomitant acceptance of responsibility on the part of institutions and their leaders and especially on the part of working scientists. This is a responsibility to *do* something about scientific misconduct. Perhaps the most difficult responsibility is to report misconduct perpetrated by colleagues; small wonder so many authors recommend protection for whistle-blowers.[6,44]

Institutionalization of investigative procedures for handling cases of alleged misconduct is often recommended. On moral and legal grounds, due process is essential to an institutional review process in the same way that informed consent is an essential part of medical research. Fair and public investigative procedures provide a structure for judging the facts of the case so that appropriate penalties – the "treatment" – can be meted out.[45] Kassirer[29] mentioned "how much trouble and disgrace are entailed in misconduct investigations," effects that apply not only to those found guilty but also to those wrongly accused.[46,47] The regular reports of the Office of Research Integrity detail a common sanction against those convicted of misconduct: ineligibility for federal funding, a serious punishment for any scientist whose livelihood depends upon outside funds. At least one journal has published sanctions to be meted out to authors involved in inappropriate acts;[48] fabrication, for example, brings a penalty of "two years to life" during which time the author may not submit a manuscript to that journal for consideration. A recent legal case involving theft of intellectual property resulted in a monetary award of just over $3 million to the plaintiff.[49]

Problems Emerging within a Framework of Secondary Prevention

As in the case of primary prevention, there are some problems in approaching scientific misconduct from the perspective of secondary prevention. If any form of increased surveillance occurs (including formal auditing procedures or the less formal approach of encouraging scientists to take seriously their responsibility to report misconduct), then we can expect an increase in the number of cases of scientific misconduct detected. However, such an increase may represent not a true change in the underlying incidence of events, but rather an apparent change due solely to more intense surveillance. This is a well-known phenomenon in programs designed to detect disease early. For the early detection of scientific misconduct, the inevitable increase in numbers of misconduct cases arising from increased surveillance could be misconstrued by commentators, the press, legislators, and others as indicative of a larger problem than truly exists.

A second problem involves the effects of financial penalties and other sanctions. The extent to which sanctions prevent further incidents of scientific misconduct is an unexplored empirical question. Institutional investigational procedures, monetary and publishing disincentives, and other strategies, such as firing the guilty party, may have a preventive effect by engendering second thoughts about committing misconduct among both would-be repeat offenders and would-be first offenders.[29]

Summary

Disease prevention frameworks sometimes include a category of tertiary prevention, which typically involves rehabilitation and other aspects of long-term care. Tertiary prevention can also be applied to scientific misconduct, inasmuch as those who commit such misconduct may require rehabilitation before they return to scientific practice. A more complete analysis will likely lead, as it did in the case of primary and secondary prevention, to questions with answers based on relatively little empirical information. Indeed, in the foregoing analysis, a host of such questions have emerged. Answers will be difficult to obtain, especially if precise scientific methodologies are to be employed. But then, we are scientists, and solving difficult empirical problems is what we do best. Perhaps the essential question is less methodological than motivational: Are we as scientists willing to study our conduct as scientists? If so, then one day we may discover why we suffer from an important and sometimes disabling professional affliction and what works to prevent it.

I am not suggesting, however, that we should postpone interventions until we fully understand the etiology, including the underlying biological, behavioral, and social mechanisms involved in the range of activities we call scientific misconduct. We need fair investigative procedures. We can accept (perhaps on faith) that the discussion of the role of ethics in the conduct of science and medicine[50] should be expanded. Those of us who act as mentors can and should conduct ourselves virtuously.[25] For the sake of those we train, and especially for those whose lives are improved by our scientific results, we must exhibit excellence, self-effacement, and, perhaps above all, an unwavering commitment to the truth.

References

 1. Gunsalus CK. Institutional structure to ensure research integrity. *Acad Med*. 1993;68 (suppl):S33–S38.
 2. Schachman HK. What is misconduct in science? *Science*. 1993;261:148–149.
 3. Buzzelli DE. The definition of misconduct in science: a view from NSF. *Science*. 1993;259:584–585,647–648.
 4. Klein DF. Should the government assure scientific integrity? *Acad Med*. 1993;68(suppl):S56–S59.
 5. Rennie D, Gunsalus CK. Scientific misconduct: new definition, procedures and office—perhaps a new leaf. *JAMA*. 1993;269:915–917.
 6. *Integrity and Misconduct in Research: Report of the Commission on Research Integrity*. Washington, DC: US Dept of Health and Human Services: 1995. USGPO 1996–746–425.
 7. Ryan KJ. Commission on Research Integrity report sparks debate on science and ethics. *Professional Ethics Rep*. 1996;9:1,6–7.
 8. Kaiser J. Scientific misconduct: panels look for common ground. *Science*. 1996;272:476.
 9. Bailar JC. The real threats to the integrity of science. *Chron Higher Educ*. April 21. 1995:B1.
10. Chalmers I. Underreporting research is scientific misconduct. *JAMA*. 1990; 263:1405–1408.
11. Huth EJ. Irresponsible authorship and wasteful publication. *Ann Intern Med*. 1986;104:257–259.
12. Kennedy TJ. Scientific fraud. *J. Med Educ*. 1988;63:806–808.
13. Woolf P. Fraud in science: how much, how serious? *Hastings Center Rep*. 1981;11:9–14.
14. Dealing with deception. *Lancet*. 1996;347:843. Editorial.
15. deLacey G, Record C, Wade J. How accurate are quotations and references in medical journals? *BMJ*. 1985;291:884–886.
16. Sekas G, Hutson WR. Misrepresentation of academic accomplishments by applicants for gastroenterology fellowships. *Ann Intern Med*. 1995;123:38–41.
17. Gurudevan SV, Mower WR. Misrepresentation of research publications among emergency medicine residency applicants. *Ann Emerg Med*. 1996;27:327–330.
18. Lock S. Misconduct in medical research: does it exist in Britain? *BMJ*. 1988;297:1531–1535.

19. Anderson C. Survey tracks misconduct, to an extent. *Science*. 1993;262:1203–1204.
20. Swazey JP, Anderson MS, Lewis KS. Ethical problems in academic research. *Amer Scientist*. 1993;81:542–553.
21. Shapiro MF, Charrow RP. Scientific misconduct in investigational drug trials. *N Engl J Med*. 1985;312:731–736.
22. Shapiro MF, Charrow RP. The role of data audits in detecting scientific misconduct: results of the FDA program. *JAMA*. 1989;261:2505–2511.
23. Rennie D. Breast cancer: how to mishandle misconduct. *JAMA*. 1994;271:1205–1207.
24. Angell M, Kassirer JP. Setting the record straight in the breast-cancer trials. *N Engl J Med*. 1994;330:1448–1450.
25. Pellegrino ED. Character and the ethical conduct of research. *Accountability Res*.1992;2:1–11.
26. Mishkin L. Fraud is a symptom of a deeper flaw. *Scientist*. 1988:9,12.
27. Angell M, Relman AS. Fraud in biomedical research: a time for congressional restraint. *N Engl J Med*. 1988;318:1462–1463.
28. *Fraud and Misconduct in Medical Research: Causes, Investigation, and Prevention*. London, England: Royal College of Physicians; 1991.
29. Kassirer JP. The frustrations of scientific misconduct. *N Engl J Med*. 1993;1634–1636.
30. Dingell JD. Shattuck Lecture: Misconduct in medical research. *N Engl J Med*. 1993;328: 1610–1615.
31. Angell M. Publish or perish: a proposal. *Ann Intern Med*. 1986;104:261–262.
32. Woolf PK. Pressure to publish and fraud in science. *Ann Intern Med*. 1986;104:254–256.
33. Andersen D, Attrup L, Axelsen N, Riis P. *Scientific Dishonesty and Good Scientific Practice*. Copenhagen, Denmark: Danish Medical Research Council; 1992.
34. Danforth WH, Schoenhoff DM. Fostering integrity in scientific research. *Acad Med*. 1992;67: 351–356.
35. Petersdorf RG. The pathogenesis of fraud in medical science. *Ann Intern Med*. 1986;104: 252–254.
36. Alberts B, Shine K. Scientists and the integrity of research. *Science*. 1994;266:1660–1661.
37. Beauchamp TL. Moral foundations. In: Coughlin SS, Beauchamp TL, eds. *Ethics and Epidemiology*. New York, NY: Oxford University Press; 1996:24–52.
38. Peach L. An introduction to ethical theory. In: Penslar RL, ed. *Research Ethics*. Bloomington, Ind: Indiana University Press; 1995:13–26.
39. MacIntyre A. *After Virtue*. 2nd ed. Notre Dame, Ind: University Press of Notre Dame; 1984.
40. Pellegrino ED. Toward a virtue-based normative ethics for the health professions. *Kennedy Inst Ethics J*. 1995;5:253–277.
41. Soskolne CL, McFarlane DK. Scientific misconduct in epidemiologic research. In: Coughlin SS, Beauchamp TL, eds. *Ethics and Epidemiology*. New York, NY: Oxford University Press; 1996;274–289.
42. Collingwood RG. *An Essay on Metaphysics*. Oxford, England: Clarendon: 1969.
43. Poole C. Exposure opportunity in case-control studies. *Am J Epidemiol*. 1986;123:352–358.
44. Edsall JT. Two aspects of scientific responsibility, *Science*. 1981;212:11–14.
45. Friedman PJ. Research ethics, due process, and common sense. *JAMA*. 1988;260:1937–1938.
46. Silbergeld EK. Protection of the public interest, allegations of scientific misconduct, and the Needleman case. *Am J Public Health*. 1995;85:165–167.
47. Needleman HC. Salem comes to the NIH: notes from inside the crucible of scientific integrity. *Pediatrics*. 1992;90:977–981.
48. Specific inappropriate acts in the publication process. *Am J Obstet Gynecol*. 1996;174:1–9.
49. Taubes G. Scientific misconduct: plagiarism suit wins; experts hope it won't set a trend. *Science*. 1995;268:1125.
50. Reiser SJ. Overlooking ethics in the search for objectivity and misconduct in science. *Acad Med*. 1993;68(suppl):S84–S87.

Questions for Discussion

1. How do personal values influence you as a scientist? What values do you hold as most important in your scientific work?
2. How does scientists' work-related honesty compare with that of other professions?
3. What is the role of intuition in science? How does this role fit with the importance of rationality and objectivity in research?
4. Can scientists have different legitimate interpretations of the same data? How should they resolve such differences?
5. In an effort to prevent misconduct through education, in December 2000 the Office of Research Integrity mandated training in the responsible conduct of science for all researchers supported by Public Health Service funding. For you, how best should such training take place? How can universally required training be most useful?

Recommended Supplemental Reading

National Academy of Sciences, Institute of Medicine. *The Responsible Conduct of Research in the Health Sciences*. Washington, D.C.: National Academy Press; 1989.

National Academy of Sciences, National Academy of Engineering, Institute of Medicine. *On Being a Scientist: Responsible Conduct in Research*. 2d ed. Washington, D.C.: National Academy Press; 1995.

National Academy of Sciences, Panel on Scientific Responsibility and the Conduct of Research. *Responsible Science, Volume I: Ensuring the Integrity of the Research Process*. Washington, D.C.: National Academy Press; 1992.

National Academy of Sciences, Panel on Scientific Responsibility and the Conduct of Research. *Responsible Science, Volume II: Background Papers and Resource Documents*. Washington, D.C.: National Academy Press; 1992.

Sigma Xi, The Scientific Research Society. *Honor in Science*. New Haven, CT: Sigma Xi; 1984.

SECTION IV

The Ethics of Authorship and Publication

Ethical Practices in the Publication of Research Results

Ruth Ellen Bulger

Science is a cumulative process in which the studies of each laboratory or scientist build upon the research done by others. Therefore, all scientific experiments need to be trustworthy and trusted. If there were no trust in the validity of the experiments done by others, the nature of the scientific effort would be forced to change. Scientists would have to spend excessive time repeating the work previously completed by others, severely limiting the overall progress of the entire scientific enterprise.

Why Do Scientists Publish?

First, scientists need to trust each other. Next, for scientists to be able to build on the work of others, there needs to be a method of knowing what scientific questions have been *asked and tested* by others and what data have been found. Also, there must be a way for investigators to be able to *assess the work* of others who may have tested the results of a prior experiment in various ways – that method is publication. Although scientists do give talks and publish abstracts, these methods generally do not have the stamp of authenticity provided by the peer-review process manuscripts that undergo prior to publication. It is publication of science that results in scientific progress. If the results are not published, doing the experiments was only wasted effort.

Publication accomplishes many purposes. First, publication disseminates the results found in scientific experiments, and, in so doing, it establishes the priority of the observation. It is not the first person to discover a phenomenon who gets the primary credit but the first to publish the results. Other scientists can readily evaluate the publication of any given scientific investigation if that work is described in an article with an introduction to place the work in perspective with that of other scientists who previously have worked on the topic under consideration, a section explaining the methods by which the hypothesis was tested, the results that were found by doing the experiments, and a discussion of the meaning of the results. Readers are then able to decide whether they agree with the author's interpretation.

To gain acceptance for publication in most journals, the manuscript first must undergo the process of peer review in which one or more scientists selected by the journal editor evaluates the manuscript to determine credibility and suitability for publication. Reviewers generally evaluate the manuscript on forms that are shared with the author, and reviewers may also give a second written confidential opinion to the editor about acceptability for publication, what changes they feel would be required before the manuscript would be ready to be published, or both. It is the role of the editor to consider the various opinions of the reviewers and decide the fate of the manuscript. (See the later section in this chapter on the role of authors, reviewers, and editors in the peer review process.)

Publication serves as a standard not only for *credit* but for the *responsibility* of the study as well. That is why the scientific output in terms of publications, especially their quality, is used by others as factors when the scientist applies for jobs, grant money, advancement at his or her institution, or for tenure decisions.

What Kind of Work Should Be Published?

Published science must follow all of the precepts of the responsible conduct of science. A recent definition of research misconduct defines it as fabrication, falsification, or plagiarism in proposing, performing, or reviewing research or *in reporting research results.*[1] *These inaccuracies get into the public's view by fraudulent publication.* Although this policy applies to research done or funded by the government, most institutional misconduct policies include under their policies all research done at their institutions. "Fabrication is making up data or results and recording or reporting them. Falsification is manipulating research materials, equipment, or processes, or changing or omitting data or results *such that the research is not accurately represented in the research record.*" "Plagiarism is the appropriation of another person's ideas, processes, results, or words without giving appropriate credit." [1] To ensure that one is ethical in the use of the intellectual property of others, it is important to do a careful *literature search when designing experiments, and again just prior to submitting a manuscript for publication*, to ascertain whether some important related but recently published findings might have been missed. Scientists consider it essential to give proper credit to others for any ideas important in the designing and the outcome of the work being published.

What Forms Do Publications Take?

The first step in preparing a manuscript for publication is to select the appropriate journal, one that will reach the scientific audience likely to be interested in the results. In choosing a journal for publication, scientists most often consider the journals that they customarily read and those that have published studies similar in content to the one they wish to publish. One needs to review several journals to see the kinds of material that they publish and their exact publication styles. A section entitled "Instructions to Authors" (periodically published in the journal or accessed on the journal's home page) provides the publication style requirements of that particular journal.

Publications can take several forms. Full-length *articles* report original research in the field covered by the publication and are the most common. *Rapid communications* of important new research findings on topics of immediate interest are sometimes given priority with respect to the time it takes to publish them. Certain journals publish *brief reports* on current topics. Other journals will publish *review articles* or important *technical notes*. Most journals have a section for publishing *letters to the editor*, in which authors can communicate opinions or criticisms of articles published in previous editions of the journal.

Over 500 journals have agreed to use the standards laid out in a document called "Uniform Requirements for Manuscripts Submitted to Biomedical Journals" prepared by the International Committee of Medical Journal Editors (ICMJE).[2] The Requirements were significantly revised and updated in October 2001, and the new version can be accessed on the ICMJE website (http://www.icjme.org). The document provides excellent guidance to authors. Because the Requirements include detailed discussions of many key issues about publication, readers are encouraged to obtain the most recent version from the ICMJE website or a participating journal for careful review.

Authorship Issues

Wasteful Publications

It is important to publish studies based on experimental findings only after they have been repeated an adequate number of times to ensure that the results are reproducible. The manuscript should describe a complete study that deals with the hypothesis being tested; it should not be a redundant or duplicated manuscript nor should the study be unnecessarily divided into small reports. Some investigators inappropriately divide a research study into a series of small studies instead of publishing an entire experiment as a whole. Broad[3] has dubbed this use of divided publications as the abuse of the "least publishable unit" or LPU. Huth[4] calls this practice of dividing a study into smaller pieces "salami science" and points out that the disreputable practice of slicing publications as thin as possible "does not always equal baloney" but is an abuse of publication. Huth also identifies another abuse that he dubs "meat extenders," in which data are added to the author's previously published data, and the new total of the data is published a second time without reaching any new conclusions.[4] Sigma Xi's *Honor in Science* defines other bad practices, such as "trimming," the smoothing of irregularities to make data look accurate and precise, and "cooking," retaining only the results that fit the theory while discarding the others.[5]

Furthermore, in the biological sciences, simultaneous submission to two different journals is not an acceptable practice. If the article is rejected by the first journal, one might rewrite it using the valid criticisms of the reviewers and then submit it to a second journal.

It is easy to understand the temptation to publish many short articles – particularly when one believes that, in the evaluative process for academic advancement, one's publications are counted or weighed instead of being read. To the extent that faculty share such perceptions, the incentives are presently aligned against doing the right thing. Some institutions have tried to remedy the incentive problem by allowing investigators to submit only a limited number of their best papers to be used in determining tenure.

One should not attempt to publish a paper that has previously been or is being published elsewhere. This does not apply to a paper for which there has been a previously published abstract but is germane to a paper that is substantially similar to an earlier publication. Any abstract on the same work should be cited in the manuscript. Publishing more than one manuscript on a given study is wasteful and expensive. In some cases, when an author submits a manuscript, he or she might have a paper with a similar title in press, but the contents may not be repetitious. Under these circumstances, it is useful to explain to the editor how the paper being submitted differs from the previous one. It is often useful to include a copy of the earlier manuscript that is in press with the new submission so that the reviewer can determine whether they are different. When an author publishes articles that are closely related to others he or she has published, these articles need to be referenced to avoid what has been identified as self-plagiarism. Authors are also responsible for identifying materials copyrighted elsewhere (even one's own material) and obtaining written permission from the editors of the journal in which an article was published for the reuse of the material. Then proper credit must be given.

Pigman and Carmichael[6] state that, to be published, science must be of good quality (e.g., the methodology is up to date and sound and has been applied in a rigorous manner with results appropriately examined for statistical significance). Science should be original in content (i.e., something new that has not been done before and that is not just a repetition of the work of others). It should be done and then described in a fashion that allows repetition by others. The science must consider prior work, and proper references to the work must be cited.

Who Deserves to Be an Author?

Defining who are the appropriate authors can be a difficult issue. However, at present there are several excellent analyses of the issue. One must consider which people fulfill the criteria for authorship and which people who may have lent assistance do not need to be considered for authorship. The criteria usually include sufficient participation in aspects of the work and willingness to take public responsibility for the whole work or for sections as indicated in the manuscript. There are a variety of accepted ways, such as the use of footnotes, to give appropriate credit to those who have provided some assistance for the research but do not meet the criteria for authorship.

Some institutions have written authorship policies to help their faculty make authorship decisions. Wilcox[7] discusses how an Ombuds Office at an institution may help with working out disagreements on authorship issues. Each laboratory should also have its own policy on how to determine the appropriate authors for studies within that laboratory, and the policy should be discussed with possible collaborators early in the work – optimally before the work begins. Authorship policy should be discussed with graduate students or postdoctoral fellows when they are considering joining a laboratory group. Because the ongoing research findings can cause change in direction of the research, the policy needs flexibility to change if the research emphasis or procedures themselves change.

The ICMJE policy states that each author should have participated sufficiently in the work to take public responsibility for it. The following three conditions indicate sufficient participation: "(1) substantial contributions to conception and design, or acquisition of data, or analysis and interpretation of data; (2) drafting the article or revising it critically for important intellectual content; and (3) final approval of the version to be published."[2]

Teich and Frankel[8] had previously proposed that, to be a legitimate author, each person should (1) have made substantial and significant contributions to the research study and (2) accept responsibility for the integrity in whole or in part as specified in the article. Significant contributions by an author could be in many areas such as in the conceptualization and design of the study, the execution of the work, the analysis and interpretation of the work, and the review, correction, and improvement of the manuscript. All authors should give final formal approval for the draft to be submitted.

Authors must know the ethical codes and standards of their discipline, ensure the quality and integrity of the research described (unless they state that they are responsible for only a specified part of the work), and must not falsify or fabricate their credentials or publications. Journals often require that the authors certify that they have followed proper Institutional Review Board regulations, regulations for laboratory animal care and use, and conflict of interest policies. Conflicts of interest can exist for a manuscript when an author, reviewer, or editor has financial or intellectual ties that could unduly influence the judgment about whether a manuscript should be published.

What Does Not Justify Authorship?

There are a variety of ways to acknowledge individuals who have provided assistance but do not fulfill criteria for authorship. Credit can be given in acknowledgments or in footnotes. Credit should be given in this way for exceptional technical help, data collection, access to patient material, advice, critical review, donation of reagents or special animals, and financial or material support. There are some areas, such as help with statistical analysis, that could either qualify for authorship or for acknowledgment, depending on the degree that the statistician was involved with other aspects of the work such as the experimental design or in making significant improvements in the manuscript. According to the ICMJE *Guidelines*, acquisition of funding, the collection of data, or general supervision of the research group alone do not justify authorship.

Honorary and Ghost Authorship

In previous years, individuals who provided monetary support, laboratory space for research, technical advice, and routine technical work, as well as department chairs or mentors who had little to do with the research, well-known scientists who might give prestige to the study may have been included as authors. This has been called honorary or gift authorship, and it is no longer considered appropriate behavior.

Equally inappropriate is the failure to name a person as an author who does qualify as an author by having made substantial contributions to the publication. This practice has been called ghost authorship. Flanagin et al.[9] studied the prevalence of articles with honorary or ghost authors in six peer-reviewed medical journals. Using a survey technique and the ICMJE criteria for authorship, they analyzed 809 articles and determined that there was evidence of honorary authorship in 19% of the articles (range in the six journals was 11–25%), evidence of ghost authorship in 11% (range 7–16%), and evidence of both practices in 2% of the articles.

How to Determine Order of Authorship

As scientific research has become more complex and more collaborative, the number of authors on manuscripts has increased. This makes the problem of deciding the order of authorship increasingly difficult. The ICMJE suggests that the authorship order should be a joint decision of the coauthors and the authors; all of them should be able to explain the rationale for the listed order. More commonly, it is the laboratory director responsible for assigning the work within the group who determines the order of authorship. Generally, the first author has been responsible for undertaking the major part of the work and its interpretation, and has written the first draft of the manuscript.

The senior author is generally the leader of the group and most often is not the person collecting the majority of the data. However, the senior author should review the data periodically with each of the laboratory group members and hence, along with the first author, is one of the persons most responsible for the integrity of the paper. The name of the senior author often appears last in the author list. All of the authors for any study should meet on a regular basis to follow the developing results and to discuss possible directions and interpretations of the research. Either the first author or the senior author usually coordinates the manuscript submission process and, if necessary, the changes to be made in the manuscript as part of the manuscript review process. Differing conventions exist about how to list the other coauthors of a paper. Often they are listed in order of the importance of their contributions to the work, but in some cases the names are alphabetized. As studies become more interdisciplinary, decisions about coauthor order become more complicated.

How Should Authors Deal with the Media Prior to Publication?

Dealing with the media prior to the publication of the manuscript can be a contentious issue upon which various journal editors and representatives of the news media disagree. The *New England Journal of Medicine* historically has not allowed preliminary release to the media of material prior to publication of the manuscript in its journal (this is the so-called Ingelfinger rule).[10]

Most journal editors believe that scientific articles should be assessed for quality by the process of formal peer review and editorial evaluation prior to publication and that the entire study with full disclosure of methods used and results obtained must be available for evaluation by the reader.[11] The *Journal of the American Medical Association* has recently set forth its policies regarding release of information to the public.[12] This policy describes why the journal will only consider a scientific manuscript for publication if it has not been published previously (or is not presently under consideration for publication by another journal). Certain exceptions are cited: information can be disseminated during open scientific meetings, information can be released during testimony before government agencies, consideration of clinically useful information that is part of the public domain can be used, and information can be released in situations in which there is an urgent public health need. For these situations in which the health of the public will be adversely affected by the delay (the time between acceptance of an article and its publication) in public release, provisions have been made for the results to be distributed to health care providers. For example, the NIH can issue a clinical alert via the National Library of Medicine to notify physicians and the public about NIH-funded studies that might have a significant effect on morbidity and mortality of disease states (http://www.nlm.nih.gov/databases/alerts).

Questions by members of the press asking for more data or information can arise at scientific meetings based on program abstracts in which the data have been presented orally prior to the publication of the full paper. It is often helpful for scientists to put *published* information into context for reporters but not to give unpublished information to them. It is important to know the policy of one's institution on giving information to reporters. Institutional communication offices can be extremely helpful in these situations.

The Review of Manuscripts

Earlier, this chapter discussed the responsibilities of authors. After authors have chosen an approriate journal, have written the manuscript in the proper publication style of the journal, and have had it approved by all of the coauthors, the manuscript can be submitted to the journal for peer review. What are reasonable expectations for authors and peer reviewers selected by the journal editor?

The journal editor will select the possible reviewers from the journal's editorial board or from ad hoc reviewers who are experts in the area of the manuscript to be reviewed. Often a person from the journal staff will call or fax material to a potential reviewer and inquire if the potential reviewer has the time and the knowledge to review the manuscript within the short time window allowed (usually from 2 weeks to a month). The reviewer is given the manuscript title and, sometimes, the names of the authors. This is the time when you as a reviewer must decide several things. Do you have the time and the knowledge for the subject being offered? Do you have any real or apparent financial conflicts of interest that would affect or could be seen to affect your judgment, either positively (perhaps by receiving money from the industry involved with producing the drug) or negatively (perhaps by receiving money from some competitor). Do you have an intellectual conflict of interest (perhaps you are working on an experiment that is too similar and you would have reason for not wanting the manuscript to be published rapidly)? Have you worked too closely with this author in the past to be objective in your review? Can you meet the timetable requested for returning the manuscript?

Let us assume that, after consideration of these issues, one decides to be the reviewer. The reviewer is now committed to write a knowledgeable, timely, honest, objective, and, it is hoped, courteous critique. The reviewer is generally told not to duplicate the manuscript (or any part of it) for personal records and not to share the manuscript with anyone without explicit permission of the journal editor (this includes others in the laboratory). The reviewer also does not discuss the article with the author. The reviewer has been entrusted with privileged materials that are unavailable to others and therefore must not be discussed or shared with others. Initially, a scientist has the right to privacy of the findings until the work is published. Before publication of experiments by the author, any unfair use of grant applications or manuscripts is considered stealing of intellectual property. After publication, the article can be quoted with appropriate citations, and data and research materials should then be shared by the author with qualified colleagues on request.

The reviewer is undertaking a service for science and is not to make use of the materials for personal purposes until after publication.

A quick, computer-driven literature review by the reviewer should reveal whether this material is original to the author and the field and can be quite useful. The reviewer is generally expected to give a clear, understandable critique of the manuscript indicating the strengths and weaknesses for the author and to submit a second opinion to the editor on whether the material should be published as is, with modifications, or not at all. Remember that these comments should be polite and helpful.

When the editor has received the critiques from all of the reviewers, a decision is made to accept, accept with modifications, or reject the manuscript. That decision is transmitted to the authors with the comments of the reviewers. The author can then benefit from the reviewer's comments to revise the manuscript as suggested or the author can justify disagreements with the reviewer's comments to the editor, or both, when deemed necessary. With the revisions, the manuscript is returned to the journal for reconsideration. If the article had been rejected by the original journal, the improved manuscript can be sent to a different journal for its consideration.

The review process can be a learning experience for the reviewer as well as the author if the editor chooses to send each original reviewer the opinions that were submitted by other reviewers along with the decision about the disposition of the manuscript. What did the other reviewers see that you did not? Was their review helpful for improving the manuscript?

Seeing your work in print can be a thrill, and it will be especially so if you have considered and met all of the appropriate ethical challenges.

References

1. Federal Policy on Research Misconduct, 65 *Federal Register*, 76260–76264 (2000).
2. International Committee of Medical Journal Editors. Uniform requirements for manuscripts submitted to biomedical journals. Available at: http://www.icmje.org. Accessed October 2001.
3. Broad WJ. The publishing game: getting more for less. *Science*. 1981;211:1137–1139.
4. Huth EJ. Irresponsible authorship and wasteful publication. *Ann Intern Med*. 1986;104:257–259.
5. Sigma Xi. *Honor in Science*. New Haven, CT: Sigma Xi; 1984.
6. Pigman W, Carmichael EB. An ethical code for scientists. *Science*. 1950;111:643–649.
7. Wilcox LJ. Authorship: the coin of the realm, the source of complaints. *JAMA*. 1998;280:216–217.
8. Teich AH, Frankel MS. AAAS–ABA National Conference of Lawyers and Scientists, AAAS, Washington, DC; March 1992.
9. Flanagin A, Carey L, Fontanarosa PB, et al. Prevalence of articles with honorary authors and ghost authors in peer-reviewed medical journals. *JAMA*. 1998;280:222–224.
10. Altman LK. The Ingelfinger Rule, embargoes, and journal peer review. *Lancet*. 1996;347:1382–1386.
11. Fontanarosa PB, Flanagin A. Prepublication release of medical research. *JAMA*. 2000;284:2927–2929.
12. Fontanarosa PB, Flanagin A, DeAngelis CD. The Journal's policy regarding release of information to the public. *JAMA*. 2000;284:2929–2931.

An Ethical Code for Scientists

Ward Pigman and Emmett B. Carmichael

A new phenomenon of our present-day society is the obviously important role played by science. Only a short time ago science was considered by many "practical" men as a plaything of inconsequential importance in contributing to the welfare of society. Although the significance of science was becoming more generally evident before World War II, this war demonstrated to the public in general and to legislators and businessmen in particular that science, especially basic science, is much more than a scholarly pursuit – that it is a vital force for the advancement or destruction of society. Science is now "big business." As a result, the scientist cannot and must not remain a scholarly recluse divorced from the remainder of society. His behavior and that of society toward him will greatly influence the progress of science and, to an increasing extent, that of society itself.

During its long period of development, science has evolved a code of professional tradition and ethics, largely in an unwritten form. This code, really the foundation of the scientific method in many of its aspects, has to a considerable extent been responsible for the achievements of science. Polanyi's (*12*) description of the effect of disregard for scientific traditions is applicable to many of our modern industrial and research organizations:

> Those who have visited the parts of the world where scientific life is just beginning, know of the backbreaking struggle that the lack of scientific tradition imposes on the pioneers. Here research work stagnates for lack of stimulus, there it runs wild in the absence of any proper directive influence. Unsound reputations grow like mushrooms: based on nothing but commonplace achievements, or even on mere empty boasts. Politics and business play havoc with appointments and the granting of subsidies for research. However rich the fund of local genius may be, such environment will fail to bring it to fruition.

The important achievements of science and its contributions to our civilization seem adequate proof of the basic validity of these traditions. On the other hand, conditions of scientific work have changed greatly, and obviously the traditions must be interpreted in terms of prevailing conditions. Science has emerged from a period in which the predominant effort was made by individuals, sometimes of almost an amateur status, to a period marked by the development of large research groups, many in the pursuit of research for profit. As a result, it is timely for the scientist to consider his professional traditions and to relate them in terms of the structure of modern scientific work.

These traditions are essentially an unwritten code of professional ethics. As pointed out by Leake (*9*), the term "professional ethics" as used generally includes the attitude of the

From *Science*, 1950, 111, pp. 643–647. © AAAS.

individual scientist to society and to other scientists. It will be so used here. This concept of professional ethics inextricably involves social obligations, questions of etiquette, and adherence to accepted traditions. Claude Bernard (*1*) has contributed one of the better discussions of the ethical qualities needed in scientists, and the relationship of these qualities to the scientific method, although his remarks apply in the main to medicine and physiology.

Some of our professional organizations have established formal written codes of professional ethics.* In the medical field numerous papers and books have been written on the subject. One of the first extensive codifications was that of Percival (*9*) (1803), but the general precepts of Hippocrates (circa 500 B.C.) have modern acceptance. A major consideration at the first meeting of the American Medical Association in 1847 was the formulation of a code of professional ethics (*9*). The present code provides means for enforcement by its members. There has been some discussion of the professional responsibilities of industrial chemists (*6*) and a code has been proposed for this group (*7*). Scientific groups generally, however, have not formalized their traditions but have passed them on by example and by word of mouth as an informal part of the graduate student's training.

This failure of scientists as a group to consider ethics is revealed in the fact that *Chemical Abstracts*, since it was founded in 1907, listed only four references under ethics in its indices. It is true that professional codes at best can only express an ideal; their acceptance and application will depend upon the individual scientists. We believe, however, that the scientist's position in the world today makes it extremely important that his time-proved traditions be reconsidered in terms of modern circumstances and possibly written into a formal code. We believe that such an action would maintain the advance of science, increase its public support, and improve the professional relations of scientists. Improved professional relations would better morale and increase productivity among research men. Mills (*10*) has pointed out the social implications of ethical behavior in the distribution of research grants.

The planning of an ethical code for scientists should take into account first the scientist's general obligations as a member of society, and beyond that his special obligation as a scientist to protect society – here, there are many problems related to warfare, to the health and general well-being of mankind, and to nationalism versus internationalism. Such a code should preserve the scientist's ethical traditions and incorporate the scientific method. It should state the scientist's obligation to explain the nature and purposes of science, and the policies in dealing directly with the public. It should clarify the scientist's attitudes toward patents and secrecy restrictions. It should affirm the scientist's obligations to individuals – to his employer, his associates, other scientists, and his assistants and graduates – and scientists' obligation as a group to other professions.

We have merely indicated the scope of the problem. To deal with it fully in all its phases would require the efforts of scientists in many different fields of study and kinds of employment. Some of these phases have already received considerable attention. Because the results of atomic research have such unmistakable implications for society, attention has

---

*   American Medical Association, *Principles of Medical Ethics* (14); American Dental Association, *Principles of Ethics* (15); American Association of University Professors, *Statements of Principle in Academic Freedom and Tenure* (16); American Institute of Chemical Engineers, *Constitution*, Article VIII (17); Engineers' Council for Professional Development, *Canons of Ethics for Engineers* (18). "The Geneticists' Manifesto" adopted at the Seventh International Congress of Genetics, held at Edinburgh in 1939. Published in *The Journal of Heredity*, September, 1939. Reprints distributed by American Genetics Association (19).

been paid to the scientist's attitude on the use of his discoveries, particularly for military purposes, and to the necessity of his being socially conscious (*3, 4, 5, 8, 10, 13*). Other phases of the problem have received little or no public consideration.

Many of the scientist's obligations are reciprocal in the sense that the scientist has grown to expect certain conditions for his work, and to a considerable extent these conditions affect the quality of his work. Sometimes his obligations are conflicting. He may at times be faced with the dilemma of obligations to his employer that conflict with obligations to the public as a whole. What should his attitude be when his employer's immediate interest causes harm to the general public? Suppose that his employer is a company that is pouring waste products into a stream and he knows that at a reasonable cost this pollution could be greatly minimized. Should he assume, as a lawyer does, that his primary obligation is to his client, and become an automatic defender of the company's position? Or should he consider that he has duties to society greater than those to the company?

A group of very pressing problems is presented in the application of traditions related to the authorship and publication of scientific researches. In the early days of science most articles carried the name of only one worker, whereas multiple authorship is now most common and sometimes ten or more persons may be involved. As a detailed example of the need for a code of professional ethics, we will discuss some of the problems involved in authorship.

General Obligations of Authors

Quality of Papers

Everyone will agree that scientific articles should be of good quality, should be original in content, and should describe all work in a reproducible fashion. These are fundamental requirements of the scientific method and yet most scientists would admit that many research articles are published that are deficient in some or all of these respects.

Claude Bernard (*2*) has described the importance of adequate details:

> In scientific investigation, minutiae of method are of the highest importance. The happy choice of an animal, an instrument constructed in some special way, one reagent used instead of another, may often suffice to solve the most abstract and lofty questions. . . . the greatest scientific truths are rooted in details of experimental investigation which form, as it were, the soil in which these truths develop.

Even casual inspection will show that many articles are not written so that the work can be repeated. Traditional procedure is often ignored in reporting new compounds; occasional articles will not give analyses of new compounds or the compounds will be poorly described so that their identity is questionable. Scientific journals lack space to print all the good material they receive today, and understandably urge authors to shorten their articles, but great care is needed to avoid eliminating important details.

Direct Responsibility to Prior Work

The traditions of science demand that any report of scientific work must consider prior work, integrate it in the general subject, and cite proper references to it. Frequent violations of this principle must be familiar to all scientists. One of us has previously called attention to an instance of this type, particularly in relation to the naming of methods (*11*).

The basic concept behind this principle, even more fundamental than professional courtesy, is that frequently the solution to a problem may already be in the literature and needless repetition is economic waste. Thorough literature searching can be defended from an economic standpoint alone. In order to speed the incorporation of new work into the general body of basic knowledge, each author has the responsibility of assisting in the integration of his work with that of previous workers.

To many scientists, establishment of priority for new discoveries is important, and organizations that seek patent protection for their work may set up involved and expensive procedures to establish the date of discovery. Is this a tradition that should be continued? Some scientific journals do not carry the date a manuscript was submitted, and few indicate whether essential changes of content have been made after that date. "Letters to the Editor" may require careful controls to prevent abuses.

Criticism and Disagreement

The scientific method requires that all research work be open to critical examination and testing by researchers in the field. It also requires that dissenting theories and results be treated with tolerance, and not suppressed merely because they disagree with currently accepted ideas. Many scientists would add that mistakes and errors should be publicly acknowledged.

The widespread violation of these principles today is affecting not only the progress of science but our economy as well. Many commercial research organizations keep closed files of their researches as a matter of policy, in the belief that they will have an advantage over their competitors. Most of them do not realize that lack of criticism of the worker by qualified colleagues in his own field fosters the carrying out and perpetuation of poor or erroneous work, the continued employment and promotion of unqualified workers, and the perpetuation of poor research policies. Criticism by members of the worker's organization and by consultants is usually inadequate because of the influence of personal motives and lack of knowledge in the specific field. Objections to excessive secrecy in military research should take into account this principle as a primary consideration.

Classical examples of the value of scientific controversy are well known. When properly conducted, such debates lead to clarification and advancement of knowledge. But improperly conducted, they lead to enduring feuds, and because of this possibility, there is a tendency among editors of journals to suppress scientific polemics. A continuation or extension of this trend will be a severe blow to the scientific method. However, as stated by Wise (*13*),

the research worker should not permit himself to become embittered or involved in useless polemics. . . . It simply means that his criticisms must be objective and that they must not descend to the plane of personalities. He must show that he is dealing with a set of data, not with an enemy.

Property Rights of the Scientist in His Work

A currently controversial problem of the application of scientific tradition involves the rights of a researcher to his work. The decision to try to publish or reveal his research once was the sole right of the scientist. Now, with the investigator receiving financial support from others in most cases, the final decision is tending to fall on the provider of the funds. In the extreme case, what is there to prevent someone in authority from taking over the work of an associate and passing it off as his own work? What should an editor of a scientific journal do if he receives for publication a suitable manuscript from an established worker and simultaneously a letter from the supporting group saying that it should not be published? Should the supporting group be required to provide satisfactory and convincing grounds? By tradition and perhaps even by legal mandate, the rights of an artist to certain phases of the disposition of his work have been affirmed. Should these not apply equally to the scientist, whose application of his science is often an art?

At least one established graduate institution has the policy that all doctoral theses are published solely in the names of the individual graduate students. In certain instances, the idea was suggested by a member of the faculty, who carried out some preliminary work, supervised the principal research, drew or helped draw the conclusions, rewrote the thesis and wrote the final published version. Is this an example of acceptable ethics?

Publicity

Some scientists violently oppose general publicity and popularization of their work. Others seek publicity, and some even condone or support erroneous and misleading publicity. What should be the attitude of the scientist? Does he owe the public a duty to attempt to explain the purpose and significance of his work? Should chicanery and excessive or misleading publicity on the part of scientists and nonscientists be exposed as a function of scientific societies? It is of interest that the *Principles of Medical Ethics* includes a considerable discussion of the impropriety of advertising and publicity, seeking and that AMA members are required to advise the public against misrepresentation. A firm stand on this issue by scientists generally might be of considerable help in establishing the professional status of the scientist in the public mind.

Multiple Authorship

With the change in status of research, owing to its being produced not by independent individuals but by several dependent workers or even large groups, the scientific tradition in respect to the etiquette of authorship needs reinterpretation or extension. The responsibilities involved in multiple authorship or group research must be analyzed.

"Senior" Authorship and Order of Names

To many scientists, the order of the authors' names on a publication has a significance. Is this a tradition that should be preserved, clarified, and enforced, or is it an outmoded, unessential form of etiquette? In current publications, the application seems uncertain and haphazard. Should the concept of the "senior author" (the first one listed) be preserved? If so, should the senior author be the person highest in the administrative rank, the one who has done most of the laboratory work, the one who has written the paper, the one who furnished the original idea, or the one whose technical skill and thoughts have carried along the research?

Administrators and Financial Supporters

In publications, what consideration should be given to administrators and financial supporters? Some scientists might say that they should be indicated as authors only when their contribution to the actual solution of the problem has been substantial, continuous, and of a high level. Probably most scientists would agree that mere general administrative supervision of a project or even the suggestion of the original idea for the project is insufficient for an authorship. Certainly no one should be granted authorship of any type merely because he has seniority or is in charge of a laboratory. We cite as an example a man serving as technical liaison between a company and a research organization who insisted that his name be included as an author before he would ask for supporting funds for the research, although his total contribution was limited to this action.

Graduate Students and Technical Assistants

Criteria are necessary for assessing the role of graduate students and technical assistants in relation to authorship. Should not senior authorship for a graduate student be limited to those instances in which a real contribution, beyond adequate laboratory work, has been made? On the other hand, is it not the duty of the directing professor to encourage the student to his maximum performance rather than use him as a laboratory assistant? If a technical assistant is to be given authorship of any type, more than an adequate performance of routine methods should be required of him.

Group Projects

An example of the large group projects that characterize modern science is the penicillin research during World War II. Industrial organizations provide many more examples. Frequently there is no attempt on the part of administrators to set up the program so that the work of individual investigators is kept discrete. The improved quality of work resulting from the establishment of definite responsibility might be the basis for making a definite statement in regard to this problem. The interpretation of the scientific tradition in terms of modern group research is an extremely important and as yet unexplored field.

Preparation of Manuscripts

The published paper is the final record of the finished research work, and the medium through which the information is made generally available and useful. With the present shortage of publication space, the preparation of the manuscript becomes more important than ever. Rigid adherence to established scientific traditions on the part of authors and editors becomes increasingly essential.

To many persons, the preparation of a research paper may seem to be a routine matter, but actually it requires a high order of skill and technical knowledge and an acquaintance with scientific traditions. In many researches the actual preparation of the manuscript, the integration of the findings with the prior related work, consideration of the significance of the data, and arrangements for publication may require a considerable portion of the time and skill required for the entire project. Possibly the actual preparation of the manuscript should be a factor in defining the responsibilities of the senior author. Laboratory workers without a good background of knowledge, and research administrators without close daily contact with the laboratory work and a thorough knowledge of the field probably should be discouraged from actual preparation of the manuscript. On the other hand, simple manuscript revision, in spite of the poor writing ability of many scientists, should not generally be made the basis for authorship of a research paper. Still another problem is determining the duties and responsibilities of the referees of scientific articles.

The interpretation of scientific traditions, and their formal codification, if that is to be accomplished, are essentially a task for scientists. As this discussion demonstrates, the problems of interpretation are manifold and if they are not solved they may severely hinder the progress of science. The harm done may not only be general but may apply particularly to industrial research of the group type. Incidental effects of the code, but of considerable importance, would be the great improvement in morale among scientific workers, the improvement in the quality of scientific work, the assistance it would give to editors of scientific journals and research administrators, and the basis it would provide for exposing poor work and even instances of chicanery. It would be of great assistance in the training of graduate students in the scientific method. The preparation of a formal code of professional ethics should be of considerable value in establishing the professional status of the scientist in the public mind. It seems more than a coincidence that the groups that already have formal statements of their social and professional responsibilities and have definite rules of professional behavior are those definitely accepted by the public as having professional status.

As we have pointed out, violations of professional ethics on the part of scientists are frequent and familiar to all scientists. Sometimes they are deliberate violations for personal power or gain. Frequently, they are the results of carelessness or unfamiliarity of research administrators or research workers with the established traditions. They may even result from excessive pressure of work, a condition that appears common in industrial research. Some violations are the result of misguided attempts by editors and reviewers of scientific journals to shorten articles.

Is not the time opportune for our scientific organizations, or some agency of UNESCO, to consider the manner of the application of scientific traditions to the newly developed conditions of scientific research? We suggest that the establishment of a definite code of professional ethics and conduct by our major scientific groups would have profound and favorable effects for science, society, and the scientist.

A mere statement of principles would be of help. An extensive codification and attempt to discipline or expose gross violations might be desirable. Our societies have various ways and means of enforcing regulations. Exclusion from membership and control of publications and means of publicity are powers that could be used to control unscrupulous and continuous violations. There may appear to be an anomaly in scientists' establishing a formal code of ethics to preserve traditions that include independence in their work, but this merely reflects an anomaly in present conditions of scientific work. It seems far better for scientists to affirm such a code positively than to be regimented to an increasing extent without any control over the conditions under which they must work. A. V. Hill(8) puts the problem as follows:

The important thing is not a creed "which except a man believe faithfully he cannot be saved." What matters is that scientific men should argue and discuss the matter of scientific ethics as one of infinite importance to themselves and the rest of mankind with the same honesty, humility and resolute regard for the facts they show in their scientific work.

If they do, then something will surely crystallize out from their discussion, and I have faith enough in the goodness and wisdom of most scientific men to believe that the result on the whole will be good and wise. It may in the end be embodied in a new Hippocratic Oath; or it may be absorbed in trade union rules for the scientific profession; or ethical behavior in science may just come to be accepted as an honorable obligation as unbreakable as that of accuracy and integrity.

We add that all problems will not be solved, but science is expanding and moving. The rate of progress will be profoundly affected by the consideration that is given to the maintenance and proper application of time-proved scientific traditions as the conditions of scientific work change.

References

1. Bernard, Claude. *An introduction to the study of experimental medicine*. Trans. by H. C. Greene. New York: Macmillan Co., 1927.
2. *Ibid.*, p. 14.
3. Blakeslee, A. F. *Science*, 1940, **92,** 589.
4. Carlson, A. J. *Science*, 1946, **103,** 377.
5. Condon, E. U. *Science*, 1946, **103,** 415.
6. Fernelius, W. C. *Chem. Eng. News*, 1946, **24,** 1664.
7. Gehrke, W. H., Aneshansley, C. H., and Rothemund, P. *Chem. Eng. News*, 1947, **25,** 2562.
8. Hill, Archibald V. *Chem. Eng. News*, 1946, **24,** 1343.
9. Leake, C. D. (Ed.) *Percival's medical ethics*. Baltimore: Williams & Wilkins, 1927.
10. Mills, C. A. *Science*, 1948, **107,** 127.
11. Peoples, S. A. and Carmichael, E. B. *Science*, 1945, **102,** 131.
12. Polanyi, M. *Sci. Mon.*, 1945, **60,** 141.
13. Wise, L. E. *Paper Industry & Paper World*, 1946, **28,** 1299.
14. *A.M.A. Directory*, 1942, p. 14.
15. *A.D.A. Directory*, 1947, p. 2.
16. *Bull. A. A. U. P.*, 1949, **35,** 66.
17. *A. I. C. E. Constitution*, Art. VIII.
18. Engineers' Council for Professional Development, Oct. 25, 1947.
19. *J. Hered.*, Sept. 1939.

Irresponsible Authorship and Wasteful Publication

Edward J. Huth

Fraud in scientific publication is a dramatic abuse and it readily catches the eye of the popular press and the public. But there are abuses that because of their frequency and ubiquity should concern us more than the extreme of fraud. These are abuse of two kinds: irresponsible authorship and wasteful publication.

Public evidence of these abuses is scanty and largely anecdotal, although they have been discussed in the literature (1,2). Aside from May's study (3) of duplicate papers in one small corner of mathematics, however, I do not know of any thorough and quantitative studies of the extent and frequency of these problems.

Irresponsible Authorship

I take authorship to mean that an author who is the sole author of a paper has been solely responsible for the work it reports and that all coauthors in a multiauthor paper have been sufficiently involved in the reported work and in the writing of the paper to be able to take public responsibility for its contents (4).

The first species of irresponsible authorship is *unjustified authorship*. There are the authors who simply made technical suggestions and did not take part in the research, did not help write the paper, and did not see the final version submitted to the journal. There is the departmental chairman who did not take part in the research. There is the laboratory technician who did routine work that would have been done regardless of the study and who could not defend the paper's content. There is the principal author's spouse listed as second author on a paper about bowel disease who has a degree in library science and gathered numbers from clinical records.

Unjustified authorship is not simply a problem of numbers. Growing numbers of authors per paper may be justified by growing complexity of research, but editors are seeing numbers that seem disproportionately large for the work the papers seem to represent.

Incomplete authorship, the second species of irresponsible authorship, is probably rare. This abuse is a failure to include as authors persons who had responsibility (5) for critical content of a paper.

From *Annals of Internal Medicine*, 1986, 104, pp. 257–259. Reproduced by permission.

Wasteful Publication

Abuses of authorship rarely seem to damage the efficiency of science or seriously sap its resources. But they do undermine the ethic of honesty. Abuses that may be doing more damage involve wasting the resources of scientific publication.

The abuse of *divided publication* is the breaking down of findings in a single piece of research into a string of papers, each of which is what Broad (1) has tagged as the "LPU" or "Least Publishable Unit." The research could probably have been reported in a single paper. But why should the investigators confine themselves to one paper when they can slice up data and interpretations into two, three, four, five, or more papers that will better serve their needs when they face promotion or tenure committees? "Salami science" does not always equal baloney, but such divided publication is often an abuse of scientific publication.

When five papers report findings that could have been reported in one, the editorial process, including peer review, has been turned on five times instead of once. Peer review is expensive in time and in money, for journal offices and for reviewers. Divided publication produces unnecessary press and postage costs for journals and the costs of multiple indexing and abstracting for what should have been represented once. Should we squander the resources of science in such multiplied costs?

Repetitive publication – republishing essentially the same content in successive papers or in chapters, reviews, and papers – also wastes resources. In one episode involving this journal about 2 years ago, we published a paper about a serious adverse pulmonary effect due to a new cardiovascular drug. A paper published in a radiological journal five months later described the same effect in apparently the same patients. The authors of the two papers were different but the papers came from the same medical school. Case details strongly suggested that the same cases had been reported twice. At least one author of the second paper must have been aware of the first paper because that author had been acknowledged for reviewing it. An excuse for this duplication might have been to get the message to two audiences unlikely to see each other's journals. But is the cost of duplicating the message for two audiences justified? For some decades the cost for searching through secondary services for information in a journal not usually seen by the searcher might have justified such duplicative publication. Now, the ease, speed, and relatively low cost of searching scientific literature through online bibliographic services discredit this excuse. One good reason to object to the repetition in this episode is that the re-reporting of the four cases misrepresents the incidence of the reported adverse drug effect. A literature search would turn up eight cases instead of four. A closely related abuse is producing the papers I call "meat extenders," papers that add data to the authors' previously reported data, without reaching new conclusions.

None of these abuses is dramatically unethical in the sense that fakery and fraud are. The scientific community might not even agree on whether repetitive and duplicative publication are unethical. Wasteful publication might be seen as justified by needs to compete for institutional and financial support to ensure academic survival. Scientists do not realize that they help pay the excessive costs for peer reviewers, editors, professional societies, bibliographers, and libraries if they subscribe to journals or use any of these services.

Possible Remedies

These abuses arise from the value publishing brings to individuals and particularly to their institutions. Publications are accomplishments that lead to income and power. I am skeptical that enunciating standards for scientific publication, no matter how rational, will readily influence what is in essence an economic problem. Science involves big money and attracts highly competitive career seekers. Short of a basic change in how science is rewarded and rewards itself, what might be done about abuses of authorship and wastes in publication? Dr. Angell proposes in her paper (6) what might be the best remedy; let me suggest some others.

A first major step could be wide and public acceptance among all scientific disciplines of clearly defined and specific criteria for authorship. Very few disciplines appear to have such criteria. The American Psychological Association has developed criteria (7); the Council of Biology Editors has published a short statement, not full criteria, on authorship (8); and the American Chemical Society has published a statement (9) on ethics of publication that covers authorship. The International Committee of Medical Journal Editors has recently issued several short statements defining authorship (10–12).

A second step could be specific requirements on authorship by scientific journals: an acknowledgment or footnote in every co-authored paper could state the exact contribution by each author that has justified authorship. Alternatively, the statement might be required in an accompanying letter. This procedure might reduce the number of abuses by at least forcing application of some kind of criteria.

A third step, one *Annals* took a few years ago, could cut back the abuse of naming persons as authors who have not seen the final version of the paper. We require that each author sign a "Conditions of Publication" form before we publish the paper. Each author thus affirms having seen the final version and agrees to its publication. Such a form could also require authors to indicate their particular contributions to the paper, such as study design, analysis of data, writing the first draft. Even if such required forms did not eliminate all abuses, they might at least raise awareness that authorship implies having taken on responsibilities and not just willingness to accept credit.

Divided publication may be more difficult for editors to deal with. When a piece of work has been chopped up for two or more papers, they are usually submitted to different journals at about the same time. Unless the authors are honest enough to cite the other papers, the peer reviewers and editors are not likely to be aware of the divided pieces. Editors who become aware of the multiple papers may face problems in asking the authors to withdraw one or more papers from the other journals and to combine them.

Editors can probably do more about repetitive publication. Editors can ask peer reviewers to call attention to any prior publication of the content of the paper under review. Many reviewers do this now, some even checking through online bibliographic searchers, but more might do so if asked specifically.

Editors can require authors to affirm by signature on an appropriate form that the present paper or the essence of its content has not been accepted for publication or already published elsewhere. This procedure could raise authors' awareness that editors are alert to such abuses.

Editorial offices could search bibliographic databases to see whether a similar if not identical paper has already been published. A few years ago this procedure would have been too costly in time and money for most journals when the search had to be carried out with paper indexes that often were not current. Now that we have relatively cheap and up-to-date online services, most journals could probably afford to use such searches for papers to be accepted.

All of us in science have ethical obligations to maintain honest authorship and to prevent wasting space in the expensive vehicles that are scientific journals. Our resources are not unlimited and must be shared.

References

1. Broad WJ. The publishing game; getting more for less. *Science*. 1981;**211:**1137–9.
2. Kronick DA. *The Literature of the Life Sciences: Reading, Writing, Research*. Philadelphia: ISI Press; 1985:67.
3. May KO. Growth and quality of the mathematical literature. *Isis*. 1968;**59:**363–71.
4. [Huth EJ]. Authorship from the reader's side [Editorial]. *Ann Intern Med*. 1982;**97:**613–4.
5. Relman AS. Responsibilities of authorship: Where does the buck stop? *N Engl J Med*. 1984;**310:**1048–9.
6. Angell M. Publish or perish: A proposal. *Ann Intern Med*. 1986;**104:**261–2.
7. *Publication Manual of the American Psychological Association*. Washington, D.C.: American Psychological Association; 1983:20–1.
8. Ethical conduct in authorship and publication. In: CBE Style Manual Committee. *CBE Style Manual: A Guide for Authors, Editors, and Publishers in the Biological Sciences*. 5th ed. Bethesda, Maryland: Council of Biology Editors; 1983:1–6.
9. American Chemical Society. ACS ethical guidelines to publication of chemical research. In: *The ACS Style Guide*. Washington, D.C.: American Chemical Society; 1986:217–22.
10. Editorial consensus on authorship and other matters. *Lancet*. 1985;**2:**595.
11. International Committee of Medical Journal Editors. Guidelines on authorship. *Br Med J*. 1985;**291:**722.
12. Huth EJ. Standards on authors' responsibilities [Editorial]. *Ann Intern Med*. 1985;**103:**797.

Reporting Provocative Results

Can We Publish "Hot" Papers without Getting Burned?

James L. Mills

In April 1981, *JAMA* published an article reporting an association between spermicide use around conception and congenital disorders (1). The authors were careful to note that "the results should be considered tentative until confirmed by other data." Nevertheless, their findings were taken up by the media and lawyers and treated as if they were established facts. Pregnant women who had used spermicides around conception became alarmed, and spermicide manufacturers were sued by former users who had had malformed infants.

Some journals publish exciting positive findings but are loath to publish subsequent negative investigations that contradict them. *JAMA*, to its credit, published an editorial the following year explaining why the association should be considered tentative or preliminary (2), along with several studies (3,4) that did not find any association between spermicides and birth defects. Subsequently, a number of negative studies appeared in other journals (5), and Food and Drug Administration hearings determined that there was insufficient evidence for an association between spermicides and birth defects to warrant a warning label (6).

However, the damage was done. Ortho Pharmaceutical Corp (Raritan, NJ), a major spermicide manufacturer, lost a $4.7 million suit brought by a spermicide user whose child was born with limb anomalies (7). *The Wall Street Journal* (May 20, 1986, p. 5) reported that Ortho was considering removing spermicides from the market, a claim other company spokesmen later denied (*Wall Street Journal*, May 21, 1986, p. 5). Today, spermicide manufacturers face numerous lawsuits despite a Food and Drug Administration statement that spermicides do not cause birth defects (8) and a statement from a distinguished teratologist and coauthor of the original paper that condemned the use of their data to prove that spermicides cause birth defects (9). This sad story demonstrates what can happen when a provocative or "hot" paper is published in a major journal despite the best efforts of the authors and editors to present the data in proper perspective.

What makes a paper provocative? Provocative papers present exciting new ideas or results. Provocative papers have a major impact on the public or the scientific community. Sometimes they are preliminary or tentative, but not always. When they are correct, such as the report identifying the molecular structure of nucleic acids (10), they can dramatically accelerate the progress of medical research. When they are incorrect, they can lead investigators down blind alleys, as happened when nickel poisoning was suggested as the cause of Legionnaires' disease (11,12). In the extreme case, they can cause great damage. The study demonstrating that diethylstilbestrol prevented toxemia, fetal death, and other bad

The author wishes to thank Mark Klebanoff, M.D., and George Rhoads, M.D., for reviewing the manuscript and Diane Wetherill for technical assistance.

From *Journal of the American Medical Association*, 1987, 258(23), pp. 3428–3429.

pregnancy outcomes (13) led to several million women being placed at increased risk for vaginal cancer for no real benefit (14). Today, we face the same challenge of determining which provocative findings will lead to great advances in our understanding of disease and which will lead to disaster. For example, will lymphokine-activated killer cells and inter-leukin 2 (15) join the ranks of the great advances in cancer therapy or will they be a false alarm?

In our current litigious and socially volatile climate, it is increasingly difficult for authors and editors to know what to do with hot findings. Can major medical journals afford to publish such papers? Certainly, if the study results are correct, they need to be disseminated as quickly as possible. If incorrect, the studies need to be repeated, and the evidence that they are not reproducible also needs to be reported as quickly as possible, preferably in the same journal. In either case, it seems desirable to have provocative findings appear in high-visibility journals.

How, then, can hot studies be handled? The primary responsibility must fall on the authors. They have four options: A finding may be (1) discarded, (2) "buried" in a small-circulation journal, (3) reported as a letter to the editor, or (4) published by a major journal. First, the authors must decide whether or not the findings are reasonable. I once uncovered an association between a very popular analgesic and malformations. Even after using a second data set to confirm the findings, I was not certain that the malformations were not the result of the infections for which the analgesics were taken. I put this study into the trash. Discarding data has its disadvantages, however. It can result in important findings being withheld from the scientific community, and it can damage the career of a young investigator. Despite these dangers, investigators must be encouraged to do it when they do not have complete confidence in their findings. The analgesic issue, incidentally, has never been resolved.

A colleague asked me to review a paper that reported an association between birth defects and a controversial contraceptive. I asked what he planned to do with it. "We're not sure if it's true," he replied. "We're going to bury it." "Burial" is researchers' slang for publication in a journal that is read by only a small group of specialists in the field. This makes it possible to present data to a select group of colleagues without attracting undue public attention. Unfortunately, burial can be too effective a method of concealing data. Fetal alcohol syndrome was actually reported five years before its discovery by Jones et al. (16). The data were published in a little known French journal (17) and would probably never have reached the public had it not been for the independent observations of the U.S. investigators. With the increasing popularity of computer literature searches, burial may not be as safe an option in the future.

Letters to the editor serve to disseminate information quickly and provide a forum for raising questions. They are viewed as less than definitive by the media. Unfortunately, they are usually not peer reviewed, leave little room for describing study design, and earn their authors little credit in the academic world.

Finally, there is the major medical journal. When the authors choose this option, the hot paper becomes the editor's responsibility. The traditional review process provides several methods for evaluating provocative papers. A rigorous review will identify many flawed studies; however, unpaid volunteer reviewers will not always provide high-quality reviews. As a reviewer, I can attest to the fact that papers with novel or unexpected results are the most difficult to assess. One looks for flaws, but frequently none are evident even in studies one knows from other sources to be of poor quality. Errors in study design may be concealed or may simply not be mentioned in the methods section. Where no problems in design or analysis are evident and no additional information is available, the reviewer is forced to base the decision to accept or reject on intution: do the results make sense?

Next comes the editorial board's review. The editors may abdicate their responsibilities and take the reviewers' suggestions without question. More properly, they can add their own wisdom to the reviewers'. Where doubts remain about the validity of a paper, the conservative approach calls for rejection. This approach can have embarrassing consequences for the editor. I recall Dr. Rosalyn Yalow's address to the Endocrine Society after she won the Nobel Prize. She announced with obvious glee that she still had the rejection letter from a well-known journal (which she mentioned by name), turning down the research that was to win her the prize. The editor's other option is to publish the article with a cautionary editorial, but there are limits to this approach. Each paper requires a skilled editorial writer and space in the journal.

One would hope that the best efforts of authors, reviewers, and editors would result in provocative papers being published in the appropriate journals, but far too often these traditional methods are proving ineffective. New approaches are needed in a society where the paper published today will be the six o'clock news tonight and the basis for a lawsuit in the morning.

It has been suggested (9) that hot findings not be published until they have been reported at meetings and other investigators have had the opportunity to review the results. This suggestion has the major advantage of not putting questionable results before the public. It would also permit other investigators with similar data sets to try to confirm the findings. Yet, it could prove impractical in a system in which rewards come with publication and where there is the risk that others will duplicate the work and publish first.

Journals could create a separate category for provocative results that require confirmation. Authors might object, but such studies would be more clearly identified. Epidemiologists identify studies that test for a variety of possible associations by the term *hypothesis-generating*. Positive results from hypothesis-generating studies are not automatically assumed to be causal. It may be hard to identify speculative papers, but some rules of thumb are helpful. Studies without a clear a priori hypothesis, those where positive results appear to be due to multiple comparisons, and those reporting chance observations are strong candidates for the speculative category.

Often the tentative nature of a study is obvious to the expert but not to the general scientific or lay reader. The expert's knowledge could be passed along without making the review and publication process too cumbersome by adding a section to the reviewer's comments designated for publication immediately following the study. These commentaries could be published anonymously (encouraging candor) or with the reviewer's name (encouraging quality) at the editor's discretion. When the editor deems it appropriate, this approach could be expanded into a formal discussion among reviewers.

The final and, perhaps, the most difficult step toward publishing hot papers without courting disaster is education. The academic community, the legal profession, and the media must recognize their responsibilities. Universities should place less emphasis on number of publications when deciding on promotions. This would eliminate some marginal papers and allow investigators the luxury to "sit on" questionable results until they can be confirmed. Lawyers must recognize that one paper rarely provides a final, definitive answer. The concept that consistency of findings across studies is needed to prove causality should make its way into the courtroom. Journalists must restrain their natural desire for an exciting story. It does the public no service to report that spermicides are related to birth defects without also noting that the investigators consider their results tentative. Journalists, like lawyers, should be given a better appreciation of the process of scientific investigation.

The spermicide experience demonstrates the risks that we take when we publish provocative findings in America today. Nonetheless, provocative studies should be published. Authors, editors, those who report medical findings to the public, and those who use them in courts of law must recognize the potential danger inherent in reporting tentative results and must accept new responsibilities to minimize that danger. As never before, hot findings must be handled with care.

References

1. Jick H, Walker AM, Rothman KJ, et al.: Vaginal spermicides and congenital disorders. *JAMA* 1981;245:1329–1332.
2. Oakley GP: Spermicides and birth defects. *JAMA* 1982;247:2405.
3. Shapiro S, Slone D, Heinonen O, et al.: Birth defects and vaginal spermicides. *JAMA* 1982;247:2381–2384.
4. Mills JL, Harley EE, Reed GF, et al.: Are spermicides teratogenic? *JAMA* 1982;248:2148–2151.
5. Bracken MB: Spermicidal contraceptives and poor reproductive outcomes: The epidemiologic evidence against an association. *Am J Obstet Gynecol* 1985;151:552–556.
6. National Center for Drug and Biologics: *Minutes of the Fertility and Maternal Health Drugs Advisory Committee Meeting*. Bethesda, MD, Food and Drug Administration, 1983.
7. *Wells v Ortho Pharmaceutical Corp*, 788 F2d 741 (11 Cir 1986).
8. Data do not support association between spermicides, birth defects. *FDA Drug Bull* 1986;16:21.
9. Holmes L: Vaginal spermicides and congenital disorders: The validity of a study. *JAMA* 1986;256:3095.
10. Watson JD, Crick FHC: Molecular structure of nucleic acids: A structure of deoxyribose nucleic acid. *Nature* 1953;171:737–738.
11. Chen JR, Francisco RB, Miller TE: Legionnaires' disease: Nickel levels. *Science* 1977;196:906–908.
12. Sunderman FW: Perspectives on Legionnaires' disease in relation to acute nickel carbonyl poisoning. *Ann Clin Lab Sci* 1977;7:187–200.
13. Smith OW, Smith G van S: The influence of diethylstilbestrol on progress and outcome of pregnancy as based on a comparison of treated with untreated primagravidas. *Am J Obstet Gynecol* 1949;58:994–1009.
14. Brackbill Y, Berendes HW: Dangers of diethylstilbestrol: Review of a 1953 paper. *Lancet* 1978;2:520.
15. Rosenberg SA, Lotze MT, Muul LM, et al.: Observations on the systemic administration of autologous lymphokine-activated killer cells and recombinant interleukin–2 to patients with metastatic cancer. *N Engl J Med* 1985;313:1485–1492.
16. Jones KL, Smith DW, Ulleland CN, et al.: Patterns of malformations in offspring of chronic alcoholic mothers. *Lancet* 1973;1:1267–1271.
17. Lemoine P, Harousseau H, Borteyru JP, et al.: Les enfants de parents alcooliques: Anomalies observées à propos de 127 cas. *Ouest Med* 1968;21:476–482.

ORI Provides Working Definition of Plagiarism

Office of Research Integrity

Although there is widespread agreement in the scientific community on including plagiarism as a major element of the PHS definition of scientific misconduct, there is some uncertainty about how the definition of plagiarism itself is applied in ORI cases.

As a general working definition, ORI considers plagiarism to include both the theft or misappropriation of intellectual property and the substantial unattributed textual copying of another's work. It does not include authorship or credit disputes.

The theft or misappropriation of intellectual property includes the unauthorized use of ideas or unique methods obtained by a privileged communication, such as a grant or manuscript review.

Substantial unattributed textual copying of another's work means the unattributed verbatim or nearly verbatim copying of sentences and paragraphs which materially mislead the ordinary reader regarding the contributions of the author. ORI generally does not pursue the limited use of identical or nearly-identical phrases which describe a commonly-used methodology or previous research because ORI does not consider such use as substantially misleading to the reader or of great significance.

Many allegations of plagiarism involve disputes among former collaborators who participated jointly in the development or conduct of a research project, but who subsequently went their separate ways and made independent use of the jointly developed concepts, methods, descriptive language, or other product of the joint effort. The ownership of the intellectual property in many such situations is seldom clear, and the collaborative history among the scientists often supports a presumption of implied consent to use the products of the collaboration by any of the former collaborators.

For this reason, ORI considers many such disputes to be authorship or credit disputes rather than plagiarism. Such disputes are referred to PHS agencies and extramural institutions for resolution.

From *ORI Newsletter*, 1994; 3(1): 6–7. Reprinted by permission.

Questions for Discussion

1. You overhear scientists from another laboratory discussing results from a manuscript they are reviewing that can be of great use to you in your present work. What can you ethically do in this situation?
2. In a highly competitive area of research, is it better to be the first to publish an important but incomplete finding or to have a later paper that is complete and accurate?
3. One aspect of a publication of a multidisciplinary study group on which you were an author has been criticized as containing falsified data in one specialized area of expertise. You had not participated in that area of research. If the data are determined to be false, are you guilty of scientific misconduct? How should this situation have been handled during the preparation of the manuscript?

Recommended Supplemental Reading

Baue AE. Peer and/or peerless review: Some vagaries of the editorial process. *Arch Surg.* 1985;120 (August):885–8.

Grossman J. *The Chicago Manual of Style: The Essential Guide for Writers, Editors, and Publishers, 14th ed.* Chicago, IL: University of Chicago Press; 1993.

International Committee of Medical Journal Editors. *The Uniform Requirements for Manuscripts Submitted to Biomedical Journals.* Available at: http://www.icmje.org

Mattews JR, Bowen JM, Matthews RW. *Successful Scientific Writing, 2d ed.* New York: Cambridge University Press; 2001.

Research with Human Beings

Research with Human Beings

Ruth Ellen Bulger

Chiseled into the stone wall where I went to graduate school was the famous Hippocratic aphorism, "Life is short, the art long, experience fleeting, experiment perilous, judgment uncertain."[1] In the time of Hippocrates there was no real clinical research. Patients were treated according to the traditions of that time. However, Hippocrates did observe the outcomes of his treatments and recorded the results. Even if he wasn't doing clinical research in the sense that we do today, his aphorism well states some of the problems encountered with human experimentation. The occasional tragic death of a human volunteer in a research study, which occurs even today, reminds us of the truth of the aphorism that extending the frontiers of knowledge by clinical investigation involving human subjects is fraught with difficulties, can be perilous, and is filled with uncertain and difficult judgments.[2]

The history of clinical research using human volunteers started centuries later with the work of scientists such as Claude Bernard. This history, even up to the present time, has been characterized not only by great achievements but also by significant ethical lapses.

The heinous experiments that the Nazis undertook on humans during World War II were one of the most horrible atrocities in history. The Nuremberg Code (published in 1949) was written so that the Nuremberg Military Tribunal had standards to judge the physicians and scientists involved with these wartime atrocities.[3] The code consisted of 10 basic, required principles to be observed when one used human volunteers in clinical research. The principles included such requirements as *knowledgeable, voluntary consent* as absolutely essential without coercion, fraud, duress, or deceit and with the clear understanding that the subject could discontinue participation at any time; *qualified investigators* sufficiently experienced and capable to judge when an experiment should be terminated; undertaking the *research first on animals* as well as having knowledge of the natural history of the disease when experiments are done using human volunteers; the stipulation that experiments provide useful *results not procurable by other means* and be conducted in such a way as to avoid, to the extent possible, all unnecessary physical and mental suffering and injury; and insistence that the degree of *risk should never exceed that of the humanitarian importance of the problem.* However, the responsibility for action was left solely with the physician or scientist doing the experiment.[4]

Another code relating to human experimentation proposed by the medical community in 1964 was called the Declaration of Helsinki because the meeting at which it was adopted by the 18th World Medical Assembly occurred in Helsinki, Finland.[3] One important part of the early document recommended that the investigator solicit independent guidance about the human experimentation protocol, but the declaration provided no real means of enforcing this recommendation except for the stipulation that the work should not be accepted for publication if external review were not used. Again, the responsibility to accept the findings of the outside review was left solely with the investigator.[4]

The Declaration of Helsinki has been frequently updated, most recently in 2000.[5] The latest revision introduces several new positions. For example, research is justified only if it offers real benefit to the participant. The update also requires investigators to disclose potential conflicts of interest to research review committees and in publications. It also discourages the use of placebo-controlled trials and mandates investigators to give the "best proven" treatment to all participants after the trial. However, without a placebo control in a trial, the new therapy may be compared with an ineffective, unproven standard therapy, and thus neither the standard nor the new therapy may be effective. The new provisions about placebo-controlled trials may bring the revised Declaration into conflict with Food and Drug Administration expectations that new drugs to be approved by them be tested using placebo-controlled trials.

Despite these codes, flagrant abuses in research with human volunteers continued to occur in the United States. One problem was that the codes for healthy volunteers were not uniformly being applied to patient volunteers in clinical research. For example, physicians at the Brooklyn Jewish Chronic Disease Hospital injected live cancer cells into aged, sometimes comatose patients, without their informed consent, to see if the cells would be rejected.[6] At Willowbrook Home for retarded children, the institutionalized children were given hepatitis so that physicians could study the natural course of the disease.[7–9]

A study that began in 1932 in Macon County, Alabama (usually referred to as the Tuskegee Study because it occurred in Tuskegee, Alabama), which was supported by the United States Public Health Service, examined the natural course of untreated syphilis only in disadvantaged, poor African American men even though the disease was not limited to that group.[10] The study, which continued until it was exposed in the 1970s, deprived the men of treatment long beyond the time in 1949 when penicillin had been proven effective for the treatment of this disease. Over an extended period, the subjects were deceived, misled, and deprived of treatment for their disease by the physicians who were doing the study.

In 1966, Henry Beecher exposed 22 instances from the published literature in which serious ethical lapses in research with human volunteers occurred, including the lack of informed consent or misuse of disadvantaged or vulnerable subjects.[11]

The first tangible governmental steps to ensure the ethical treatment of human volunteers were taken at the National Institutes of Health Clinical Center in 1953 when it was required that a review of human subjects' protocols be done by an external committee. In 1966, the Surgeon General of the United States Public Health Service (PHS) expanded this mandate into federal guidelines for all of the studies supported by the PHS.[12] The membership of the review committees was to include scientists, clinicians, ethicists, and community representatives.

In 1972–73, the public gained some insight into the ethical problems relating to clinical research when congressional hearings about human experiments involving sterilization of mentally retarded people, research on human fetuses, and research on prisoners were conducted by the U.S. Senate Committee on Labor and Public Welfare and broadcast on television.[13]

All of these factors led to Congress's passing the National Research Act of 1974 (PL 93–348), which made two important advances. First, it required the use of institutional committees to review PHS-supported clinical studies with human volunteers. Institutional Review Boards (IRBs) remain to this day as one of the primary mechanisms to protect human volunteers. The role of IRBs will be discussed below.

Second, the National Research Act of 1974 established the National Commission for the Protection of Human Subjects of Biomedical and Behavioral Research and gave it the task of formulating principles and guidelines for including human volunteers in clinical research. The National Commission (with members coming mainly from the disciplines of philosophy, law, or religion), staff, and those consultants chosen to write background papers for the commissioners initiated the new discipline of bioethics in the United States. After writing 14 reports over 4 years on various aspects of research using human studies, the commissioners summarized, in a paper called the Belmont Report,[14] the basic ethical principles that should inform research involving human volunteers. The Belmont Report identified three comprehensive basic principles: *respect for persons, beneficence, and justice*.

Respect for Persons

Respect for persons incorporates two ethical convictions. The first is that individuals be *treated as autonomous agents capable of self-determination*. They are capable of thinking about their own goals and making rational choices. The second is that persons with diminished autonomy are entitled to protection.

The implications of the first conviction – that human research subjects are autonomous agents in the research – are threefold. First, to make a choice to become a participant in clinical research, the prospective volunteer must have *adequate information* about what is being asked of him or her. This is provided by the process called *informed consent*, which entails an explanation of the research and, generally, the signing of an informed consent document. To give informed consent, the subject must have information about the procedure, its purpose, the risks and benefits involved, and other accepted procedures that could be used instead to accomplish the aims of the experiment. Human subjects must have time to ask questions and must understand that they can withdraw from the research whenever they choose. Second, the subjects must comprehend what is being asked. Both the oral presentation and the written form should be in the native language of the individual being asked to participate. To aid understanding, the material is generally written at no more than an eighth-grade level, explaining all of the material using lay language (e.g., number of teaspoons, not milliliters, of blood to be removed). The IRBs of the institutions approving the research not only review these translations as part of their overseeing the informed consent process and documents but also have the material translated back into English to ensure that the original informed consent document has been translated accurately. Third, all persons must enter voluntarily, free of any coercion or undue influence, and understand that they can withdraw at any time. They must be informed that they will not lose any rights to which they are entitled or incur any penalties if they withdraw.

If an individual with diminished autonomy is incapable of self-determination – either because of age, maturation, illness, mental disability, or circumstances that severely restrict liberty – he or she may require protection. The Belmont Report says that the extent of protection should depend on the risk of harm and the likelihood of benefit.

Beneficence

Beneficence requires that relevant positive efforts are made to secure the well-being of persons (do good, beneficence) and protect them from harm (do no harm, nonmaleficence). Before the research is approved, it must be justified by a favorable risk-benefit ratio.

To do this, one needs to evaluate the magnitude and probability of harms and risks and balance them with the anticipated benefits. Risks should always be reduced to the absolute minimum. Harms, which can be physical, psychological, social, or legal, should be understood. Benefits should be maximized. When risks are too great, then benefits should be forgone. The risks and benefits of any research proposal must be carefully explained in the informed consent process.

Justice

Justice requires that there be fair procedures and outcomes in the selection of research subjects. Burdens and benefits of research should be equally distributed. Classes of people must not be systematically selected on the basis of easy availability, compromised position, or susceptibility to manipulation. In earlier times, the burdens of research fell largely on poor ward patients, while the benefits went to private patients.

More recently, it has been realized that not only risks but also benefits are gained for classes of people who participate in clinical trials. In recent years, women of child-bearing age, pregnant women, and minorities have not been included in certain clinical trials as frequently as white, middle-aged, 70-kg Caucasian males. Hence, more is known about how pharmaceutical agents act in males. Justice then requires that attention be given to including individuals of both genders, of different ages, and of various racial and ethnic groups in clinical trials.

The three Belmont Report principles form an analytical framework within which to judge the ethics of proposed human participant research. Review of these principles as they relate to any proposed research will help the investigator understand the ethical issues inherent in research involving human volunteers and what is required in the experiment. The Belmont Report includes a careful distinction between what is research and what is patient care. Health care is for the well-being of the particular individual or group of individuals. Research is an activity with a hypothesis that is tested to develop generalizable knowledge.

In 1981 the Department of Health, Education, and Welfare revised its human volunteer guidelines as 45 CFR 46. The guidelines were again updated in 1991 and have been adopted by 17 federal agencies and departments that conduct, support, or otherwise regulate research involving human subjects.[15] Some agencies have not only incorporated provisions of 45 CFR 46 into their regulations but also have additional regulations.

Protections for special subjects requiring additional safeguards form three further subparts of 45 CFR 46. They have been accepted by many of the agencies and departments as well. These include protections for fetuses, pregnant women, and human in vitro fertilization (subpart B), prisoners (subpart C), and children (subpart D). Subpart B has just been modified and announced as a final rule.

In general, these regulations for special populations allow IRBs to approve research with these groups only under certain conditions, such as in a protocol with only minimal risks to the subject and a direct subject benefit. The NIH has released policy and guidelines that NIH-supported investigators must consider concerning the inclusion of women and minorities as subjects of clinical research[16] as well as children as participants in research involving human subjects.[17] In addition, NIH now requires documentation of education on protection of human research participants for all key personnel in NIH-funded grants funded before an award is issued. Several computer-based training programs concerning protection of human subjects are now available on the Internet and are listed among the recommended supplemental reading on page 152.

As noted certain advantages can accrue to classes of people who are involved as subjects in clinical trials. Yet women in general, women of child-bearing age, and pregnant women have not been included as subjects in several large-scale prevention trials, such as the Physicians' Health Study of 1989,[18] which evaluated aspirin in the prevention of heart attacks, or the Multiple Risk Factor Intervention Trials of 1977 (MRFIT), which investigated the relationships among lifestyle, cholesterol levels, and heart disease.[19]

Moreover women have not been treated as aggressively as men in certain medical conditions. Tobin et al.[20] had shown that only 4% of women with chest pain and abnormal exercise test results were referred for coronary arteriography, while 40% of men with similar results were referred. Khan et al.[21] found that differences in later referral for coronary bypass surgery and greater age, rather than gender, could account for the higher mortality of women in coronary bypass surgery.

The lack of research on women's health compromised the health information available about women. This was well documented by the 1985 USPHS Task Force on Women's Health.[22] In spite of a 1986 NIH policy to encourage inclusion of women in clinical research, public attention was focused on the lack of any real change in the involvement of women in clinical research by a General Accounting Office (GAO) report in 1990.[23] To help rectify the situation, William Raub, acting director of the NIH at that time, created the Office of Research on Women's Health in 1990, and the NIH and the Alcohol, Drug Abuse, and Mental Health Administration (ADAMHA) instructed grant applicants to include women in clinical trials unless "clear and compelling reasons" were given for their omission.[24] A second GAO report in 1992 demonstrated that women were still not being equitably included. The report disclosed that, for 60% of drugs, the number of women in the trials was less than the number of women in the population with the disease under study. And even when women were included, gender differences frequently were not analyzed from the trial data.

Pressure from women, women's rights groups, and women in Congress finally led to the 1993 NIH Revitalization Act (PL 103–43) requiring that, for all NIH-funded trials, women and members of minority groups be included as subjects in each project of such research. The trials were to be designed and carried out to provide a *valid analysis* of whether the variables being studied affect women or members of minority groups *differently than other subjects* in the trial. The NIH has guidelines on how this act is to be followed in research supported by the NIH. The NIH is diligent in obtaining feedback from investigators in the annual research progress reports, thus seeking to ensure that investigators are following this law. The Defense Authorization Act for Fiscal Year 1994 (PL 103-160) has the same inclusion requirements for women and minorities for research that is supported by the Department of Defense.

The Institute of Medicine Report on Women and Health Research concluded that, in most situations addressed so far, women and men did not react differently to treatments if data were normalized for factors such as body size.[25] Therefore, including both genders in clinical trials is reasonable, for treatment effects should not differ. However, when there are reasons to believe that differences between women and men, or between members of various ethnic or racial groups, might occur with respect to a particular treatment being investigated, then it would make sense to include members of both sexes, or members of affected ethnic or racial groups, in the trials in sufficient numbers to test for differences.

45 CFR 46 and Institutional Review Boards

It is 45 CFR 46 that describes the role of the IRB in the review of research involving human participants. This regulation details information concerning the IRB such as its membership, functions and operations, criteria for review and approval, and the general requirements and documentation of informed consent. The IRB must review, approve, modify, or disapprove research involved with human volunteers covered by the federal policy at the institution. The IRB will ensure that the risks of the research are minimized and are reasonable in relation to anticipated benefits and the importance of the expected results, that the selection of the subjects is equitable, that adequate informed consent is obtained, that the subject knows that the study is research and not health care, that it is entered voluntarily, and the subject can withdraw any time at will without the loss of any benefits to which he or she is entitled.

It is the IRB system and staff that oversee the human protection programs ensuring the ethical conduct of clinical research. However, in the last few years, the Office of Protections from Research Risks, subsequently elevated and renamed as the Office of Human Research Protections, has found problems with the IRB system at certain universities. Each of these two agencies has recently stopped research involving human participants at several universities until the problems identified at these institutions were rectified.

The regulations define three types of review process that may be used by the university offices that protect human volunteers. They are classified as exempt, expedited, or full review. Because there is some variation in which of the processes are used by an institution, it is important that all investigators know what kinds of research must be reviewed at their institution by their human protection programs.

Exempt review is discussed in 45 CFR 46.101(b) (available at http://ohrp/osophs/dhhs. gov/humansubjects/guidance/exempt-pb.htm). Certain research activities involving human subjects may not require IRB review. However, the decision about whether a proposal requires review is generally made by the personnel protecting human participants at the institution, not by the investigator. Some institutions ask to be notified by investigators according to institutional procedures whenever there is a question so that an appropriate decision can be made about whether the study is to be reviewed or should be placed in an exempt category and the records kept by that office. Research that the institution could put in an exempt category includes the collection or study of existing data, documents, pathological specimens, or diagnostic specimens if the information is kept in such a manner that subjects cannot be identified directly or through identifiers that can be linked to the subjects. Studies that do not require any review include those being done strictly for quality assurance purposes or those involving normal educational practices if they are not being done as research for ultimate publication of the results. Universities disagree over what requires exempt review. For example, the use of established human cell lines is reviewed as exempt by some universities; at others it does not fall into a category that requires any IRB review.

An *expedited review procedure* is a review of research with human participants by the IRB chair or by one or more knowledgeable reviewers designated from among the members of the IRB, following the requirement of 45 CRF 46.110 or 21 CFR 56.101. The Secretary of the Department of Health and Human Services has established and published a notice in the *Federal Register* that lists the categories of research that may be reviewed by the IRB using an expedited review procedure. To be eligible for expedited review, the research activities must constitute no more than minimal risk to human subjects and involve procedures listed in certain categories found in the most recent document released in November 1998 (http://ohrp.osophs.dhhs.gov). These include research requiring the collection of blood samples by finger stick or venipuncture from healthy, nonpregnant adults; the prospective collection of biological specimens for research purposes by noninvasive means; or the collection of data through noninvasive procedures (not involving anesthesia or sedation) routinely employed in clinical practice, excluding X-ray procedures. The standard informed consent procedures still apply to expedited research. The categories are precisely described and, depending on the circumstance, might be classified as exempt; thus investigators should consult with the human protection office at their institution for advice on the type of review necessary for each research proposal they are contemplating. The IRB must be kept informed of the expedited reviews that have been administratively approved.

For the process of *full review*, the research proposal will be reviewed at a convened meeting at which a quorum of the members of the IRB are present, including at least one member whose primary concerns are in a nonscientific area. To be approved, the IRB must determine that the risks are minimal and reasonable in relation to anticipated benefits, if any, to the subjects, and that the knowledge reasonably expected to be gained is important, the selection of subjects is equitable, informed consent will be sought and appropriately documented, data will be appropriately monitored to ensure subject safety, and privacy and confidentiality of data will be ensured. The proposal must receive the approval of a majority of the members present at the meeting.

The Public Health Service Office of Human Subjects Research provides decisional charts that help the investigator decide what review is appropriate (http://ohrp.osophs.dhhs.gov/humansubjects/guidance/decisioncharts.htm). The NIH has developed a user-friendly brochure to help investigators understand the regulations for using human subjects.

Food and Drug Administration Regulations (21 CFR 50, 56)

Thalidomide, a drug once used for nausea during pregnancy in many countries, was not approved for use in the United States. Yet in many other countries, many serious limb malformations were seen in children of women who had taken the drug during pregnancy, and these birth defects were associated with the use of the drug.

Diethylstilbesterol (DES) was given to pregnant women in the 1940s and 1950s to prevent miscarriage, although a small clinical trial had demonstrated that the drug was ineffective for that purpose. About 20 years later, children of mothers who had taken this drug were noted to develop a rare adenocarcinoma of the vagina.

These two terrible experiences with pharmaceutical drug administration – in the context of the Kefauver–Harris amendment to the drug approval laws of 1962 mandating that manufacturers of drugs demonstrate the safety and efficacy of the drug, that the Food and Drug Administration (FDA) collect adverse reactions reports, and that investigators of experimental drugs obtain formal informed consent from human volunteers – have led to promulgation of another set of regulations, this time for clinical trials of drugs and devices regulated by the FDA.[26]

The FDA released guidelines in 1977 recommending that women of child-bearing age not be admitted to early-phase drug trials unless those trials were for life-threatening conditions.[27] These guidelines remained in force until 1993, when women's rights groups had exerted sufficient pressure to be included in trials so that more would be learned about their diseases and the treatment of women as well as men with pharmaceuticals.[28] The new guideline recommends that subjects for clinical trials reflect the proportion of people that would receive the drug if it were marketed and that both women and men be included so that results can be directly compared across genders. The guideline encouraged but did not require that women of child-bearing age be included. Pharmacokinetic studies of women in various estrogen states were also suggested.

Former President Clinton appointed the National Bioethics Advisory Commission (NBAC) (http://bioethics.gov/) to again look at several areas of concern related to the use of human volunteers or their tissues. The charge to the NBAC included a new look at the way that human subject protections are being undertaken. The commission has published several reports on the ethical issues in research related to human stem cell research, human biological materials, persons with mental disorders that may affect decision-making capacity, cloning of human beings, and oversight of human research in the United States and in international settings.[29]

Conclusions

This is a time of change for how human volunteers are to be protected as participants in research, and yet the basic principles of respect for persons, beneficence (and nonmaleficence), and justice have remained constant. It is important that research investigators understand the IRB system of protections and obtain appropriate advice and review for their studies.

References

1. Selections from the Hippocratic Corpus. In: Reiser, SJ, Dyke, AJ, Curran, WJ, eds. *Ethics in Medicine: Historical Perspectives and Contemporary Concerns*. Cambridge, MA: Massachusetts Institute of Technology Press; 1989.
2. Bulger RE. New paradigms in clinical research. In: Proceedings for the International Conference on Human Clinical Research: Ethics and Economics, Naples, Italy, September 15–17, 1997.
3. The Nuremberg Code. In: *Trials of War Criminals Before the Nuremberg Military Tribunals Under Control Council Law No. 10*. Vol 2. Washington, DC: U.S. Government Printing Office; 1949:181–182.
4. World Medical Association. Declaration of Helsinki: Recommendations Guiding Medical Doctors in Biomedical Research Involving Human Subjects. Adopted by the 18th World Medical Assembly, Helsinki, Finland, 1964.
5. World Medical Association. Declaration of Helsinki: Ethical Principles for Medical Research Involving Human Subjects. Adopted by the 52nd World Medical Association General Assembly, Edinburgh, Scotland, October 2000.
6. Katz J. The Jewish chronic disease case. In: *Experimentation with Human Beings*. New York: Russell Sage Foundation; 1972.
7. Levine RJ. *Ethics and Regulations of Clinical Research*. 2nd ed. Baltimore, MD: Urban and Schwarzenberg; 1986.
8. Faden R, Beauchamp TL. *A History and Theory of Informed Consent*. New York: Oxford University Press; 1986.

9. Rothman DJ. *Strangers at the Bedside: A History of How Law and Bioethics Transformed Medical Decision Making*. New York: Basic Books; 1991.
10. *Final Report of the Tuskegee Syphilis Study Ad Hoc Advisory Panel*. Washington, DC: Public Health Services; 1973.
11. Beecher HK. Ethics and clinical research. *N Engl J Med*. 1966;274:1354–1360.
12. USPHS, Division of Research Grants, memo PPO#129, February 8, 1966, and supplement, April 7, 1966.
13. Senate Committee on Labor and Public Welfare, Quality of Health Care – Human Experimentation: Hearings Before the Subcommittee on Health, 93rd Congress (February 21–23, March 6–8, April 30, June 28–29, July 10). Washington, DC: U.S. Government Printing Office; 1973.
14. National Commission for the Protection of Human Subjects of Biomedical and Behavioral Research. *The Belmont Report: Ethical Principles and Guidelines for the Protection of Human Subjects of Research*. Washington, DC: U.S. Government Printing Office; 1979. Available at: http://ohrp.osophs.dhhs.gov/humansubjects/guidance/belmont.htm.
15. Department of Health and Human Services, 45 Code of Federal Regulations, Part 46, Protection of Human Subject, amended *Federal Register* 56, 28012, June 28, 1991, (http://ohrp.osophs.dhhs.gov/ humansubjects/guidance/45CFR46.htm).
16. National Institutes of Health. Guidelines on the inclusion of women and minorities as subjects in clinical research. *Federal Register* 59(59):14508–14513, 1994, (http://www4.od.nih.gov/orwh/overview.html).
17. National Institutes of Health. *Policy and guidelines on the inclusion of children as participants in research involving human subjects*. Bethesda, MD: NIH; 1998. Available at: http://www.nih.gov/grants/guide/notice-files/not98-024.html.
18. Steering Committee of the Physicians Health Study Research Group. Health Study Research Group: final report on the aspirin component of the ongoing physician's health study. *N Engl J Med*. 1989;321:129–135.
19. Multiple Risk Factor Intervention Trial Group. Statistical design considerations in the NHLBI multiple risk factor intervention trial (MRFIT). *J Chron Dis*. 1977;30:261–275.
20. Tobin JN, Wassertheil-Smoller S, Wexler JP, et al. Sex bias in considering coronary bypass surgery. *Ann Intern Med*. 1987;107:19–25.
21. Khan SD, Nessim S, Gray R et al. Increased mortality of women in coronary artery bypass surgery: Evidence for referral bias. *Ann Intern Med*. 1990;112:561–567.
22. U.S. Public Health Service. Women's health: Report of the Public Health Service Task Force on Women's Health Issues. *Public Health Rep*. 1985;100:73–106.
23. National Institutes of Health: Problem in implementing policy on women in study populations. GAO–HRD–90–80. Statement of Mark Nadel, June 18, 1990.
24. National Institutes of Health and Alcohol, Drug Abuse, and Mental Health Administration (ADAMHA). NIH/ADAMHA policy concerning inclusion of women in study populations. *NIH Guide*. August 24, 1990(31):18–19.
25. Mastroianni AC, Faden R, Federman D, eds. *Women and Health Research*: *Ethical and Legal Issues of Including Women in Clinical Studies*. Vol 1. Washington, DC: National Academy Press; 1994.
26. Food and Drug Administration, 21 Code of Federal Regulations, Parts 50 FDA Regulations; Protection of human subjects amended, *Federal Register* 62: 39440, July 23, 1997 and 56: FDA Regulations; IRB, amended, *Federal Register* 162, 51529, October 2, 1996.
27. Food and Drug Administration. *General Consideration for the Clinical Evaluation of Drugs*. Washington, DC: U.S. Government Printing Office; 1977.
28. Food and Drug Administration. Guideline for the Study and Evaluation of Gender Differences in the Clinical Evaluation of Drugs: Notice. *Federal Register* 58(139):39406–39416, 1993.
29. National Bioethics Advisory Commission. Reports available at: http://bioethics.gov.

The Nuremberg Code

The Proof as to War Crimes and Crimes against Humanity

Judged by any standard of proof the record clearly shows the commission of war crimes and crimes against humanity substantially as alleged in counts two and three of the indictment. Beginning with the outbreak of World War II criminal medical experiments on non-German nationals, both prisoners of war and civilians, including Jews and "asocial" persons, were carried out on a large scale in Germany and the occupied countries. These experiments were not the isolated and casual acts of individual doctors and scientists working solely on their own responsibility, but were the product of coordinated policy-making and planning at high governmental, military, and Nazi Party levels, conducted as an integral part of the total war effort. They were ordered, sanctioned, permitted, or approved by persons in positions of authority who under all principles of law were under the duty to know about these things and to take steps to terminate or prevent them.

Permissible Medical Experiments

The great weight of evidence before us is to the effect that certain types of medical experiments on human beings, when kept within reasonably well-defined bounds, conform to the ethics of the medical profession generally. The protagonists of the practice of human experimentation justify their views on the basis that such experiments yield results for the good of society that are unprocurable by other methods or means of study. All agree, however, that certain basic principles must be observed in order to satisfy moral, ethical and legal concepts:

　1. The voluntary consent of the human subject is absolutely essential.

　This means that the person involved should have legal capacity to give consent; should be so situated as to be able to exercise free power of choice, without the intervention of any element of force, fraud, deceit, duress, over-reaching, or other ulterior form of constraint or coercion; and should have sufficient knowledge and comprehension of the elements of the subject matter involved as to enable him to make an understanding and enlightened decision. This latter element requires that before the acceptance of an affirmative decision by the experimental subject there should be made known to him the nature, duration, and purpose of the experiment; the method and means by which it is to be conducted; all inconveniences and hazards reasonably to be expected; and the effects upon his health or person that may possibly come from his participation in the experiment.

From *Trials of War Criminals before the Nuernberg Military Tribunals under Control Council Law* No. 10, Vol. 2 (Washington, D.C.: U.S. Government Printing Office, 1949), pp. 181–182.

The duty and responsibility for ascertaining the quality of the consent rests upon each individual who initiates, directs or engages in the experiment. It is a personal duty and responsibility which may not be delegated to another with impunity.

2. The experiment should be such as to yield fruitful results for the good of society, unprocurable by other methods or means of study, and not random and unnecessary in nature.

3. The experiment should be so designed and based on the results of animal experimentation and a knowledge of the natural history of the disease or other problem under study that the anticipated results will justify the performance of the experiment.

4. The experiment should be so conducted as to avoid all unnecessary physical and mental suffering and injury.

5. No experiment should be conducted where there is an *a priori* reason to believe that death or disabling injury will occur; except, perhaps, in those experiments where the experimental physicians also serve as subjects.

6. The degree of risk to be taken should never exceed that determined by the humanitarian importance of the problem to be solved by the experiment.

7. Proper preparations should be made and adequate facilities provided to protect the experimental subject against even remote possibilities of injury, disability, or death.

8. The experiment should be conducted only by scientifically qualified persons. The highest degree of skill and care should be required through all stages of the experiment of those who conduct or engage in the experiment.

9. During the course of the experiment the human subject should be at liberty to bring the experiment to an end if he has reached the physical or mental state where continuation of the experiment seems to him to be impossible.

10. During the course of the experiment the scientist in charge must be prepared to terminate the experiment at any stage, if he has probable cause to believe, in the exercise of the good faith, superior skill, and careful judgment required of him that a continuation of the experiment is likely to result in injury, disability, or death to the experimental subject.

The Belmont Report

Ethical Principles and Guidelines for the Protection of Human Subjects of Research

The National Commission for the Protection of Human Subjects of Biomedical and Behavioral Research

Agency: Department of Health, Education, and Welfare.

Action: Notice of Report for Public Comment.

Summary: On July 12, 1974, the National Research Act (Pub. L. 93–348) was signed into law, there-by creating the National Commission for the Protection of Human Subjects of Biomedical and Behavioral Research. One of the charges to the Commission was to identify the basic ethical principles that should underlie the conduct of biomedical and behavioral research involving human subjects and to develop guidelines which should be followed to assure that such research is conducted in accordance with those principles. In carrying out the above, the Commission was directed to consider: (i) the boundaries between biomedical and behavioral research and the accepted and routine practice of medicine, (ii) the role of assessment of risk–benefit criteria in the determination of the appropriateness of research involving human subjects, (iii) appropriate guidelines for the selection of human subjects for participation in such research and (iv) the nature and definition of informed consent in various research settings.

The Belmont Report attempts to summarize the basic ethical principles identified by the Commission in the course of its deliberations. It is the outgrowth of an intensive four-day period of discussions that were held in February 1976 at the Smithsonian Institution's Belmont Conference Center supplemented by the monthly deliberations of the Commission that were held over a period of nearly four years. It is a statement of basic ethical principles and guidelines that should assist in resolving the ethical problems that surround the conduct of research with human subjects. By publishing the Report in the Federal Register, and providing reprints upon request, the Secretary intends that it may be made readily available to scientists, members of Institutional Review Boards, and Federal employees. The two-volume Appendix, containing the lengthy reports of experts and specialists who assisted the Commission in fulfilling this part of its charge, is available as DHEW Publication No. (OS) 78-0013 and No. (OS) 78-0014, for sale by the Superintendent of Documents, U.S. Government Printing Office, Washington, D.C. 20402.

Unlike most other reports of the Commission, the Belmont Report does not make specific recommendations for administrative action by the Secretary of Health, Education, and Welfare. Rather, the Commission recommended that the Belmont Report be adopted in its entirety, as a statement of the Department's policy. The Department requests public comment on this recommendation.

From *The Belmont Report: Ethical Principles and Guidelines for the Protection of Human Subjects of Research.* (Washington, D.C.: U.S. Government Printing Office, 1979).

Ethical Principles and Guidelines for Research Involving Human Subjects

Scientific research has produced substantial social benefits. It has also posed some troubling ethical questions. Public attention was drawn to these questions by reported abuses of human subjects in biomedical experiments, especially during the Second World War. During the Nuremberg War Crime Trials, the Nuremberg code was drafted as a set of standards for judging physicians and scientists who had conducted biomedical experiments on concentration camp prisoners. This code became the prototype of many later codes (1) intended to assure that research involving human subjects would be carried out in an ethical manner.

The codes consist of rules, some general, others specific, that guide the investigators or the reviewers of research in their work. Such rules often are inadequate to cover complex situations; at times they come into conflict, and they are frequently difficult to interpret or apply. Broader ethical principles will provide a basis on which specific rules may be formulated, criticized and interpreted.

Three principles, or general prescriptive judgments, that are relevant to research involving human subjects are identified in this statement. Other principles may also be relevant. These three are comprehensive, however, and are stated at a level of generalization that should assist scientists, subjects, reviewers and interested citizens to understand the ethical issues inherent in research involving human subjects. These principles cannot always be applied so as to resolve beyond dispute particular ethical problems. The objective is to provide an analytical framework that will guide the resolution of ethical problems arising from research involving human subjects.

This statement consists of a distinction between research and practice, a discussion of the three basic ethical principles, and remarks about the application of these principles.

Part A: Boundaries Between Practice and Research

A. Boundaries Between Practice and Research

It is important to distinguish between biomedical and behavioral research, on the one hand, and the practice of accepted therapy on the other, in order to know what activities ought to undergo review for the protection of human subjects of research. The distinction between research and practice is blurred partly because both often occur together (as in research designed to evaluate a therapy) and partly because notable departures from standard practice are often called "experimental" when the terms "experimental" and "research" are not carefully defined.

For the most part, the term "practice" refers to interventions that are designed solely to enhance the well-being of an individual patient or client and that have a reasonable expectation of success. The purpose of medical or behavioral practice is to provide diagnosis, preventive treatment or therapy to particular individuals (2). By contrast, the term "research" designates an activity designed to test an hypothesis, permit conclusions to be drawn, and thereby to develop or contribute to generalizable knowledge (expressed, for example, in theories, principles, and statements of relationships). Research is usually described in a formal protocol that sets forth an objective and a set of procedures designed to reach that objective.

When a clinician departs in a significant way from standard or accepted practice, the innovation does not, in and of itself, constitute research. The fact that a procedure is "experimental," in the sense of new, untested or different, does not automatically place it in the category of research. Radically new procedures of this description should, however, be made the object of formal research at an early stage in order to determine whether they are safe and effective. Thus, it is the responsibility of medical practice committees, for example, to insist that a major innovation be incorporated into a formal research project (3).

Research and practice may be carried on together when research is designed to evaluate the safety and efficacy of a therapy. This need not cause any confusion regarding whether or not the activity requires review; the general rule is that if there is any element of research in an activity, that activity should undergo review for the protection of human subjects.

Part B: Basic Ethical Principles

B. Basic Ethical Principles

The expression "basic ethical principles" refers to those general judgments that serve as a basic justification for the many particular ethical prescriptions and evaluations of human actions. Three basic principles, among those generally accepted in our cultural tradition, are particularly relevant to the ethics of research involving human subjects: the principles of respect of persons, beneficence and justice.

1. Respect for Persons

Respect for persons incorporates at least two ethical convictions: first, that individuals should be treated as autonomous agents, and second, that persons with diminished autonomy are entitled to protection. The principle of respect for persons thus divides into two separate moral requirements: the requirement to acknowledge autonomy and the requirement to protect those with diminished autonomy.

An autonomous person is an individual capable of deliberation about personal goals and of acting under the direction of such deliberation. To respect autonomy is to give weight to autonomous persons' considered opinions and choices while refraining from obstructing their actions unless they are clearly detrimental to others. To show lack of respect for an autonomous agent is to repudiate that person's considered judgments, to deny an individual the freedom to act on those considered judgments, or to withhold information necessary to make a considered judgment, when there are no compelling reasons to do so.

However, not every human being is capable of self-determination. The capacity for self-determination matures during an individual's life, and some individuals lose this capacity wholly or in part because of illness, mental disability, or circumstances that severely restrict liberty. Respect for the immature and the incapacitated may require protecting them as they mature or while they are incapacitated.

Some persons are in need of extensive protection, even to the point of excluding them from activities which may harm them; other persons require little protection beyond making sure they undertake activities freely and with awareness of possible adverse consequence. The extent of protection afforded should depend upon the risk of harm and the likelihood of benefit. The judgment that any individual lacks autonomy should be periodically reevaluated and will vary in different situations.

In most cases of research involving human subjects, respect for persons demands that subjects enter into the research voluntarily and with adequate information. In some situations, however, application of the principle is not obvious. The involvement of prisoners as subjects of research provides an instructive example. On the one hand, it would seem that the principle of respect for persons requires that prisoners not be deprived of the opportunity to volunteer for research. On the other hand, under prison conditions they may be subtly coerced or unduly influenced to engage in research activities for which they would not otherwise volunteer. Respect for persons would then dictate that prisoners be protected. Whether to allow prisoners to "volunteer" or to "protect" them presents a dilemma. Respecting persons, in most hard cases, is often a matter of balancing competing claims urged by the principle of respect itself.

2. Beneficence

Persons are treated in an ethical manner not only by respecting their decisions and protecting them from harm but also by making efforts to secure their well-being. Such treatment falls under the principle of beneficence. The term "beneficence" is often understood to cover acts of kindness or charity that go beyond strict obligation. In this document, beneficence is understood in a stronger sense, as an obligation. Two general rules have been formulated as complementary expressions of beneficent actions in this sense: **(1)** do not harm and **(2)** maximize possible benefits and minimize possible harms.

The Hippocratic maxim "do no harm" has long been a fundamental principle of medical ethics. Claude Bernard extended it to the realm of research, saying that one should not injure one person regardless of the benefits that might come to others. However, even avoiding harm requires learning what is harmful; and, in the process of obtaining this information, persons may be exposed to risk of harm. Further, the Hippocratic Oath requires physicians to benefit their patients "according to their best judgment." Learning what will in fact benefit may require exposing persons to risk. The problem posed by these imperatives is to decide when it is justifiable to seek certain benefits despite the risks involved, and when the benefits should be foregone because of the risks.

The obligations of beneficence affect both individual investigators and society at large, because they extend both to particular research projects and to the entire enterprise of research. In the case of particular projects, investigators and members of their institutions are obliged to give forethought to the maximization of benefits and the reduction of risk that might occur from the research investigation. In the case of scientific research in general, members of the larger society are obliged to recognize the longer term benefits and risks that may result from the improvement of knowledge and from the development of novel medical, psychotherapeutic, and social procedures.

The principle of beneficence often occupies a well-defined justifying role in many areas of research involving human subjects. An example is found in research involving children. Effective ways of treating childhood diseases and fostering healthy development are benefits that serve to justify research involving children – even when individual research subjects are not direct beneficiaries. Research also makes it possible to avoid the harm that may result from the application of previously accepted routine practices that on closer investigation turn out to be dangerous. But the role of the principle of beneficence is not always so unambiguous. A difficult ethical problem remains, for example, about research that presents more than minimal risk without immediate prospect of direct benefit to the children involved. Some have argued that such research is inadmissible, while others have pointed out that this limit would rule out much research promising great benefit to children in the future. Here again, as with all hard cases, the different claims covered by the principle of beneficence may come into conflict and force difficult choices.

3. Justice

Who ought to receive the benefits of research and bear its burdens? This is a question of justice, in the sense of "fairness in distribution" or "what is deserved." An injustice occurs when some benefit to which a person is entitled is denied without good reason or when some burden is imposed unduly. Another way of conceiving the principle of justice is that equals ought to be treated equally. However, this statement requires explication. Who is equal and who is unequal? What considerations justify departure from equal distribution? Almost all commentators allow that distinctions based on experience, age, deprivation, competence, merit and position do sometimes constitute criteria justifying differential treatment for certain purposes. It is necessary, then, to explain in what respects people should be treated equally. There are several widely accepted formulations of just ways to distribute burdens and benefits. Each formulation mentions some relevant property on the basis of which burdens and benefits should be distributed. These formulations are (1) to each person an equal share, (2) to each person according to individual need, (3) to each person according to individual effort, (4) to each person according to societal contribution, and (5) to each person according to merit.

Questions of justice have long been associated with social practices such as punishment, taxation and political representation. Until recently these questions have not generally been associated with scientific research. However, they are foreshadowed even in the earliest reflections on the ethics of research involving human subjects. For example, during the 19th and early 20th centuries the burdens of serving as research subjects fell largely upon poor ward patients, while the benefits of improved medical care flowed primarily to private patients. Subsequently, the exploitation of unwilling prisoners as research subjects in Nazi concentration camps was condemned as a particularly flagrant injustice. In this country, in the 1940's, the Tuskegee syphilis study used disadvantaged, rural black men to study the untreated course of a disease that is by no means confined to that population. These subjects were deprived of demonstrably effective treatment in order not to interrupt the project, long after such treatment became generally available.

Against this historical background, it can be seen how conceptions of justice are relevant to research involving human subjects. For example, the selection of research subjects needs to be scrutinized in order to determine whether some classes (e.g., welfare patients, particular racial and ethnic minorities, or persons confined to institutions) are being systematically selected simply because of their easy availability, their compromised position, or their manipulability, rather than for reasons directly related to the problem being studied. Finally, whenever research supported by public funds leads to the development of therapeutic devices and procedures, justice demands both that these not provide advantages only to those who can afford them and that such research should not unduly involve persons from groups unlikely to be among the beneficiaries of subsequent applications of the research.

Part C: Applications

C. Applications

Applications of the general principles to the conduct of research leads to consideration of the following requirements: informed consent, risk/benefit assessment, and the selection of subjects of research.

1. Informed Consent

Respect for persons requires that subjects, to the degree that they are capable, be given the opportunity to choose what shall or shall not happen to them. This opportunity is provided when adequate standards for informed consent are satisfied.

While the importance of informed consent is unquestioned, controversy prevails over the nature and possibility of an informed consent. Nonetheless, there is widespread agreement that the consent process can be analyzed as containing three elements: information, comprehension and voluntariness.

Information. Most codes of research establish specific items for disclosure intended to assure that subjects are given sufficient information. These items generally include: the research procedure, their purposes, risks and anticipated benefits, alternative procedures (where therapy is involved), and a statement offering the subject the opportunity to ask questions and to withdraw at any time from the research. Additional items have been proposed, including how subjects are selected, the person responsible for the research, etc.

However, a simple listing of items does not answer the question of what the standard should be for judging how much and what sort of information should be provided. One standard frequently invoked in medical practice, namely the information commonly provided by practitioners in the field or in the locale, is inadequate since research takes place precisely when a common understanding does not exist. Another standard, currently popular in malpractice law, requires the practitioner to reveal the information that reasonable persons would wish to know in order to make a decision regarding their care. This, too, seems insufficient since the research subject, being in essence a volunteer, may wish to know considerably more about risks gratuitously undertaken than do patients who deliver themselves into the hand of a clinician for needed care. It may be that a standard of "the reasonable volunteer" should be proposed: the extent and nature of information should be such that persons, knowing that the procedure is neither necessary for their care nor perhaps fully understood, can decide whether they wish to participate in the furthering of knowledge. Even when some direct benefit to them is anticipated, the subjects should understand clearly the range of risk and the voluntary nature of participation.

A special problem of consent arises where informing subjects of some pertinent aspect of the research is likely to impair the validity of the research. In many cases, it is sufficient to indicate to subjects that they are being invited to participate in research of which some features will not be revealed until the research is concluded. In all cases of research involving incomplete disclosure, such research is justified only if it is clear that (1) incomplete disclosure is truly necessary to accomplish the goals of the research, (2) there are no undisclosed risks to subjects that are more than minimal, and (3) there is an adequate plan for debriefing subjects, when appropriate, and for dissemination of research results to them. Information about risks should never be withheld for the purpose of eliciting the cooperation of subjects, and truthful answers should always be given to direct questions about the research. Care should be taken to distinguish cases in which disclosure would destroy or invalidate the research from cases in which disclosure would simply inconvenience the investigator.

Comprehension.   The manner and context in which information is conveyed is as important as the information itself. For example, presenting information in a disorganized and rapid fashion, allowing too little time for consideration or curtailing opportunities for questioning, all may adversely affect a subject's ability to make an informed choice.

Because the subject's ability to understand is a function of intelligence, rationality, maturity and language, it is necessary to adapt the presentation of the information to the subject's capacities. Investigators are responsible for ascertaining that the subject has comprehended the information. While there is always an obligation to ascertain that the information about risk to subjects is complete and adequately comprehended, when the risks are more serious, that obligation increases. On occasion, it may be suitable to give some oral or written tests of comprehension.

Special provision may need to be made when comprehension is severely limited – for example, by conditions of immaturity or mental disability. Each class of subjects that one might consider as incompetent (e.g., infants and young children, mentally disabled patients, the terminally ill and the comatose) should be considered on its own terms. Even for these persons, however, respect requires giving them the opportunity to choose to the extent they are able, whether or not to participate in research. The objections of these subjects to involvement should be honored, unless the research entails providing them a therapy unavailable elsewhere. Respect for persons also requires seeking the permission of other parties in order to protect the subjects from harm. Such persons are thus respected both by acknowledging their own wishes and by the use of third parties to protect them from harm.

The third parties chosen should be those who are most likely to understand the incompetent subject's situation and to act in that person's best interest. The person authorized to act on behalf of the subject should be given an opportunity to observe the research as it proceeds in order to be able to withdraw the subject from the research, if such action appears in the subject's best interest.

Voluntariness.   An agreement to participate in research constitutes a valid consent only if voluntarily given. This element of informed consent requires conditions free of coercion and undue influence. Coercion occurs when an overt threat of harm is intentionally presented by one person to another in order to obtain compliance. Undue influence, by contrast, occurs through an offer of an excessive, unwarranted, inappropriate or improper reward or other overture in order to obtain compliance. Also, inducements that would ordinarily be acceptable may become undue influences if the subject is especially vulnerable.

Unjustifiable pressures usually occur when persons in positions of authority or commanding influence – especially where possible sanctions are involved – urge a course of action for a subject. A continuum of such influencing factors exists, however, and it is impossible to state precisely where justifiable persuasion ends and undue influence begins. But undue influence would include actions such as manipulating a person's choice through the controlling influence of a close relative and threatening to withdraw health services to which an individual would otherwise be entitled.

2. Assessment of Risks and Benefits

The assessment of risks and benefits requires a careful arrayal of relevant data, including, in some cases, alternative ways of obtaining the benefits sought in the research. Thus, the assessment presents both an opportunity and a responsibility to gather systematic and comprehensive information about proposed research. For the investigator, it is a means to examine whether the proposed research is properly designed. For a review committee, it is a method for determining whether the risks that will be presented to subjects are justified. For prospective subjects, the assessment will assist the determination whether or not to participate.

The Nature and Scope of Risks and Benefits. The requirement that research be justified on the basis of a favorable risk/benefit assessment bears a close relation to the principle of beneficence, just as the moral requirement that informed consent be obtained is derived primarily from the principle of respect for persons. The term "risk" refers to a possibility that harm may occur. However, when expressions such as "small risk" or "high risk" are used, they usually refer (often ambiguously) both to the chance (probability) of experiencing a harm and the severity (magnitude) of the envisioned harm.

The term "benefit" is used in the research context to refer to something of positive value related to health or welfare. Unlike, "risk," "benefit" is not a term that expresses probabilities. Risk is properly contrasted to probability of benefits, and benefits are properly contrasted with harms rather than risks of harm. Accordingly, so-called risk/benefit assessments are concerned with the probabilities and magnitudes of possible harm and anticipated benefits. Many kinds of possible harms and benefits need to be taken into account. There are, for example, risks of psychological harm, physical harm, legal harm, social harm and economic harm and the corresponding benefits. While the most likely types of harms to research subjects are those of psychological or physical pain or injury, other possible kinds should not be overlooked.

Risks and benefits of research may affect the individual subjects, the families of the individual subjects, and society at large (or special groups of subjects in society). Previous codes and Federal regulations have required that risks to subjects be outweighed by the sum of both the anticipated benefit to the subject, if any, and the anticipated benefit to society in the form of knowledge to be gained from the research. In balancing these different elements, the risks and benefits affecting the immediate research subject will normally carry special weight. On the other hand, interests other than those of the subject may on some occasions be sufficient by themselves to justify the risks involved in the research, so long as the subjects' rights have been protected. Beneficence thus requires that we protect against risk of harm to subjects and also that we be concerned about the loss of the substantial benefits that might be gained from research.

The Systematic Assessment of Risks and Benefits. It is commonly said that benefits and risks must be "balanced" and shown to be "in a favorable ratio." The metaphorical character of these terms draws attention to the difficulty of making precise judgments. Only on rare occasions will quantitative techniques be available for the scrutiny of research protocols. However, the idea of systematic, nonarbitrary analysis of risks and benefits should be emulated insofar as possible. This ideal requires those making decisions about the justifiability of research to be thorough in the accumulation and assessment of information about all aspects of the research, and to consider alternatives systematically. This procedure renders the assessment of research more rigorous and precise, while making communication between review board members and investigators less subject to misinterpretation, misinformation and conflicting judgments. Thus, there should first be a determination of the validity of the presuppositions of the research; then the nature, probability and magnitude of risk should be distinguished with as much clarity as possible. The method of ascertaining risks should be explicit, especially where there is no alternative to the use of such vague categories as small or slight risk. It should also be determined whether an investigator's estimates of the probability of harm or benefits are reasonable, as judged by known facts or other available studies.

Finally, assessment of the justifiability of research should reflect at least the following considerations: (i) Brutal or inhumane treatment of human subjects is never morally justified. (ii) Risks should be reduced to those necessary to achieve the research objective. It should be determined whether it is in fact necessary to use human subjects at all. Risk can perhaps never be entirely eliminated, but it can often be reduced by careful attention to alternative procedures. (iii) When research involves significant risk of serious impairment, review committees should be extraordinarily insistent on the justification of the risk (looking usually to the likelihood of benefit to the subject – or, in some rare cases, to the manifest voluntariness of the participation). (iv) When vulnerable populations are involved in research, the appropriateness of involving them should itself be demonstrated. A number of variables go into such judgments, including the nature and degree of risk, the condition of the particular population involved, and the nature and level of the anticipated benefits. (v) Relevant risks and benefits must be thoroughly arrayed in documents and procedures used in the informed consent process.

3. Selection of Subjects

Just as the principle of respect for persons finds expression in the requirements for consent, and the principle of beneficence in risk/benefit assessment, the principle of justice gives rise to moral requirements that there be fair procedures and outcomes in the selection of research subjects.

Justice is relevant to the selection of subjects of research at two levels: the social and the individual. Individual justice in the selection of subjects would require that researchers exhibit fairness: thus, they should not offer potentially beneficial research only to some patients who are in their favor or select only "undesirable" persons for risky research. Social justice requires that distinction be drawn between classes of subjects that ought, and ought not, to participate in any particular kind of research, based on the ability of members of that class to bear burdens and on the appropriateness of placing further burdens on already burdened persons. Thus, it can be considered a matter of social justice that there is an order of preference in the selection of classes of subjects (e.g., adults before children) and that some classes of potential subjects (e.g., the institutionalized mentally infirm or prisoners) may be involved as research subjects, if at all, only on certain conditions.

Injustice may appear in the selection of subjects, even if individual subjects are selected fairly by investigators and treated fairly in the course of research. Thus injustice arises from social, racial, sexual and cultural biases institutionalized in society. Thus, even if individual researchers are treating their research subjects fairly, and even if IRBs are taking care to assure that subjects are selected fairly within a particular institution, unjust social patterns may nevertheless appear in the overall distribution of the burdens and benefits of research. Although individual institutions or investigators may not be able to resolve a problem that is pervasive in their social setting, they can consider distributive justice in selecting research subjects.

Some populations, especially institutionalized ones, are already burdened in many ways by their infirmities and environments. When research is proposed that involves risks and does not include a therapeutic component, other less burdened classes of persons should be called upon first to accept these risks of research, except where the research is directly related to the specific conditions of the class involved. Also, even though public funds for research may often flow in the same directions as public funds for health care, it seems unfair that populations dependent on public health care constitute a pool of preferred research subjects if more advantaged populations are likely to be the recipients of the benefits.

One special instance of injustice results from the involvement of vulnerable subjects. Certain groups, such as racial minorities, the economically disadvantaged, the very sick, and the institutionalized may continually be sought as research subjects, owing to their ready availability in settings where research is conducted. Given their dependent status and their frequently compromised capacity for free consent, they should be protected against the danger of being involved in research solely for administrative convenience, or because they are easy to manipulate as a result of their illness or socioeconomic condition.

Notes

(1) Since 1945, various codes for the proper and responsible conduct of human experimentation in medical research have been adopted by different organizations. The best known of these codes are the Nuremberg Code of 1947, the Helsinki Declaration of 1964 (revised in 1975), and the 1971 Guidelines (codified into Federal Regulations in 1974) issued by the U.S. Department of Health, Education, and Welfare. Codes for the conduct of social and behavioral research have also been adopted, the best known being that of the American Psychological Association, published in 1973.

(2) Although practice usually involves interventions designed solely to enhance the well-being of a particular individual, interventions are sometimes applied to one individual for the enhancement of the well-being of another (e.g., blood donation, skin grafts, organ transplants) or an intervention may have the dual purpose of enhancing the well-being of a particular individual, and, at the same time, providing some benefit to others (e.g., vaccination, which protects both the person who is vaccinated and society generally). The fact that some forms of practice have elements other than immediate benefit to the individual receiving an intervention, however, should not confuse the general distinction between research and practice. Even when a procedure applied in practice may benefit some other person, it remains an intervention designed to enhance the well-being of a particular individual or groups of individuals; thus, it is practice and need not be reviewed as research.

(3) Because the problems related to social experimentation may differ substantially from those of biomedical and behavioral research, the Commission specifically declines to make any policy determination regarding such research at this time. Rather, the Commission believes that the problem ought to be addressed by one of its successor bodies.

National Commission for the Protection of Human Subjects of Biomedical and Behavioral Research

Members of the Commission

Kenneth John Ryan, M.D., Chairman, Chief of Staff, Boston Hospital for Women.
Joseph V. Brady, Ph.D., Professor of Behavioral Biology, Johns Hopkins University.
Robert E. Cooke, M.D., President, Medical College of Pennsylvania.
Dorothy I. Height, President, National Council of Negro Women, Inc.
Albert R. Jonsen, Ph.D., Associate Professor of Bioethics, University of California at San Francisco.
Patricia King, J.D., Associate Professor of Law, Georgetown University Law Center.
Karen Lebacqz, Ph.D., Associate Professor of Christian Ethics, Pacific School of Religion.
*** *David W. Louisell, J.D., Professor of Law, University of California at Berkeley.*
Donald W. Seldin, M.D., Professor and Chairman, Department of Internal Medicine, University of Texas at Dallas.
*** *Eliot Stellar, Ph.D., Provost of the University and Professor of Physiological Psychology, University of Pennsylvania.*
*** *Robert H. Turtle, LL.B., Attorney, VomBaur, Coburn, Simmons & Turtle, Washington, D.C.*

*** *Deceased.*

False Hopes and Best Data: Consent to Research and the Therapeutic Misconception

Paul S. Appelbaum, Loren H. Roth, Charles W. Lidz,
Paul Benson, and William Winslade

Following a suicide attempt, a young man with a long history of tumultuous relationships and difficulty controlling his impulses is admitted to a psychiatric hospital. After a number of days, a psychiatrist approaches the patient, explaining that he is conducting a research project to determine if medications may help in the treatment of the patient's condition. Is the patient interested, the psychiatrist asks? The answer: "Yes, I'm willing to do anything that might help me."

The psychiatrist returns over the next several days to explain the project further. He tells the patient that two medications are being used, along with a placebo; medications and placebo are assigned randomly. The trial is double-blinded; that is, neither physician nor patient will know what the patient is receiving until after the trial has been completed. The patient listens to the explanation and reads and signs the consent form. Since the process of providing information and obtaining consent seems, on the surface, exemplary, there appears to be little reason to question the validity of the consent.

Yet when the patient is asked why he agreed to be in the study, he offers some disquieting information. The medication that he will receive, he believes, will be the one most likely to help him. He ruled out the possibility that he might receive a placebo because that would not be likely to do him much good. In short, this man, now both a patient and a subject, has interpreted, even distorted, the information he received to maintain the view – obviously based on his wishes – that every aspect of the research project to which he had consented was designed to benefit him directly. This belief, which is far from uncommon, we call the "therapeutic misconception." To maintain a therapeutic misconception is to deny the possibility that there may be major disadvantages to participating in clinical research that stem from the nature of the research process itself.

Research Risks and the Scientific Method

The unique aspects of clinical research include the goal of creating generalizable knowledge; the techniques of randomization; and the use of a study protocol, control groups, and double-blind procedures. Do these elements create a body of risks or disadvantages for research subjects? The answer lies in understanding how the scientific method is often incompatible with one of the first principles of clinical treatment – the value that the legal philosopher Charles Fried calls "personal care."[1]

The authors acknowledge the invaluable assistance of Paul Soloff, M.D., in the collection of the data described in this paper.

From the *Hastings Center Report*, 1987, 17, (April) pp. 20–24. © The Hastings Center.

According to the principle of personal care, a physician's first obligation is solely to the patient's well-being. A corollary is that the physician will take whatever measures are available to maximize the chances of a successful outcome. A failure to adhere to this principle creates at least a potential disadvantage for the clinical research subject: there is always a chance that the subject's interests may become secondary to other demands on the physician-researcher's loyalties.[2] And the methods of science inhibit the application of personal care.

Randomization, an important element of many clinical trials, demonstrates the problem. The argument is often made that comparisons of multiple treatment methods are legitimately undertaken only when the superiority of one over the other is unknown; thus the physician treating a patient in one of these trials does not abandon the patient's personal care, but merely allows chance to determine the assignment of treatments, each of which is likely to meet the patient's needs.[3]

But as Fried and others have noted, it is very unlikely that two treatments in a clinical trial will be identically desirable *for a particular patient*. The physician may have reason to suspect, for example, that a given treatment is more likely to be efficacious for a particular patient, even if overall evidence of greater efficacy is lacking. This suspicion may be based on the physician's previous experience with a subgroup of patients, the patient's own past treatment experience, the family history of responsiveness to treatment, or idiosyncratic elements in the patient's case. Subjects may have had previous unsatisfactory responses to one of the medications in a clinical trial, or may display clinical characteristics that suggest that one class of medications is more likely to benefit them than another.

Ordinarily, these factors would guide the therapeutic approach. But in a randomized study physicians cannot allow these factors to influence the treatment decision, and efforts to control for such factors in the selection of subjects, while theoretically possible, are cumbersome, expensive, and may bias the sample. Thus reliance on randomization represents an inevitable compromise of personal care in the service of attaining valid research results. There are at least two reports in the literature of physicians' reluctance to refer patients to randomized trials because of the possible decrement in the level of personal care.[4]

The use of a study protocol to regulate the course of treatment – essential to careful clinical research – also impedes the delivery of personal care. Protocols often indicate the pattern and dosages of medication to be administered or the blood levels to be attained. Even if they allow some individualization of medication, changes in time or magnitude may be limited. Thus patients who do not respond initially to a low dose of medication may not receive a higher dose, as they would if they were being treated without a protocol; on the other hand, patients experiencing side effects, which could be controlled by lowering their dosage, yet which are not so severe as to require withdrawal from the study, cannot receive the relief they would get in a therapeutic setting.

Analogously, adjunctive medications or forms of therapy, which may interfere with measurement of the primary treatment effect, are often prohibited. The exclusion of adjunctive medications, such as sleeping medications or decongestants, may increase a patient's discomfort. The requirement for a "wash-out" period, during which subjects are kept drug-free, may place previously stable patients at risk of relapse even before the experimental part of the project begins. And alternating placebo and active treatment periods may mean that a patient who responds well to a medication must be taken off that drug for the purposes of the study; conversely, patients who improve on placebo must be subject to the risks of active medication. In sum, the necessary rigidities of an experimental protocol often lead investigators to forgo individualized treatment decisions.

The need for control groups or placebos and double-blind procedures can produce similar effects. In the therapeutic setting patients will rarely receive medications that are deliberately designed to be pharmacologically ineffective; the ethics of those occasional situations when placebos are employed clinically are hotly disputed.[5] Yet, placebos are routinely employed in clinical investigations, without the intent of benefiting the individual subject.

Similarly, clinicians in a nonresearch setting will never allow themselves to remain ignorant of the treatment patients are receiving. Double-blind procedures, however, are necessary to ensure the integrity of a research study, even if they delay recognition of side effects or drug interactions, or have other adverse consequences.

Are these disadvantages so important that they should routinely be called to the attention of research subjects? That issue raises an empirical question: how prevalent is the therapeutic misconception?

Studies on Consent

Our findings suggest that research subjects systematically misinterpret the risk/benefit ratio of participating in research because they fail to understand the underlying scientific methodology.[6]

This conclusion is based on our observations of consent transactions in four research studies on the treatment of psychiatric illness, and our interviews with the subjects immediately after consent was obtained. The studies varied in the extent of the information they provided to subjects. Two of the studies compared the effects of two medications on a psychiatric disorder (one used, in addition, a placebo control group). A third study examined the relative efficacy of two dosage ranges of the same medication. And a fourth examined two different social interventions in chronic psychiatric illness, compared with a control group.

The populations in these studies ranged from actively psychotic schizophrenic patients to nonpsychotic, and in some cases, minimally symptomatic, borderline, and depressed patients. Our questions were based on information included on the consent form with regard to the understanding of randomized or chance assignment; and the use of control groups, formal protocols, and double-blind techniques. Eighty-eight patients comprised the final data pool, but since all of the issues addressed here were not relevant to each project the sample size varied for each question.

We found that fifty-five of eighty subjects (69 percent) had no comprehension of the actual basis for their random assignment to treatment groups, while only twenty-two of eighty (28 percent) had a complete understanding of the randomization process. Thirty-two subjects stated their explicit belief that assignment would be made on the basis of their therapeutic needs. Interestingly, many of these subjects constructed elaborate but entirely fictional means by which an assignment would be made that was in their best interests. This was particularly evident when information about group assignment was limited to the written consent forms and not covered in the oral disclosure; subjects filled vacuums of knowledge with assumptions that decisions would be made in their best interests.

Similar findings were evident concerning other aspects of scientific design. With regard to nontreatment control groups and placebos, fourteen of thirty-three (44 percent) subjects failed to recognize that some patients who desired treatment would not receive it. Concerning use of a double-blind, twenty-six of sixty-seven subjects (39 percent) did not understand that their physician would not know which medication they would receive; an additional sixteen of sixty-seven subjects (24 percent) had only partially understood this. Most striking of all, only six of sixty-eight subjects (9 percent) were able to recognize a single way in which joining a protocol would restrict the treatment they could receive. In the two drug studies in which adjustment of medication dosage was tightly restricted, twenty-two of forty-four subjects (50 percent) said explicitly that they thought their dosage would be adjusted according to their individual needs.

Two cases illustrate how these flaws in understanding affect the patient's ability to assess the benefits of the research. The first demonstrates the effect of a complete failure to recognize that scientific methodology has other than a therapeutic purpose. The second demonstrates a more subtle influence of a therapeutic orientation on a subject who understands the overall methodology but has certain blindspots.

In the first case, a twenty-five-year-old married woman with a high-school education was a subject in a randomized, double-blind study that compared the use of two medications and a placebo in the treatment of a nonpsychotic psychiatric disorder. When interviewed, she was unsure how it would be decided which medication she would receive, but thought that the placebo would be given only to those subjects who "might not need medication." The subject understood that a double-blind procedure would be used, but did not see that the protocol placed any constraints on her treatment. She said that she considered this project not an "experiment," a term that implied using drugs whose effects were unknown. Rather, she considered this to be "research," a process whereby doctors "were trying to find out more about you in depth." She decided to participate because, "I needed help and the doctor said that other people who had been in it had been helped," Her strong conviction that the project would benefit her carried through to the end of the study. Although the investigators rated her a nonresponder, she was convinced that she had improved on the medication. She attributed her improvement in large part to the double-blind procedures, which kept her in the dark as to which medication she was receiving, thereby preventing her from persuading herself that the medication was doing no good. She was quite pleased about having participated in the study.

In the same study, another subject was a twenty-five-year-old woman with three years of college. At the time of the interview, she had minimal psychiatric symptoms and her understanding of the research was generally excellent. She recognized that the purpose of the project was to find out which treatment worked best for her group of patients. She spontaneously described the three groups, including the placebo group, and indicated that assignment would be at random. She understood that dosages would be adjusted according to blood levels and that a double-blind would be used. When asked directly, however, how *her* medication would be selected, she said she had no idea. She then added, "I hope it isn't by chance," and suggested that each subject would probably receive the medication she needed. Given the discrepancy between her earlier use of the word "random" and her current explanation, she was then asked what her understanding was of "random." Her definition was entirely appropriate: "by lottery, by chance, one patient who comes in gets one thing and the next patient gets the next thing." She then began to wonder out loud if this procedure was being used in the current study. Ultimately, she concluded that it was not.

In this case, despite a cognitive understanding of randomization, and a momentary recognition that random assignment would be used, the subject's conviction that the investigators would be acting in her best interests led to a distortion of an important element of the experimental procedure and therefore of the risk/benefit analysis.

The comments of colleagues and reports by other researchers have persuaded us that this phenomenon extends to all clinical research. Bradford Gray, for example, found that a number of subjects in a project comparing two drugs for the induction of labor believed, incorrectly, that their needs would determine which drug they would receive.[7] A survey of patients in research projects at four Veterans Administration hospitals showed that 75 percent decided to participate because they expected the research to benefit their health.[8] Another survey of attitudes toward research in a combined sample of patients and the general public revealed the thinking behind this hope: when asked why people in general should participate in research, 69 percent cited benefit to society at large and only 5 percent cited benefit to the subjects; however, when asked why *they* might participate in a research project, 52 percent said they would do it to get the best medical care, while only 23 percent responded that they would want to contribute to scientific knowledge.[9] Back in the psychiatric setting, Lee Park and Lino Covi found that a substantial percentage of patients who were told they were being given a placebo would not believe that they received inactive medication,[10] and Vincenta Leigh reported that the most common fantasy on a psychiatric research ward was that the research was actually designed to benefit the subjects.[11]

Responding to the Problem

Should we do anything about the therapeutic misconception? It could be argued that as long as the research project has been peer-reviewed for scientific merit and approved for ethical acceptability by an institutional review board (IRB), the problem of the therapeutic misconception is not significant enough to warrant intervention. In this view, some minor distortion of the risk/benefit ratio has to be weighed against the costs of attempting to alter subjects' appreciation of the scientific methods. Such costs include time expended and the delay in completing research that will result when some subjects decide that they would rather not participate.

Whether we accept this view depends on the value that we place on the principle of autonomy that underlies the practice of informed consent. Autonomy can be overvalued when it limits necessary treatment, as it may, for example, in the controversy over the right to refuse psychotropic medications. There, we believe, patients' interests would best be served by giving claims to autonomy lesser weight.[12] But when we enter the research setting, limiting subjects' autonomy becomes a tool not for promoting their own interests, but for promoting the interests of others, including the researcher and society as a whole. We are not willing to accept such limitations for the benefit of others, particularly when, as described below, there may exist an effective mechanism for mitigating the problem.

Assuming that one agrees that distortions of the type we have described in subjects' reasoning are troublesome and worthy of correction, is such an effort likely to be effective? One might point to the data just presented to argue that little can be done to ameliorate the problem. The investigator in one of the projects we studied offered his subjects detailed and extensive information in a process that often extended over several days and included one session in which the entire project was reviewed. Despite this, half the subjects failed to grasp that treatment would be assigned on a random basis, four of twenty misunderstood how placebos would be used, five of twenty were not aware of the use of a double-blind, and eight of twenty believed that medications would be adjusted according to their individual needs. Is it not futile, then, to attempt to disabuse subjects of the belief that they will receive personal care?

Various theoretical explanations of our findings could support this view. Most people have been socialized to believe that physicians (at least ethical ones) always provide personal care.[13] It may therefore be very difficult, perhaps nearly impossible, to persuade subjects that *this* encounter is different, particularly if the researcher is also the treating physician, who has previously satisfied the subject's expectations of personal care. Further, insofar as much clinical research involves persons who are acutely ill and in some distress, the well-known tendency of patients to regress and entrust their well-being to an authority figure would undercut any effort to dispel the therapeutic misconception.

In response, more of our data must be explored. In each of the studies we observed, one cell of subjects was the target of an augmented informational process, which supplemented the investigator's disclosures to subjects with a "preconsent discussion." This discussion was led by a member of our research team who was trained to teach potential subjects about such things as the key methodologic aspects of the research project, especially methods that might conflict with the principle of personal care.

By introducing a neutral discloser, distinct from the patient's treatment team, we shifted the emphasis of the disclosure to focus on the ways in which research differs from treatment. Of the subjects who received this special education, eight of sixteen (50 percent) recognized that randomization would be used, as opposed to thirteen of the fifty-one (25 percent) remaining subjects; five of five (100 percent) understood how placebos would be employed in the single study that used them, compared with eleven of the fifteen (73 percent) remaining subjects; nine of sixteen (56 percent) comprehended the use of a double blind while only fifteen of fifty-one (31 percent) remaining subjects did so; and five of seventeen (29 percent) initially recognized other limits on their treatment as a result of constraints in the protocol compared with one of the fifty-one (2 percent) other subjects.

Our data suggest that many subjects can be taught that research *is* markedly different from ordinary treatment. Other efforts to educate subjects about the use of scientific methodology offer comparably encouraging results.[14] There is no reason to believe that subjects will refuse to hear clear-cut efforts to dispel the therapeutic misconception.

Novel approaches such as we employed may be one thing, of course, while routine procedures are something else. Perhaps our data derive from an unusually gifted group of patient-subjects. Will the complexity of explaining the principle of the scientific method defy understanding by most research subjects?

Undercutting the therapeutic misconception, thereby laying out some of the major disadvantages of any clinical research project, is probably much simpler than it seems. About the goals of research, subjects could be told: "Because this is a research project, we will be doing some things differently than we would if we were simply treating you for your condition. Not all the things we do are designed to tell us the best way to treat *you*, but they should help us to understand how people with your condition *in general* can best be treated." About randomization: "The treatment you receive of the three possibilities will be selected by chance, not because we believe that one or the other will be better for you." About placebos: "Some subjects will be selected at random to receive sugar pills that are not known to help the condition you have; this is so we can tell whether the medications that the other patients get are really effective, or if everyone with your condition would have gotten better anyway."

One can quibble about the wording of specific sections, and complexities can arise with particular projects, but the concepts underlying scientific methodology are in reality quite simple. And as long as subjects understand the key principles of how the study is being conducted, investigators can probably omit some of the detail that currently clogs consent forms and confuses subjects about the minor risks that accompany the experimental procedures, such as blood drawing. Overall, then, we may end up with a much simpler consent process when we focus on the issue of personal care.

Who should have the task of explaining the therapeutic misconception to subjects? Clearly, investigators should be encouraged to discuss such issues with subjects and to include them on consent forms, but several problems arise here. First, it is decidedly *not* in investigators' self-interest for them to disabuse potential subjects of the therapeutic misconception. Experienced investigators, as we have reported elsewhere,[15] view the recruitment of research subjects as an intricate and extended effort to win the potential subject's trust. One of our subjects in this study described the process in these words: "It was almost as if they were courting me. . . . everything was presented in the best possible light." One could argue that it is unrealistic to expect investigators to raise additional doubts about the benefits that subjects can expect; any effort in that regard will result in resistance by investigators, particularly those who have yet to internalize the justifications for informed consent in general.

Second, even investigators who recognize the desirability of subjects' making informed decisions may have great trouble conveying this particular information. When a researcher tells subjects that he or she is not selecting the treatment that will be given or that the medications being used may be on more effective than a placebo, the researcher is confessing uncertainty over the best approach to treatment, as well as the likely outcome. Harold Bursztajn and colleagues have argued that the essential uncertainty of all medical practice is precisely what physicians need to convey in *both* research and treatment settings.[16] Yet, as Jay Katz points out, physicians have been systematically socialized to underplay or ignore uncertainty in their discussions with patients.[17] In a recent report of physicians' reluctance to enter patients in a multicenter breast cancer study, 22 percent of the principal investigators cited as a major obstacle to enrolling subjects difficulty in telling patients that they did not know which treatment was best.[18]

Third, few researchers who are also clinicians feel comfortable acknowledging, even to themselves, that the course of treatment may not be optimally therapeutic for the patient. Thus, there appear such statements as the following, which recently was published in *The Lancet*: "A doctor who contributes to randomized treatment trials should not be thought of as a research worker, but simply as a clinician with an ethical duty to his patients not to go on giving them treatments without doing everything possible to assess their true worth."[19] The author concludes that since randomized trials are not really research, there is no need to obtain *any* informed consent from research subjects. Although this conclusion may be extreme, the example emphasizes the difficulties of getting investigators to admit to themselves, much less to their patient-subjects, the limits they have accepted on the delivery of personal care.

If there is concern with particular protocols, IRBs might consider supplementing the investigators' disclosure and the "courtship" process with a session in which the potential subject reviews risks and benefits with someone who is not a member of the research team. (John Robertson has proposed a similar approach, albeit out of other concerns.[20]) The neutral explainer would be responsible to the IRB and would be trained to emphasize those aspects of the research situation about which the IRB has the greatest concern. This approach might be especially appropriate when the investigator is also the subject's treating physician and the methodology used is likely to be interpreted as therapeutic in intent. The model we employed of using a trained educator (nurses are natural candidates for the job) worked well. It is certainly more manageable and less disruptive than the oftheard suggestions that patient advocates or consent monitors sit in on every interaction between subject and investigator.

There may be advantages to using a trained, neutral educator, apart from aiding subjects' decision-making. Subjects' perceptions of the research team as willing to "level with them," even to the point of explaining why it might not be in subjects' interests to participate in the study, may increase their trust and cooperation. On the other hand, failure to deal with the therapeutic misconception during the consent process could increase distrust of researchers and the health care system in general if subjects later come to feel they were "deceived," as a few did in the studies we observed. Enough experiences of this sort could further heighten public antipathy to medical research, particularly if they are publicized as some have been.[21] The scientific method is a powerful tool for advancing knowledge, but like most potent clinical procedures it has side effects that must be attended to, lest the benefits sought be overwhelmed by the disadvantages that accrue. With careful planning, the therapeutic misconception can be dispelled, leaving the subjects with a much clearer picture of the relative risks and benefits of participation in research.

References

1. Charles Fried, *Medical Experimentation: Personal Integrity and Social Policy* (New York: American Elsevier Publishing Co., 1974).
2. Arthur Schafer, "The Ethics of the Randomized Clinical Trial," *New England Journal of Medicine* 307 (Sept. 16, 1982), 719–24.
3. "Consent: How Informed?" *The Lancet* I (June 30, 1984), 1445–47.
4. Kathryn M. Taylor, Richard G. Margolese, and Colin L Soskolne, "Physicians' Reasons for Not Entering Eligible Patients in a Randomized Clinical Trial of Surgery for Breast Cancer," *New England Journal of Medicine* 310 (May 24, 1984), 1363–67; Mortimer J. Lacher, "Physicians and Patients as Obstacles to Randomized Trial," *Clinical Research* 26 (December 1978), 375–79.
5. Sissela Bok, "The Ethics of Giving Placebos," *Scientific American* 231:5 (May 1974), 17–23.
6. Paul S. Appelbaum, Loren H. Roth, and Charles W. Lidz, "The Therapeutic Misconception: Informed Consent in Psychiatric Research," *International Journal of Law and Psychiatry* 5 (1982), 319–29; Paul Benson, Loren H. Roth, and William J. Winslade, "Informed Consent in Psychiatric Research: Preliminary Findings from an Ongoing Investigation," *Social Science and Medicine* 20 (1985), 1331–41.
7. Bradford H. Gray, *Human Subjects in Medical Experimentation: A Sociological Study of the Conduct and Regulation of Clinical Research* (New York: John Wiley & Sons, 1975).
8. Henry W. Riecken and Ruth Ravich, "Informed Consent to Biomedical Research in Veterans Administration Hospitals," *Journal of the American Medical Association* 248 (July 16, 1982), 344–48.
9. Barrie R. Cassileth, Edward J. Lusk, David S. Miller, and Shelley Hurwitz, "Attitudes Toward Clinical Trials Among Patients and Public. "*Journal of the American Medical Association* 248 (August 27, 1982), 968–70.
10. Lee C. Park and Lino Covi, "Nonblind Placebo Trial: An Exploration of Neurotic Patients' Responses to Placebo When Its Inert Content is Disclosed," *Archives of General Psychiatry* 12 (April 1965), 336–45.
11. Vincenta Leigh, "Attitudes and Fantasy Themes of Patients on a Psychiatric Research Unit," *Archives of General Psychiatry* 32 (May 1975), 598–601.
12. Paul S. Appelbaum and Thomas G. Gutheil, "The Right to Refuse Treatment: The Real Issue is Quality of Care," *Bulletin of the American Academy of Psychiatry and the Law* 9 (1982), 199–202.

13. Cassileth et al., *op cit.*

14. Jan M. Howard, David DeMets, and the BHAT Research Group, "How Informed Is Informed Consent? The BHAT Experience," *Controlled Clinical Trials* 2 (1981), 287–303.

15. Paul S. Appelbaum and Loren H. Roth, "The Structure of Informed Consent in Psychiatric Research," *Behavioral Sciences and the Law* 1:3 (Autumn 1983), 9–19.

16. Harold Bursztajn, Richard I. Feinbloom, Robert M. Hamm, and Archie Brodsky. *Medical Choices, Medical Chances: How Patients, Families, and Physicians Can Cope with Uncertainty* (New York: Free Press, 1984).

17. Jay Katz, *The Silent World of Doctor and Patient* (New York: Free Press, 1984).

18. Taylor, et al., *op cit.*

19. Thurston B. Brewin, "Consent to Randomized Treatment," *The Lancet* II (Oct. 23, 1982). 919–21.

20. John A. Robertson, "Taking Consent Seriously: IRB Intervention in The Consent Process," *IRB: A Review of Human Subjects Research* 4:5 (September–October 1982), 1–5.

21. Dava Sobel, "Sleep Study Leaves Subject Feeling Angry and Confused," *New York Times* (July 15, 1980), p. C–1.

Declaration of Helsinki

Ethical Principles for Medical Research Involving Human Subjects

World Medical Association

Adopted by the 18th WMA General assembly Helsinki, Finland, June 1964 and amended by the
29th WMA General Assembly, Tokyo, Japan, October 1975
35th WMA General Assembly, Venice, Italy, October 1983
41st WMA General Assembly, Hong Kong, September 1989
48th WMA General Assembly, Somerset West, Republic of South Africa, October 1996
52nd WMA General Assembly, Edinburgh, Scotland, October 2000

A. Introduction

1. The World Medical Association has developed the Declaration of Helsinki as a statement of ethical principles to provide guidance to physicians and other participants in medical research involving human subjects. Medical research involving human subjects includes research on identifiable human material or identifiable data.

2. It is the duty of the physician to promote and safeguard the health of the people. The physician's knowledge and conscience are dedicated to the fulfillment of this duty.

3. The Declaration of Geneva of the World Medical Association binds the physician with the words, "The health of my patient will be my first consideration," and the International Code of Medical Ethics declares that, "A physician shall act only in the patient's interest when providing medical care which might have the effect of weakening the physical and mental condition of the patient."

4. Medical progress is based on research which ultimately must rest in part on experimentation involving human subjects.

5. In medical research on human subjects, considerations related to the well-being of the human subject should take precedence over the interests of science and society.

6. The primary purpose of medical research involving human subjects is to improve prophylactic, diagnostic and therapeutic procedures and the understanding of the aetiology and pathogenesis of disease. Even the best proven prophylactic, diagnostic, and therapeutic methods must continuously be challenged through research for their effectiveness, efficiency, accessibility and quality.

7. In current medical practice and in medical research, most prophylactic, diagnostic and therapeutic procedures involve risks and burdens.

8. Medical research is subject to ethical standards that promote respect for all human beings and protect their health and rights. Some research populations are vulnerable and need special protection. The particular needs of the economically and medically disadvantaged must be recognized. Special attention is also required for those who cannot give or refuse consent for themselves, for those who may be subject to giving consent under duress, for those who will not benefit personally from the research and for those for whom the research is combined with care.

9. Research Investigators should be aware of the ethical, legal and regulatory requirements for research on human subjects in their own countries as well as applicable international requirements. No national ethical, legal or regulatory requirement should be allowed to reduce or eliminate any of the protections for human subjects set forth in this Declaration.

B. Basic Principles for All Medical Research

10. It is the duty of the physician in medical research to protect the life, health, privacy, and dignity of the human subject.
11. Medical research involving human subjects must conform to generally accepted scientific principles, be based on a thorough knowledge of the scientific literature, other relevant sources of information, and on adequate laboratory and, where appropriate, animal experimentation.
12. Appropriate caution must be exercised in the conduct of research which may affect the environment, and the welfare of animals used for research must be respected.
13. The design and performance of each experimental procedure involving human subjects should be clearly formulated in an experimental protocol. This protocol should be submitted for consideration, comment, guidance, and where appropriate, approval to a specially appointed ethical review committee, which must be independent of the investigator, the sponsor or any other kind of undue influence. This independent committee should be in conformity with the laws and regulations of the country in which the research experiment is performed. The committee has the right to monitor ongoing trials. The researcher has the obligation to provide monitoring information to the committee, especially any serious adverse events. The researcher should also submit to the committee, for review, information regarding funding, sponsors, institutional affiliations, other potential conflicts of interest and incentives for subjects.
14. The research protocol should always contain a statement of the ethical considerations involved and should indicate that there is compliance with the principles enunciated in this Declaration.
15. Medical research involving human subjects should be conducted only by scientifically qualified persons and under the supervision of a clinically competent medical person. The responsibility for the human subject must always rest with a medically qualified person and never rest on the subject of the research, even though the subject has given consent.
16. Every medical research project involving human subjects should be preceded by careful assessment of predictable risks and burdens in comparison with foreseeable benefits to the subject or to others. This does not preclude the participation of healthy volunteers in medical research. The design of all studies should be publicly available.
17. Physicians should abstain from engaging in research projects involving human subjects unless they are confident that the risks involved have been adequately assessed and can be satisfactorily managed. Physicians should cease any investigation if the risks are found to outweigh the potential benefits or if there is conclusive proof of positive and beneficial results.
18. Medical research involving human subjects should only be conducted if the importance of the objective outweighs the inherent risks and burdens to the subject. This is especially important when the human subjects are healthy volunteers.

19. Medical research is only justified if there is a reasonable likelihood that the populations in which the research is carried out stand to benefit from the results of the research.
20. The subjects must be volunteers and informed participants in the research project.
21. The right of research subjects to safeguard their integrity must always be respected. Every precaution should be taken to respect the privacy of the subject, and the confidentiality of the patient's information as well as to minimize the impact of the study on the subject's physical and mental integrity and on the personality of the subject.
22. In any research on human beings, each potential subject must be adequately informed of the aims, methods, sources of funding, any possible conflicts of interest, institutional affiliations of the researcher, the anticipated benefits and potential risks of the study and the discomfort it may entail. The subject should be informed of the right to abstain from participation in the study or to withdraw consent to participate at any time without reprisal. After ensuring that the subject has understood the information, the physician should then obtain the subject's freely-given informed consent, preferably in writing. If the consent cannot be obtained in writing, the non-written consent must be formally documented and witnessed.
23. When obtaining informed consent for the research project the physician should be particularly cautious if the subject is in a dependent relationship with the physician or may consent under duress. In that case the informed consent should be obtained by a well-informed physician who is not engaged in the investigation and who is completely independent of this relationship.
24. For a research subject who is legally incompetent, physically or mentally incapable of giving consent or is a legally incompetent minor, the investigator must obtain informed consent from the legally authorized representative in accordance with applicable law. These groups should not be included in research unless the research is necessary to promote the health of the population represented and this research cannot instead be performed on legally competent persons.
25. When a subject deemed legally incompetent, such as a minor child, is able to give assent to decisions about participation in research, the investigator must obtain that assent in addition to the consent of the legally authorized representative.
26. Research on individuals from whom it is not possible to obtain consent, including proxy or advance consent, should be done only if the physical/mental condition that prevents obtaining informed consent is a necessary characteristic of the research population. The specific reasons for involving research subjects with a condition that renders them unable to give informed consent should be stated in the experimental protocol for consideration and approval of the review committee. The protocol should state that consent to remain in the research should be obtained as soon as possible from the individual or a legally authorized surrogate.
27. Both authors and publishers have ethical obligations. In publication of the results of research, the investigators are obliged to preserve the accuracy of the results. Negative as well as positive results should be published or otherwise publicly available. Sources of funding, institutional affiliations and any possible conflicts of interest should be declared in the publication. Reports of experimentation not in accordance with the principles laid down in this Declaration should not be accepted for publication.

C. Additional Principles for Medical Research Combined with Medical Care

28. The physician may combine medical research with medical care, only to the extent that the research is justified by its potential prophylactic, diagnostic or therapeutic value. When medical research is combined with medical care, additional standards apply to protect the patients who are research subjects.

29. The benefits, risks, burdens and effectiveness of a new method should be tested against those of the best current prophylactic, diagnostic, and therapeutic methods. This does not exclude the use of placebo, or no treatment, in studies where no proven prophylactic, diagnostic or therapeutic method exists.

30. At the conclusion of the study, every patient entered into the study should be assured of access to the best proven prophylactic, diagnostic and therapeutic methods identified by the study.

31. The physician should fully inform the patient which aspects of the care are related to the research. The refusal of a patient to participate in a study must never interfere with the patient–physician relationship.

32. In the treatment of a patient, where proven prophylactic, diagnostic and therapeutic methods do not exist or have been ineffective, the physician, with informed consent from the patient, must be free to use unproven or new prophylactic, diagnostic and therapeutic measures, if in the physician's judgement it offers hope of saving life, re-establishing health or alleviating suffering. Where possible, these measures should be made the object of research, designed to evaluate their safety and efficacy. In all cases, new information should be recorded and, where appropriate, published. The other relevant guidelines of this Declaration should be followed.

Questions for Discussion

1. Identify several groups of people who are often recruited for medical research but who may not be completely free to refuse to participate. What conditions might coerce them into taking part? What are the consequences of automatically excluding such groups from research?

2. Is the Nuremberg Code's statement on the individual's freedom to withdraw from a research project adequate protection from the risks of unanticipated events? How do the researcher's responsibilities to stop a study complement this safeguard?

3. What long-term protections are needed for the new class of professional human research participants who make their livelihood by taking part in human studies?

4. What are some of the difficulties inherent in relying on written consent documents to provide information on a research protocol? Who should obtain the subject's consent and how?

Recommended Supplemental Reading

Advisory Committee on Human Radiation Experiments. Research ethics and the medical profession: Report of the Advisory Committee on Human Radiation Experiments. *JAMA*. 1996;276:403–409.

Brody B. *The Ethics of Biomedical Research: An International Perspective*, New York: Oxford University Press; 1998.

Bulger RE, Bobby EM, Fineberg HV, eds. *Society's Choices: Social and Ethical Decisions in Biomedicine*. Washington, DC: National Academy Press; 1996.

Council for International Organization of Medical Sciences (CIOMS). International Ethical Guidelines for Biomedical Research Involving Human Subjects. CIOMS; 1993.

Dunn C M, Chadwick G. *Protecting Study Volunteers in Research. A Manual for Investigative Sites*. Rochester, NY: University of Rochester Medical Center; 1999.

FDA Guidance for Institutional Review Boards and Clinical Investigators. Available at: http://www.fda.gov/oc/oha/IRB.

Human Participant Protections Education for Research Teams Web site. Available at: http://cme.nci.nih.gov.

National Institutes of Health, Office of Protection from Research Risks. *Protecting Human Research Subjects*: *IRB Guidebook*. Washington, DC: U.S. Government Printing Office; 1993. Available at http://ohrp.osophs.dhha.gov/irb/irb_guidebook.htm.

National Ethics Advisory Committee Web site. Available at http://bioethics.gov.

Office for Human Research Protections. (http://ohrp.osphs.dhhs.gov/guidance).

Ethics in Epidemiologic Research

Ethical Issues in Epidemiologic Research

Elizabeth Heitman

Epidemiology is generally considered the bedrock of public health research and practice – a basic science essential to general biomedical knowledge. Nonetheless, the nature and scope of epidemiology are unfamiliar to many basic biomedical researchers outside the field of public health. The Council for International Organizations of Medical Sciences (CIOMS) defines epidemiology as "the study of the distribution and determinants of health-related states or events in specified populations, and the application of this study to control of health problems."[1] The term comes from an ancient Greek phrase meaning "upon the people," and epidemiologists' original focus was on understanding, addressing, and preventing epidemics. Epidemiology today involves the recognition, investigation, analysis, control, and prevention of health problems as they affect populations rather than individual patients.

Epidemiology is a multifaceted discipline, and its research is often complex. Epidemiologic investigation may focus on the identification of syndromes and specification of diagnostic criteria; the search for the causes and mediating factors of specific conditions; the determination of group and individual risk for disease; the historical study of a given health problem; and community assessment of the nature, distribution, and response to health problems across a population. Research in epidemiology depends on careful observation – both in the field and in clinical settings, the definition of specific conditions and the counting of clearly defined cases, and the demonstration of relationships between cases and the populations in which they occur.

Cross-sectional studies, case-control studies, and cohort studies became important forms of epidemiologic research in the first half of the twentieth century, with randomized controlled trials taking precedence in epidemiologic research at the end of the second half of the century. Community assessment is a prominent dimension of epidemiology today, whereas clinical epidemiology is also becoming increasingly important. In the past decade, genetic research has made molecular epidemiology a powerful means of identifying biological markers for disease.

Epidemiology relies on research with human subjects for most of its achievements. However, both the practice of epidemiologic research and the ethical issues it may raise often differ from the practice and ethics of interventional research. Epidemiologic research is largely observational, and the interventions common in epidemiologic research are typically limited to medical examination, laboratory testing, and the taking of medical and social histories. Both epidemiologists and ethicists maintain that epidemiologic research presents few of the risks of harm to subjects posed by more traditional biomedical research.[2,3]

Nonetheless, some of the most horrendous abuses of human subjects in research have been committed as part of epidemiologic studies. The most infamous epidemiologic research in the United States was the Tuskegee Syphilis Study, in which a group of 300 African American men in rural Alabama were unknowingly denied effective medical treatment over a 40-year period in order for U.S. Public Health Service researchers to observe the effects of their untreated disease.[4] The study was made public by an investigative reporter in 1972, decades after the availability of effective antibiotic treatment for syphilis and several years after the creation of federal requirements for informed consent and institutional ethical review of research protocols. The scandal that followed led to several additional formal safeguards for the protection of human subjects and 30 years of ethical reflection on the special demands of population-based research.

The Tuskegee syphilis trial illustrates several important ethical dimensions of epidemiologic research inherent in many population-based studies. The most widely recognized are, of course, the issues of informed consent, privacy, the prevention of harm, and the provision of benefit to research subjects. But beyond consent are ethical considerations implicit in the identification of any human experience as a health problem: the definition of illness presumes deviation from an accepted human norm shaped by moral and social values. Moreover, ethical values are evident in the definition of the variables by which health problems are assessed. In particular, the standard stratification of populations by race has been harshly criticized in recent years as being based more on social perception than scientific criteria.

The Ethics of Defining Disease and Its Variables

Whether as surveillance that identifies a health problem or as research that evaluates a course of action, epidemiology depends on a portrait of the human condition that includes a spectrum of normal and abnormal states and behaviors. Most societies understand illness in terms of a recognized norm of form and functionality. However, such norms and deviations from them may be defined differently over time and across cultures, and deviance may be understood not only in relation to health but also with respect to religious, social, political, moral, and even criminal considerations. By categorizing certain forms of deviance as issues of health or religion or morality, a society implicitly identifies their causes, advocates certain behaviors for affected individuals, and designates particular experts as having authority over the condition.

Over the past generation, a number of social scientists and ethicists have called attention to the "medicalization" of modern life in which both biological events and many expressions of human variation have been categorized as health-related problems that require expert medical intervention. The medicalization of some conditions, such as infectious diseases once thought to have supernatural or environmental causes, has relieved much physical suffering by leading to new interventions. Additionally, conceptualizing a problem as a medical one may reduce or eliminate the shame associated with some forms of deviance historically considered to be moral failings. The reclassification of alcoholism as a biological affliction rather than as a manifestation of moral weakness is one such example.

However, as H. Tristram Engelhardt points out, efforts to understand the medical connections between personal behaviors and physical signs of disease may also attribute medical ills to behaviors that society finds immoral, thus providing a seemingly scientific justification for condemning those behaviors.[5] The public response to the original epidemiologic connection between homosexual sexual contact and AIDS (initially called gay-related immune deficiency syndrome or GRIDS) illustrates how linking behaviors and disease may strengthen the stigma attached to certain "deviant" activities and those who engage in them.[6]

Epidemiologists and social scientists have also long recognized that the experience, expressions, and definitions of disease may vary markedly across cultures – even in industrialized nations that accept a common biomedical science.[7,8] But epidemiologists are only now coming to appreciate the variation in the rates of many diseases across subgroups of the population, and much is still unknown about the causes of this variability. Understanding the different experiences among populations and subgroups requires biological norms against which to define and measure health and illness. Identifying such norms raises ethical as well as scientific considerations.

Over the past two decades, women's health and minority health activists have criticized biomedical researchers for presuming that white males offered an adequate model of the full range of human health, disease, and response to treatment.[9,10] Epidemiologic observations that the incidence, manifestations, and response to treatment of many diseases vary with gender and ethnicity gave weight to activists' calls for greater representativeness in research – especially research on conditions that disproportionately affect women or minorities. In 1990 the National Institutes of Health (NIH) adopted new policy standards on the inclusion of women and minorities in biomedical research.[11] Still, efforts to include a wider spectrum of humanity in both clinical trials and epidemiologic studies pose the challenge of identifying meaningful similarities and differences among groups and classifying individuals once categories have been defined.

This challenge has been most difficult with regard to race. Health law scholar Patricia A. King has observed that both recognizing and ignoring racial differences in research and treatment may have dangerous consequences for the health of minority populations.[12] And, as Richard Cooper and Vincent L. Freeman note in their article included later in this section, while there is "tremendous variation in the rates of many chronic diseases across racial groups . . . serious technical and conceptual limitations hamper the ability of racial comparisons to illuminate the causative pathways."[13] The dilemma for epidemiologists lies in *how* to recognize the correlations between race and disease.

The study of such correlations has a tragic history. Many attempts to study differences among racial groups scientifically have been shaped by society's general views about the moral meaning of racial difference. From the beginning of the 1800s, proponents of "racial medicine" understood many diseases to have different effects on whites and nonwhites. Many ailments now associated with poverty were attributed to biological and moral flaws that medical researchers often contended were more common among persons of African heritage than among those of European descent. In the United States, the conclusions of racial medicine were also used to justify slavery on "scientific" grounds.[14] The Tuskegee syphilis trial was based on such assumptions about the different natural immunity and reactions to disease of blacks and whites and was intended to document these differences by comparison to available research data on untreated syphilis among Norwegian men.[15(p.106)]

Today, researchers investigating variations in health status among groups struggle to understand apparent differences without incorporating racist perspectives into their questions and methods. As part of this endeavor, the meaning of race as a variable has come into question as well. Critics contend that there is no adequate theoretical framework for the concept of race in health research and that the definition of racial categories is inconsistent and based on the scientifically unsound assumption that racial classification identifies key genetic differences among peoples.[16–18] Moreover, these critics note, the epidemiologic assignment of individuals to specific racial categories is arbitrary and related much more to social rather than biological characteristics.

Increasingly, epidemiologists are encouraged to interpret racial classification as a form of social organization more like ethnicity than biology. Thus, racial identification is important because it signals health-related behavioral and environmental considerations that interact with genetic and physical characteristics, not because it reveals essential biological information. Cooper and Freeman particularly stress this point with respect to the growing use of race as a variable in the study of genetic susceptibility to disease.[13] They insist that simple assumptions about racial links to genetic conditions must be replaced with rigorous criteria for the identification of genetic traits and improved understanding of gene–environment interaction. While such research is inevitably much more conceptually and technically demanding, its methodology will ultimately have greater integrity and its results will be more practically applicable to improving the health of all populations.

Epidemiologic Research, Institutional Review, and Informed Consent

Because of the ethical complexity of the conceptual issues involved in population-based studies and concern for the vulnerable populations that are often their focus, epidemiologic research demands careful consideration of the welfare of the individuals and groups under study. As with all human research, epidemiologic studies are governed by governmental standards for institutional review and informed consent and must be conducted with attention to the basic ethical principles of respect for persons, beneficence and nonmaleficence, and justice. However, the nature of informed consent for epidemiologic studies research and the scope of appropriate disclosure have been the subjects of ongoing ethical and regulatory debate. As Alexander M. Capron[2] observes in his essay in this section, epidemiologists may worry that institutional review and the growing demand for informed consent create undue obstacles for epidemiologic research, whereas ethicists and institutional review boards (IRBs) continue to insist that epidemiologic research can lead to harm and personal wrongs that necessitate the subjects' informed consent to participation.

Capron distinguishes between the risk of harms that epidemiologic research may pose for subjects and the moral wrongs that research may impose without causing direct harm.[2] Harms might include the loss of employment or social ostracism that can result from a researcher's public disclosure of sensitive personal information, whereas a researcher's review of a patient's personal medical information without his or her consent would be the moral wrong of invasion of privacy. Informed consent is essential to epidemiologic research as a means of preventing or minimizing both the inadvertent harms and wrongs that a study may foster.

IRB review ensures that the protocol does not subject the study population to any undue risk of harm and that researchers will minimize and disclose any potential actions or effects that the study population might interpret as wrongs. It is the epidemiologist's responsibility to communicate appropriate information about the research to the study population and to justify to the IRB any plan *not* to provide certain disclosures or obtain informed consent. The practical issue of how to get consent for some epidemiologic research often affects whether and what degree of disclosure and consent is necessary.

Much epidemiologic research uses health-related data or specimens that individuals have given to others in the course of diagnosis and treatment, such as the retrospective review of medical charts or the unrelated testing of blood samples collected for diagnostic purposes. Here the original collector of the data or tissue has a responsibility to disclose in advance that the material may be sought by epidemiologic researchers and to seek the subject's written consent to its use. To the greatest extent possible, members of groups that are likely to be included in epidemiologic research involving personal identifiers should be told about the project and that their information may be included in it as well as how their individual confidentiality will be protected. This disclosure should include information about which governmental or private agencies may have access to personal information gathered during the study, such as health departments, insurers, or pharmaceutical company study monitors, and how they may use the information.

Maintaining confidentiality of research data is of paramount importance in epidemiologic research, for breaches of confidentiality may cause direct harm as well as perceived moral wrongs to subjects. Many individuals are unaware of the scope of publicly maintained archives of personal health information, such as birth or death records or databases established by law as part of ongoing public health surveillance. Some governmental databases – such as state and local registries of tuberculosis, HIV/AIDS, and sexually transmitted diseases – may appear particularly intrusive, yet the collection of this information and epidemiologic research using it do not require individual informed consent.

To minimize the potential for invasion of privacy and breach of confidentiality, researchers using data collected by others should explicitly plan how they will protect privacy and confidentiality as part of any study and avoid using personal identifiers that may link individuals to their health information. Because individual disclosure is typically impossible, at times this may mean announcing the study and its safeguards publicly to the community in which the research is conducted and seeking both IRB approval and that of representatives or leaders of the community in which the data are gathered.

Reporting the results of epidemiologic research is often recognized as one of the most important benefits that researchers can offer study participants. As described in the CIOMS Guidelines for Ethical Review of Epidemiological Studies recommended for supplemental reading, "protocols should include provision for communicating such information to communities and individuals" as well as to health authorities.[1] Studies that maintain personal identifiers carry an additional responsibility to individual study participants to communicate research findings – good and bad – to them in ways that will maximize the potential benefit that the information can offer. Although studies that do not link epidemiologic data to individual participants may protect subjects from breaches of confidentiality, they also preclude researchers from providing useful health-related findings directly to those who might benefit from them. In such cases, communication of findings to relevant communities is especially important.

Communication of study results must be undertaken carefully to avoid any negative impact. The potential for harm in disclosing research findings lies not only in individuals' response to bad news in general but also in the stigma that some research findings may impose on individuals or a particular group (i.e., persons with HIV, individuals, and families with a stigmatizing genetic predisposition). When findings reveal that subjects need medical attention, including even follow-up observation, researchers should have a plan for referring them to treatment. Ideally, researchers should provide participants with relevant health care or appropriate referral throughout the course of the study. If the study population has little or no access to treatment, it may create an additional burden for researchers to identify a health problem for which effective treatment is not available. Moreover, the community may be harmed if the study creates new needs that the community cannot meet, if harmful publicity leads to economic loss, or if the social fabric of the community is disrupted by the study or its results.

Even before the advent of the Human Genome Project, questions about the benefits, harms, and role of informed consent in epidemiologic research in genetics received considerable attention from ethicists and IRBs. For much of the past decade, as the scope of genetic research has exploded, the meaning of genetic information has remained uncertain. One central ethical question involves how to distinguish between the potential harms and benefits of genetic knowledge for the individual: Does knowledge about one's genetic predispositions confer the power to prevent suffering or impose a sense of inevitable doom? Identifying the link between a genetic mutation and disease is not enough to predict who will and will not develop the associated condition, and informed consent for molecular epidemiologic studies must highlight this uncertainty for participants.

High standards of confidentiality for genetic information are widely accepted as the norm, especially in genetic disease registries, which typically require patients' consent before their names are added or identifying information is disclosed.[19] Because genetic information may be used in a discriminatory manner, particularly in the context of employment and insurance and when the predictive value of test results is unclear, health law and policy specialists have proposed legislative restrictions on employers' and insurers' access to medical records containing genetic information and prohibitions against the discriminatory use of available genetic information.[19] However, others insist that most genetic information is really no different than other medical information and that attempts to maintain a higher than normal level of confidentiality for genetic information will only make genetic discrimination more likely.

The demand for epidemiologic research in genetics also raises new procedural ethical questions related to databases and tissue banks. Hospitals across the United States preserve many kinds of tissue samples, and patients typically give blanket consent to research using "extra" blood and tissue originally obtained in the process of diagnosis and treatment. As one of this section's cases portrays, research on the prevalence of specific mutations can be accelerated by the use of banked tissue samples from the general hospital population as well as from specific patient groups. However, whether and how meaningful consent can be obtained for unspecified genetic research on banked tissue is the subject of debate.

The proposed practice of seeking blanket consent for future research with banked genetic material clearly places more responsibility on IRBs to safeguard the welfare of patients who will not be contacted for specific consent to individual projects using their tissue. However, while concern for confidentiality may suggest a need to bank samples without personal identifiers, the potential benefit of providing genetic information to tissue donors suggests that coded identifiers be retained so that researchers may attempt to contact individuals affected by the findings of as-yet-undefined genetic research. Whether individuals contacted are likely to remember or understand the ramifications of their original blanket consent and how they will respond to findings of research in which they took part unknowingly are also subjects for future research.

Ethical Controversies over International Research

During much the same period in which genetic research gained prominence, epidemiologic research also became increasingly international, particularly as a result of efforts to track and control the international spread of HIV. The CIOMS guidelines on epidemiologic studies were intended specifically to address the emerging ethical conflicts raised by international epidemiologic research. The guidelines maintain that, while provisions of ethical review in any society are "influenced by economic and political considerations, the organization of health care and research, and the degree of independence of investigators," all epidemiologic research should take into account the provisions of the Declaration of Helsinki[20] and the CIOMS International Guidelines for Biomedical Research Involving Human Subjects.[21] The CIOMS guidelines established a benchmark for international research ethics by asserting that researchers' ethical standards in developing countries should be "no less exacting" than would be expected if the research were in their own or their sponsors' countries; included in these standards are requirements for informed consent and the provision of no less than the standard of care in all research.

CIOMS' ground rules led to serious controversy, particularly in HIV research in Africa and Southeast Asia, and debate soon spread to the United States and Europe. HIV researchers grew frustrated with the paradoxical requirement for informed consent for populations that neither believed in personal autonomy nor had any real option for medical treatment outside of international research protocols. By the middle of the decade, both biomedical researchers and ethicists were calling for careful and extensive global discussion of how researchers should address international differences in standards of care and the limited applicability of informed consent in developing countries.

The World Medical Association and CIOMS had begun to revise the Declaration of Helsinki and the guidelines on biomedical research when, in 1997, the *New England Journal of Medicine* published a report denouncing several placebo-controlled studies on the perinatal transmission of HIV in developing countries, which its authors found highly unethical.[22] While the original researchers and the studies' sponsors maintained that control groups' inclusion in a purely observational arm of the prevention trials with AZT represented an improvement over the community's standard of care, *New England Journal* editor Marcia Angell drew parallels between this justification for denying known effective treatment to control groups and the arguments used to support nontreatment in the Tuskegee syphilis study.[23] The heads of NIH and the Centers for Disease Control and Prevention in turn maintained that the studies met accepted ethical principles and guidelines,[24] but debate continued over placebo-controlled trials – particularly regarding their use in communities and nations in which the notion of informed consent was largely incomprehensible.

The World Medical Association adopted revisions during the General Assembly in October 2000 that call for every patient-subject to receive "proven effective prophylactic, diagnostic, and therapeutic methods" instead of "the best proven ... methods"[21] in recognition of the variable quality of available treatment worldwide. The new draft also includes a provision for the use of placebos when no proven diagnostic or therapeutic method exists. Revision of the CIOMS guidelines is ongoing, although the process has been significantly more closed than that of the Declaration of Helsinki. Advocates for a single ethical standard for biomedical research worldwide contend that the information that has been made available suggests that CIOMS will weaken current ethical protections for populations in developing countries.[25]

Conclusions

Epidemiologic research provides invaluable knowledge about the diagnosis, prevention, and control of many human health problems. Epidemiology's research methods typically pose less risk of immediate harm to individuals than do other forms of biomedical research.

Nonetheless, epidemiologic studies are subject to the requirements for ethical review and informed consent in light of the power of epidemiologic data to categorize diseases and people in significant ways. Epidemiology's population-based perspective on health and illness creates additional needs for the protection of individuals through ethical safeguards on the use of medical data, and biological samples collected by researchers and governmental agencies so serve the public's health. As the growth and integration of the biomedical sciences draw increasingly upon epidemiology to identify and portray new conditions, the need to understand the commonalities and distinctions between epidemiologic research and other types of human studies will almost certainly expand the ethical discourse in this field.

References

1. Council for International Organizations of Medical Sciences. International guidelines for ethical review of epidemiological studies. *Law, Medicine and Health Care.* 1991;19:247–258.
2. Capron AM. Protection of research subjects: Do special rules apply in epidemiology? *J Clin Epidemiol.* 1991:44(suppl 1):81S–89S.
3. Coughlin SS. Ethically optimized study designs in epidemiology. In: Coughlin SS, ed. *Ethics in Epidemiology and Public Health Practice. Collected Works.* Columbus, Ga: Quill Publications; 1997:87–102.
4. Tuskegee Syphilis Study Ad Hoc Advisory Panel. *Final Report.* Washington, DC: U.S. Public Health Service; 1973.
5. Engelhardt HT Jr. The disease of masturbation, values and the concept of disease. *Bull Hist Med.* 1974;48:234–248.
6. Sontag S. *AIDS and Its Metaphors.* New York: Farrar, Straus, & Giroux; 1989.
7. Mechanic D. Social psychological factors affecting the presentation of bodily complaints. *N Engl J Med.* 1972;286:1132–1139.
8. Payer L. *Medicine and Culture: Varieties of Treatment in the United States, England, West Germany, and France.* New York, NY: Penguin; 1988.
9. Dresser R. Wanted: Single, white male for medical research. *Hastings Center Report.* 1992; 22:24–29.
10. Mastroianni AC, Faden R, Federman D, eds. Committee on the Ethical and Legal Issues Relating to the Inclusion of Women in Clinical Studies. *Women and Health Research: Ethical and Legal Issues of Including Women in Clinical Studies.* Vols. 1 & 2. Washington, DC: National Academy Press; 1994.
11. National Institutes of Health and Alcohol, Drug Abuse, and Mental Health Administration. *Special Instruction to Applicants Using Form PHS 398 Regarding Implementation of the NIH/ADAMHA Policy Concerning Inclusion of Women and Minorities in Clinical Research Study Populations.* Washington, DC: NIH; 1990.
12. King PA. The dangers of difference. *Hastings Center Report.* 1992;22(Nov-Dec):35–38.
13. Cooper RS, Freeman VL. Limitations in the use of race in the study of disease causation. *J Natl Med Assoc.* 1999;91:379–383.
14. Jones J. Race and medicine. In: Reich WT, ed. *Encyclopedia of Bioethics.* Vol 4. New York, NY: The Free Press; 1978:1405–1410.
15. Jones J. *Bad Blood: The Tuskegee Syphilis Experiment.* New York, NY: The Free Press; 1993.
16. Cooper R, David R. The biological concept of race and its application to public health and epidemiology. *J Health Polit Policy Law.* 1986;11:97–116.
17. Sheldon TA, Parker H. Race and ethnicity in health research. *J Public Health Med.* 14;2:104–110.
18. Hahn RA, Stroup DF. Race and ethnicity in public health surveillance: Criteria for the scientific use of social categories. *Public Health Rep.* 1994;109:7–15.

19. Institute of Medicine. *Assessing Genetic Risks: Implications for Health and Social Policy.* Washington, DC: National Academy Press; 1994.

20. World Medical Association. *Declaration of Helsinki:Recommendations Guiding Medical Doctors in Biomedical Research Involving Human Subjects.* Geneva: WMA; 1964;1975;1983; 1989;1996;2000.

21. World Health Organization. *International Ethical Guidelines for Biomedical Research Involving Human Subjects.* Geneva: Council for International Organizations of Medical Science; 1993.

22. Lurie P, Wolfe SM. Unethical trials of interventions to reduce perinatal transmission of the human immunodeficiency virus in developing countries. *N Engl J Med.* 1997;337:853–856.

23. Angell M. The ethics of clinical research in the third world. *N Engl J Med.* 1997;337:847–849.

24. Varmus H, Satcher D. Ethical complexities of conducting research in developing countries. *N Engl J Med.* 1997;337:1003–1005.

25. Lurie P, Wolfe SM. Scientists seek to justify and continue unethical research by gutting international ethical guidelines. *Public Citizen* press release, 1999 (Aug11). Available at http://www.citizen.org/hrg/publications/1493.htm.

Protection of Research Subjects

Do Special Rules Apply in Epidemiology?

A. M. Capron

Introduction

Imagine, if you will, a place where health, hospitalization, education, military, employment, law enforcement, housing, tax and financial records, as well as disease registries and the data sources for the census, vital statistics, and all aspects of people's private activities, are meticulously kept, fully linked together, and easily accessible to qualified researchers. What is that place? Epidemiologists' heaven.

Of course, formidable problems face epidemiologists trying to reach heaven. The data sources on many aspects of our lives are incomplete and the means of linking them are typically non-existent or partial at best. But even if the data all existed, there would be a further "catch": epidemiologists would probably find themselves facing great obstacles in gaining access to the data.

Epidemiologists sometimes think of "ethics" as the source of those obstacles, which are believed to be embodied in the federal rules for the protection of research subjects – colloquially called 45 *CFR* Part 46 – especially as they are interpreted by some institutional review boards (IRBs). It has even been suggested by Dr Rothman that review procedures and consent requirements could render epidemiology impossible [1]. This seems a strange result, not the least because many of the concerns that justify prior scrutiny of research protocols by IRBs are simply absent for most epidemiological research. Thus, not surprisingly, epidemiologists cry foul when they find – as two Harvard investigators did a few years ago – their research being burdened by the requirement that they obtain written informed consent from subjects who would merely be asked to answer a few questions in an interview [2–4]. I suspect that a major cause for confusion – despite provisions in the federal regulations intended to avoid (or the very least, to speed up) inappropriate or unnecessary reviews – is that most IRBs, being used to reviewing clinical research, may impose expectations that are poorly suited to epidemiological research.

Yet before we dismiss ethics as nothing more than a cause of confusion and needless worry, I think we need to take a careful look at epidemiologists' ethical obligations to research subjects. In doing so, we should pay particular attention to three points: first, the difference between harming someone and wronging them; second, the role of informed consent in protecting against such wrongs; and third, the steps that can be taken to avoid or minimize particular harms associated with breaches of privacy and confidentiality.

The Ethical Tension

The aspect of epidemiology addressed in this essay is that involving research on the association of a population's health status with particular genetic and environmental factors, rather than studies involving prospective, manipulative interventions, such as clinical trials of drugs or devices, on the one hand, or officially authorized or mandated surveillance for public health purposes, on the other hand. Yet an adequate description of epidemiological research must locate it within moral – not merely factual – terrain because it rests on competing ethical orientations about research involving human beings, roughly involving the competition between deontology and utilitarianism.

A good exposition of a conservative deontological tradition can be found in the writings of philosopher Hans Jonas [5]. He argues that research is usually warranted only when those who are exposed to risk have knowingly agreed to bear that risk; otherwise, the prospect of improving the social condition does not justify imposing a sacrifice on anyone. In his words, "progress is an optional goal, not an unconditional commitment" [5, p. 255]. Since such sacrifices fall outside the social contract, only activities necessary for the continued existence of society can command something from us beyond what we choose to give.

Such a deontological view would strictly limit researchers, including epidemiologists. At the opposite pole is the position that investigators have not merely a duty but also a right to advance human knowledge [6–8]. Rather than either extreme, I think society accepts the more modest notion that scientists have an obligation which extends beyond non-maleficence (not harming others) to beneficience (the positive duty to remove existing harms and produce social benefits when that is within their powers).

The prospect of providing much needed benefits exists for epidemiology today as never before. Beyond its past role in studying the incidence of infectious disease – a role that remains vital in the area of AIDS – the field has much to contribute to our understanding of environmental and occupational risks, of the relative effectiveness of health care interventions, and of the role genetics plays in both human illness and human capabilities [9]. Therefore, while never doubting that the present discussion turns on a conflict of values, I would submit that this conflict does not admit of absolute resolution. That is, we will be required to weigh the value of knowledge (both for its own sake and as a means for improving life) against many other values, prime among them autonomy, beneficience and justice.

The Difference Between Harms and Wrongs

Traditional Concerns in Biomedical Research

At the heart of the protection of research subjects – through the federal regulations and the institutional review process – is concern for the physical well-being of the human beings who become involved in research projects. While everyday biomedical research, conducted by responsible investigators in approved projects, seems to be at least as safe as medical care itself, the history of research has been marked by some horrific examples of harm to subjects. (In this discussion, I am referring to what is often termed "harms to interests" rather than "moral harm," which "is inflicted on someone when some course of action produces in that person a greater propensity to commit wrongs" [10, p. 178]). Most of these harms have involved injury to, or even loss of, health and life. Beyond physical harm have been instances of psychological harm, especially among subjects who were deceived about the purpose of a study or the nature of their participation in it. Finally, in some instances, the requirements of research design – such as the use of a control group that receives a placebo – involve a reverse risk to subjects, viz. that they will find themselves in the less beneficial arm of the protocol. Hence the need for protection, both through IRB approval of the benefit/harm ratio and through the requirement of informed consent from research subjects.

Risks Created by Epidemiological Research

Epidemiologic research can also involve the risk of harm, but it is typically of a different sort. Since, in most cases, investigators do not intervene physically with the subject and may not even have direct contact of any sort, physical and psychological injuries are unlikely. Yet other sorts of harm may occur. First, if data dealing with sensitive matters – either raw data or final results – can be linked to subjects, they may suffer social harm, such as ostracism or loss of employment. Second, even when individuals cannot be linked to information that is embarrassing (or worse), findings that paint an adverse picture of an entire population may eventuate in harm to that group, either directly or as a result of the adoption of laws or policies that have a negative impact on the welfare of group members.

Despite these risks, the harms entailed in epidemiological research seem less grave, seldom touching on matters of physical or even emotional well-being; moreover, their avoidance either seems simpler (e.g. merely taking care to disguise any facts that could be linked to a particular subject) or may, in fact, seem inappropriate where group harms are involved, since a group can hardly claim any right to a preferential social policy rather than one based on an accurate understanding of the true facts.

Wrongs Beyond Harms

The argued unfairness of binding epidemiology to the same Procrustean bed as biomedical research rests largely on this perception of different, and markedly less significant, risks. This argument is fine as far as it goes, but it fails to note another, less tangible but no less significant, concern: people may have been wronged even when they have not suffered harm. Some things are both harms and wrongs, while others amount to harming another's interest (as, for example, when one seller takes business away from another) without committing a wrong (as when no duty exists to avoid the harm) [10, p. 177]. My concern in this essay is with situations in which the consequence of an epidemiological study might be characterized as a wrong even though subjects' interests (material as well as physical) have not been harmed.

Consider the following example: suppose that I enter your house (through an unlocked back door) while you were away. Suppose that I not only leave everything undisturbed but also that I do not even know your identity. Have you suffered a harm? Not in the usual sense – as you would if I took something from the house or if you come home while I was still there and I surprised or, even worse, injured you. But I have wronged you. And that wrong is not overcome if I happen to be a scientist studying dustballs in their native habitat (viz. under sofas) rather than a mere Nosey Parker. The wrong is the invasion of your privacy without your consent, what is known in the law as trespass.

Wrongs of this type may clearly be implicated in epidemiological research. If I have allowed information to be gathered about me – e.g. by my personal physician, in the course of being evaluated and treated by the physician – and a researcher goes through that information, a wrong has been done even if I do not know about the intrusion. Information about me is an aspect of myself, just as is a physical space that I occupy, and someone looking through it has intruded on me as surely as if he or she had entered my home. The gravity of the wrong *will* depend on several factors. How personal is the information – data on one's sex life is not the same as height and weight – and to what extent would a person have a reasonable expectation that the information would not be known to people beyond those rendering care?

Wrongs may occur in other ways besides trespasses. Treating people solely as means to an end not chosen by them wrongs them even when it does not harm them. It is a wrong because it treats them as an instrument not as a person [11]. For an epidemiologist to commit a wrong against a person would thus violate two ethical principles: respect for autonomy (i.e. respecting persons and allowing them to make choices about their lives rather than having choices imposed upon them) and non-maleficience (i.e. the duty to avoid injuring a person). Accordingly, the risk that epidemiological studies could wrong people explains why one ought not simply to dismiss ethical guidelines as irrelevant, even if one believes that the risk of direct harm to subjects is negligible.

The Basic Role of Informed Consent

Consent as a Means of Minimizing Harm

How, then, have the law and ethics dealt with the risk of subjects being harmed? Primarily through two requirements: first, research must undergo review by a properly constituted body – usually called an IRB – which is supposed to foreclose studies that entail an unfavourable benefit-risk ratio, that are unfair in the distribution of risk in the population, or that do not provide for an adequate consent process.

The second means of protecting against harm is through requiring that investigators obtain the informed and voluntary consent of subjects before studying them. Since everyone has his or her own particular sense of what constitutes harm, the agreement of each subject to participate in a study – based upon disclosure of all information material to an informed choice – is necessary if the harm caused by the study is to be minimized. Simply put, if I tried to decide for you whether participation was acceptable and my sense of what constitutes a harm and how grave it is differs markedly from yours, the presumed maximization of benefit-to-risk from the research could be very erroneous.

The same principle applies to studies that involve potential wrongs to subjects rather than harms; indeed, a wrong is entailed in a study that would make use of some aspect of a person without consent. The question then is whether the potential of wronging subjects erects an absolute barrier to a study, or whether there are circumstances when research may proceed without subjects' consent nonetheless, perhaps because of other benefits expected to be derived from the research.

Several Additional Functions of Informed Consent

To answer this question requires a closer – albeit still brief – look at the functions that informed consent serves in research. Four stand out: promoting autonomy and self-determination, improving research, regularizing relationships between investigators and subjects, and protecting privacy [12]. If these purposes can be met without individual subjects giving informed consent, then the omission of consent may be more ethically acceptable.

Promoting Autonomy and Self-Determination

In the brief sketch of informed consent offered above, I viewed consent primarily in pragmatic terms: that respect for self-determination is necessary in order that the harm generated by research be minimized, since potential subjects are the best judges of the gravity of any prospective harm. The first purpose I want to argue for now expands on that, viz. that the requirement of informed consent manifests the human desire "to be conscious of [oneself] as a thinking, willing, active being, responsible for his choices and able to explain them by reference to his own ideas and purposes," as Sir Isaiah Berlin put in [13]. In other words, the requirement of informed consent protects the human status of research subjects by reminding everyone involved in a research project of the Kantian imperative against using human beings merely as means. A subject who has truly consented to participate has thereby become a collaborator with the investigators by effectively adopting the study's ends as his or her own.

Of course, to reach this goal, informed consent must be a reality, embodying both the autonomous authorization described by Faden and Beauchamp [14] (viz. a competent subject who substantially understands the circumstances and who, in the absence of significant control by others, authorizes the researcher to proceed) and the dialogic process between investigator and subject urged by Jay Katz as well as the President's Commission [15,16] (viz. a discussion in terms understandable to both parties in which both exchange information and both agree to proceed).

Improving Research

A second purpose served by informed consent relates to good research design and education. In preparing to explain a project to prospective subjects, investigators should be provoked to scrutinize it with additional care; further, the obligation of informed consent may have a beneficial "reflexive effect," as Paul Freund put it, "on the management of the experiment itself" [17]. Besides the benefits of greater thoughtfulness on the investigators' part, in some kinds of ongoing studies, the active collaboration of informed subjects may increase the accuracy and pertinence of the data collected. Finally, by educating people about both the methods and purposes of scientific investigation, the informed consent process can improve the public climate in which research is conducted and supported.

Regularizing Relationships

Third, requiring consent allows the relationship of subjects and investigators to be brought within the norms of more typical social interactions. Especially in research that involves the observation of people, or collection of disparate pieces of information about them, the investigators "have changed the normal relationship of equality between freely associating individuals in society into one which they have usurped power over aspects of their subjects' lives and personalities" [12].

Protecting Privacy

This leads into the fourth function of informed consent that I want to mention, safeguarding people from unwanted invasions of their privacy. The term privacy is today a rich and multifaceted one in ethics and the law. In addition to referring to the protection of private space, it connotes guarantees against the public disclosure of facts that falls short of defamation. "Privacy is not simply an absence of information about us in the minds of others," as Charles Fried has written, "rather it is the control we have over information about ourselves" [18].

Three Hypothetical Studies

Having in mind these varied functions of informed consent, imagine three hypothetical research projects in which an epidemiologist might argue that obtaining informed consent is undesirable (for reasons of research design), impractical, or even impossible.*

PROJECT SMOKE intends to discover whether the peer-pressure methods of reducing cigarette smoking employed among seventh graders by school officials in District 1 were more effective than the didactic techniques used in District 2 junior highs. The researchers plan to question 17-year-olds in the two school districts to determine whether they smoke 5 years after their exposure to the programs. The researchers wish to pass out anonymous questionnaires that ask a number of questions about personal habits and health status, but they do not want to explain the purpose of the study (for fear of biasing the answers) nor to obtain explicit consent in advance (for fear of lowering the participation rate and thereby biasing the results).

PROJECT FAMILY is an inquiry into the effects on juvenile delinquency of various judicial and social service interventions with families in which child abuse has occurred. The researchers would use public records to follow the course from the official response to a report of child abuse to later juvenile court dispositions involving any child in the family. These results would be compared with the prior judicial and social service involvement with the families of juvenile offenders whose families were never found to be abusive. Since there will be no direct contact with any of the families or juveniles, the researchers argue that they should not face the burden of obtaining their consent to review and link the records involved.

The third hypothetical is PROJECT HIV in which the investigators are interested in the natural history of HIV injection in a group of individuals who have been discharged from the armed services after having been identified as HIV-positive through HIV screening, which is mandatory for service personnel. In addition to linking service records with the National Death Index, VA hospitalization and death records, and CDC's AIDS registry, the investigators want to ask the HIV-positive individuals to release their post-service medical records, to fill out a questionnaire, and to submit to a clinical examination. The researchers will need access to the individuals' service records before they obtain consent from them to participate in the research.

The justifications for not seeking consent differ in these three hypotheticals, as do the risks – both of harming subjects (PROJECT FAMILY and PROJECT HIV, for example, involve information about subjects that could pose social and economic harms if known widely) and of wronging them. Let us turn, then, to consider the alternatives to informed consent that might be available to an IRB called upon to decide whether to permit these projects.

Alternatives to Prospective, Indivdiual Consent

One approach is to see whether a project falls outside the federal government's regulatory requirements in 45 *CFR* Part 46. Section 46.101 (b) (5) exempts

Research involving the collection or study of existing data, documents, records, pathological specimens, or diagnostic specimens, if these sources are publicly available or if the information is recorded by the investigator in such a manner that subjects cannot be identified, directly or through identifiers linked to the subjects.

In effect, this rule – which might apply to PROJECT SMOKE and PROJECT FAMILY – seems to be premised on the notion that subjects are not wronged when public records or anonymous data are used by researchers. I believe that the goals of good research design and minimization of harm would still be best served were such research to be reviewed by an IRB – so as to overcome the blind-spots that researchers have about their own studies – but I would agree that consent is not always the only means to serve these goals. What about the other purposes of consent we discussed earlier, such as promoting autonomy and self-determination, regularizing relationships, and protecting privacy? One's answer to the question depends upon whether one thinks that the subjects in a study using public records differ in their relationship to the investigator from that of other people and whether reasonable expectations of privacy are violated in these circumstances. It is my own view that, except in situations involving records that are truly public, there is something unique here that requires either consent or some reasonble substitute therefore.

What might such alternatives be? To place this question in context: section 46.116 (d) of the regulations provides that an IRB may approve an alternative to the usual consent procedures (including a complete waiver) when the research, which may "involve no more than minimal risk to the subjects," could not otherwise be carried out and when the "waiver or alteration will not adversely affect the rights and welfare of the subjects." We may take from this, again, that the harm-prevention goal of informed consent is met by the IRB reveiw process, but this does not, I would argue, necessarily respond to the other purposes of informed consent that we have discussed.

One alternative to individual consent might be to convene what Diana Baumrind has termed "peer consultants," selected from the study population [19]. This would symbolize the investigator's respect for the human beings involved in the study as rational agents worthy of consideration; the peers would take the place of the subjects as collaborators in the design of the research, thereby approximating "self-determination"; and the information given to peers could serve the same function as informed consent in educating and reassuring the public. Of course, for this strategy to be successful, it must be approached conscientiously and with ingenuity, making sure that those asked to serve as the peer consultants accurately represent the study population and are positioned so as to make the sort of choices one would want a proxy to make on one's behalf. This would appear to be applicable to all three hypotheticals. Peer consultants might also be used for more than proxy consent; a medical anthropological approach could provide richly detailed case studies, which might serve both to illustrate the statistical findings for eventual readers of the study and, perhaps more important, to give a human face to the nameless research subjects, thereby deepening the empathy of the epidemiologists and perhaps increasing their ability truly to understand the meaning and significance of their data.**

A related – but distinct – strategy is to obtain permission for the use of records from their custodians. In the case of PROJECT FAMILY, for example, the cooperation of officials in the judicial and social service offices would doubtless be essential. I think it is, however, misleading to say that subjects have given implied consent to the researcher's use of data about them when officials give their permission in such circumstances; rather, one could say that the goal of regularizing relationships has been fulfilled because the subjects' relationship to the researchers resembles their relationship to the judicial and social service process, since in both cases they are involuntarily entangled in a process intended to benefit society. The same cannot be said about PROJECT HIV, in which the subjects' relationship to the researchers is "irregular" compared with their relationship with the treating physicians who are the source of the initial information used by the researchers to identify and contact the HIV-infected individuals.

Another alternative to prospective informed consent is to employ after-the-fact debriefing and informed veto. This gives subjects an opportunity to exercise self-determination as to at least part of the study, it symbolizes the researchers' respect for subjects' autonomy, and it removes the implication of coercion that inheres in non-voluntary participation in research. For example, in PROJECT SMOKE, questionnaires could bear identifying numbers and each respondent could be given an envelope with a form bearing the matching number. After the questionnaires are turned in, respondents could be provided with an explanation of the true purposes of the research, and any who wished to have his or her questionnaire removed from the data set could check off on the form. This alternative is probably not feasible for PROJECT FAMILY, however, because of the difficulty of contacting all involved family members and asking for their permission. In PROJECT HIV, a veto is effectively given to subjects when they are contacted by the researchers to ask for their cooperation, provided that the researchers – at the risk of biasing the results – delete any information about non-cooperating subjects from the data set. (We shall return to this issue in the final section.)

Finally, provisions could be made to compensate subjects for any injury they suffer as a result of being studied without their advance consent. Since this entire exception is limited to situations involving negligible risk, the need for compensation for harm should be small, but providing compensation can still serve some purposes of consent, such as encouraging self-scrutiny by the investigator and providing a further incentive to choose among reasonable research designs in order to maximize subjects' welfare. We should recognize, however, that it will be much easier to measure the extent to which compensation is owed for harms to a person than for wrongs, which typically involve injury to a dignitary interest that is not easily monetizable.

The Special Problem of Groups

Obviously, this brief list does not exhaust all alternatives to consent that might be argued to be legitimate to the extent they fulfill some of the same purposes as consent. One additional purpose is sometimes attributed to the requirement of obtaining subjects' consent, viz. that it permits members of a group to prevent a study from being conducted of which they disapprove. Thus stated, the effect is descriptively accurate and normatively true, as an aspect of self-determination. But if the idea is that informed consent protects groups against studies that will reveal information that is, from some viewpoint, harmful to the group, then I believe too much is claimed for informed consent. As an ethical matter, I do not believe – outside of situations in which a group can be taken to speak as whole through duly constituted leaders – that the notion of a group veto has anything to do with informed consent; and, as a practical matter, so long as *some* members of a group are willing to participate in a study, the group as a whole has no guarantee against being affected by the results of the study.

Minimizing Breaches of Privacy and Confidentiality

The discussion of the harms and wrongs intended to be avoided by the requirement of advance informed consent should already have made apparent that personal privacy is one of the major concerns in the protection of research subjects. Related to this is the notion of confidentiality, which requires those to whom private information has been conveyed for a professional purpose not to disclose that information outside the bounds drawn by that purpose. The courts have recognized that the protection of personally identifiable information is important to the success of epidemiology and hence serves a public good that may outweigh other social goods, such as full disclosure of information in the judicial process [20, 21]. Regrettably, in the medical world today, confidentiality is often honored in the breach, which is especially ironic when one considers that medical records today probably contain more information about people than ever, thanks in large measure to the electronics revolution and to the ever-increasing demands for more data for various reimbursement and other management purposes.

When a researcher uses data collected for other purposes, it is important for the researcher – and then the IRB – to consider the privacy and confidentiality expectations that attached to the data when the subjects provided it. Especially when direct consent for the use of data is not sought from the subjects, the researchers should realize that they are, in effect, being brought into the circle of confidentiality that attaches to the data, and they are governed by the same strictures against unauthorized release that attach to the persons who originally gathered the data. Indeed, to the extent that new information has effectively been generated by the researchers having linked together data from several sources, they are under a greater obligation than that applicable to the original sources, so far as protecting their files from public disclosure.

Public disclosure is usually associated with one form or another of psychological or social (including financial) harm. But even when confidentiality is not breached by the investigator, the mere fact that the investigator has gained access to private information may constitute a wrong to the subject. In PROJECT FAMILY, for example, if the researcher has access to files maintaind by social workers who dealt with the abusing families – files that are not usually thought of as part of the *public record* – then merely reading those files (even with identifiers removed) is in some sense to intrude on the privacy of the people involved. (One can be sure that the social workers would feel that *their* privacy had been invaded were the files reviewed without their advance approval [22–24].)

It would, therefore, usually be appropriate to have the contact with the potential subject come initially from someone who is inside the circle of confidentiality before any disclosure is made to a researcher. Thus, in PROJECT HIV it would seem advisable for the treating physician, rather than the researcher, to contact the potential subject so as to have permission for enlarging the circle before any information is disclosed. There is a risk, however, that the potential subject's agreement to participate may not be truly voluntary because the request to participate in research comes from a person on whom the subject is dependent in some sense [25]. This should be less of a problem in situations like PROJECT HIV when the physician–patient relationship is not current; in any event, it is important always to make explicit to the subject that further services are not conditioned upon an agreement to participate and to be alert to the need to re-enforce this message, which subjects may have a hard time accepting or believing, perhaps for unconscious reasons. (In the context of treatment, Laurence Tancredi has noted that "the physician's predisposition will influence the way the information is presented and bias the patient toward (or away from) particular . . . options" [26].)

None of the strategies discussed previously are fully responsive to the concerns about privacy, although after-the-fact debriefing and veto rights comes closest if it means that any data involving an objecting subject will be removed from the researcher's files. Nonetheless, the use of peer consultants might at least serve to alert investigators to situations in which people in the subject population take the view that certain aspects of their lives are particularly private matters onto which the researchers should be especially reluctant to intrude. If a small modification of study design would provide a means of steering clear of such problems, the use of proxies could avoid wronging the actual subjects in a significant fashion.

Notes

* These hypotheticals were without reference to any studies that might actually be – or have been – undertaken. While any resemblance to actual studies may enhance the hypotheticals' credibility and even their usefulness in analyses, it is purely accidental, and the comments in this essay should not be taken as judgments about any actual study.

** I am indebted to Kathleen M. West, MPH, for this point.

References

1. Rothman KJ. The rise and fall of epidemiology, 1950–2000 A.D. **N Engl J Med** 1981; 304: 600–602.
2. Chann CI. Rothman KJ. IRBs and epidemiologic research: how inappropriate restrictions hamper studies. **IRB: A Journal of Human Subjects Research** 1984; 6(4): 5–7.
3. Hershey N. IRB jurisdiction and limits in IRB actions. **IRB: A Journal of Human Subjects Research** 1985; 7(2): 7–9.
4. Cann CI. Rothman KJ. Reply: Overcoming hurdles to epidemiologic research. **IRB: A Journal of Human Subjects Research** 1985; 7(2): 9.
5. Jonas H. Philosophical Reflections on Experimenting with Human Subjects. **Daedalus** 1969; 98: 219–245.
6. de Sola Pool I. The New Censorship of Social Research. **Public Interest** 1980; 59: 56–88.
7. Pattullo EL. Who risks what in social research. **IRB: A Journal of Human Subjects Research** 1980; 2(3): 1–3, 12.
8. Robertson J. The scientist's right to research: A constitutional analysis. **So Cal L Rev** 1979; 51: 1203–1281.
9. Gibbs RA, Caskey CT. The application of recombinant DNA technology for genetic probing in epidemiology. **Ann Rev Public Health** 1989; 10: 27–48.
10. MacIntyre A. Risk, harm, and benfit assessments as instruments of moral evaluation. In: Beauchamp T, Faden R, Wallace R, Walters L, Eds. **Ethical Issues is Social Science Research. Baltimore,** MD: Johns Hopkins University Press; 1982: 175.

11. Dworkin G. Must subjects be objects? In: Beauchamp T, Faden R, Wallace R, Walters L, Eds. **Ethical Issues in Social Science Research.** Baltimore, Md: Johns Hopkins University Press; 1982: 246, 247–248.

12. Capron AM. Is consent always necessary in social science research. In: Beauchamp T, Faden R, Wallace R, Walters L, Eds. **Ethical Issues in Social Science Research.** Baltimore, Md: Johns Hopkins University Press; 1982: 215, 220–229.

13. Berlin I. **Two Concepts of Liberty.** Oxford: Clarendon Press; 1958: 16.

14. Faden RR, Beauchamp TL. **A History and Theory of Informed Consent.** New York: Oxford University Press; 1986.

15. Katz J. **The Silent World of Doctor and Patient.** New Haven: Yale University Press; 1983.

16. President's Commission for the Study of Ethical Problems in Medicine and Biomedical and Behavioral Research. **Making Health Care Decisions.** Washington, D.C.: Government Printing Office; 1982.

17. Freund P. Legal frameworks for human experimentation. **Daedalus** 1969; 98: 323.

18. Fried C. Privacy. **Yale L J** 1968; 77: 482.

19. Baumrind D. Nature and Definition of Informed Consent in Research Involving Deception. In: National Commission for the Protection of Human Subjects of Biomedical and Behavioral Research. **The Belmont Report: Ethical Principles and Guidelines for the Protection of Human Subjects of Research,** DHEW Publication No. (OS) 78-0014. Washington, D.C.: Government Printing Office; 1978: Appendix, Vol. 2. 23–42.

20. Farnsworth v. Procter and Gamble Co.; 758 F. 2d 1545 (11th Cir. 1985).

21. Curran WJ. Protecting Confidentiality in Epidemiologic Investigations by the Centers for Disease Control. **N Engl J Med** 1986; 314: 1027–1028.

22. Hughes EC. Who studies whom? **Hum Organ** 1974; 33: 327–334 (threats inhere in studying people in institutions).

23. Geller JL, Lidz CW. When the subjects are hospital staff, is it ethical (or possible) to get informed consent? **IRB: A Journal of Human Subjects Research** 1987; 9(5): 4–5 (problems with obtaining informed consent from employees).

24. Pattullo EL. Exemption from review, not informed consent. **IRB: A Journal of Human Subjects Research** 1987; 9(5): 6–8 (consent to observe employees' work can be given by employer).

25. Capron AM. The law of genetic therapy. In: Hamilton M, Ed. **The New Genetics and the Future of Man.** Grand Rapids, Mich.: Eerdmans Publishing Co.; 1972: 133, 150–152.

26. Tancredi L. The new technology of psychiatry: ethics, epidemiology and technology assessment. In: Tancredi L, Ed. **Ethical Issues in Epidemiologic Research.** New Brunswick, N.J.: Rutgers University Press; 1986: 1, 16.

Limitations in the Use of Race in the Study of Disease Causation

Richard S. Cooper and Vincent L. Freeman

Tremendous variation exists in the rates of many chronic diseases across racial groups.[1] Investigators have made use of these differences for several purposes, with the most fundamental being for the understanding of etiologic relationships.[2-4] The concept of race as a biologic model providing genetic explanations for disease has made this approach particularly appealing to some for the study of genetic effects in prostate cancer.[5] While race may be useful in defining where the problem is, using it to test etiologic hypotheses is inherently problematic. Race, or ethnicity, is a proxy for determinants of disease; it alone does not represent a primary pathway or mechanism. As a result, ethnic comparisons to elucidate disease causes face major design and analytic obstacles, namely, the presence and measurement of confounders, the reasonableness and adequacy of statistical "adjustments" for race effects, interpreting the meaning of residual confounding, and accounting for interactions.

To provide examples of these technical and conceptual limitations and thus shed light on the limitations of the biologic concept of race in etiologic investigation, this article focuses on two essential areas used to measure racial effects: social class and genetics. We will identify issues that need to be resolved to move forward not only on the problem of prostate cancer but also of other chronic diseases characterized by marked ethnic differentials.

Large differences in cancer disease rates by ethnicity have been well documented.[1] Table 1 shows the ratio of cancer death rates, which are considerably higher among blacks across virtually all tumor sites and somewhat lower for Hispanics. A common alternative hypothesis proposed to explain such racial/ethnic variation in disease is that the observed differences are not due to race per se, but social class, often measured as socioeconomic status (SES).[6] Thus, race is "confounded" by social class.

Confounding is a mixing of effects.[7] Specifically, the estimate of the effect of the exposure of interest is distorted because it is mixed with the effect of a third factor. For the third factor to be a confounder, it must be a correlate of the exposure and a correlate of the outcome (although not necessarily in a causal fashion). Thus, in this context, "race" is the exposure of interest, "cancer death rate" is the outcome of interest, and "social class" is the third factor, which is a correlate of both exposure (race) and outcome (cancer death rate). However, . . . these data are not entirely consistent by our general measures of social class: on the one hand, we see a relationship between blacks and whites, and lower SES is associated with higher mortality; however, that is not true for Mexican Americans. One of the problems is that SES, like race, is not a direct measure but a proxy of certain lifestyles or patterns. Thus, if dietary

From the *Journal of the National Medical Association*, 1999; 91: 379–383. Reproduced by permission.

Table 1. *Mortality Rates* for Selected Cancers in Whites, Blacks, and Hispanics, 1990[†]*

Type of Cancer	Men			Women		
	White[‡]	Black	Hispanic	White	Black	Hispanic
Lung	83.5	116.2	56.8	39.9	34.2	20.1
Colorectal	23.3	32.4	22.8	17.5	22.9	15.0
Prostate	31.2	63.9	26.0	—	—	—
Breast	—	—	—	29.4	33.4	25.0

*Per 100,000 persons.
[†]From reference 1.
[‡]Non-Hispanic whites.

patterns are suspected to be related to cancer risk, we might see the relationship between cancer mortality and race if SES is replaced with the causal variable diet as measured by intake of fruits and vegetables.

Cross-Ethnic Comparisons

Two major assumptions are involved when making cross-ethnic comparisons. First, it is assumed that the potential operative variables of interest can be measured with comparable validity across ethnic groups, and second, the variable measured has a similar relationship within each group. As a result, it then would not be necessary to take into account interactions between race and other explanatory variables. An interaction can be thought of as the condition where the presence of one factor alters the relative effect of another.

Unfortunately, the aforementioned assumptions about measurement validity and the absence of interactions are usually quite difficult to satisfy. For example, income and education are believed to be the primary determinants of social class.[8] However, other conditions or attributes, such as accumulated wealth, may, in fact, be how income and education mediate their effects, which also may vary across racial groups. Table 2 shows that while among whites, financial assets rose significantly with education, this was not the case among blacks, where there is virtually no correlation between education and financial assets. Ultimately, it is financial assets that determine one's ability to buy a house, send children to college, etc. [In] another example of what has been referred to as an "interaction," socioeconomic status, as measured by income, is plotted against both death rates and age, creating a diagram of the relative risk of dying at different SES levels. These data show that by middle age, SES, as measured by income, is a major predictor of the risk of dying. However, by retirement age, the measure of income is a predictor neither of risk or social class. Hence, this effect of income varies across age groups, ie, exhibits an interaction with age.

In summary, ethnic comparisons are confounded by SES, a measure of social class. Socioeconomic status is multifaceted, poorly defined, and difficult to measure. Furthermore, it often is approached in categories, and there is substantial potential for interactions, ie, variation of its effects across those categories. What are the implications for the use of the biologic concept of race posed by the generic technical problems that these examples

Table 2. *Education, Income, and Financial Assets Among US Blacks and Whites**

Education	Income		Financial Assets	
	White[†]	Black	White	Black
Some high school	$11,554	$8724	$1100	$0
High school	17,328	11,534	3287	0
Some college	27,594	21,076	5500	0
College degree	35,068	28,080	17,300	5
Postgraduate	40,569	31,340	23,200	78

*Source: Oliver & Shapiro, *Black Wealth/White Wealth*, 1995.
[†]Non-Hispanic whites.

illustrate? A discussion of the standard analytic approaches used in epidemiology used to solve these problems should provide some insight into this question.

Epidemiologic Considerations

Statistical adjustments are used to account for the effects of known confounders when comparing groups. After this "adjustment," the difference that remains between the groups being compared is referred to as "residual confounding."[9] In epidemiology, when comparing blacks and whites, what is often done is to adjust for the effect of SES and other confounders, and interpret any residual difference as a "race effect." The temptation is to infer that what is left over after environmental adjustments must be genetic.

For example, one might make the argument that the racial difference observed in prostate cancer disease rates after adjusting for SES is an intrinsic attribute of blacks compared with whites. The logic of this argument, however, is fatally flawed because there are many attributes bound up in the social development of race that play out in our culture and simply cannot be removed by "adjustment." And yet, the medical literature is filled to overflowing with analyses that conclude with these arguments.[10–15] Furthermore, for a given race–disease relationship, all of the relevant environmental factors are never known. Therefore, to the extent to which these effects can be inferred in this fashion, statistical adjustments inherently overestimate the presence of genetic effects. Consequently, for the basis of ethnic comparisons, the method of statistical adjustment, which is the fundamental approach used in epidemiology and in medical science generally, is inadequate and usually unreasonable.

Gene–Environment Interactions

As has been suggested, there appears to be a formal standard in epidemiology that if there is something left over after statistical adjustments of racial comparisons, it must be a generalized attribute of race. This is analogous to what philosophers call an "essentialist" concept.[16] There is a generalized view that the force of some fundamental process underlies the exposure–disease relationship and functions as an essential matrix of the individual. Science tries to make this quantifiable and develops a set of rules and logic to evaluate and understand it. In epidemiology, the usual approach is to say that phenotypic variation, or the individual we can observe, is the product of two inputs – genes and the environment – and these are generally considered to be additive quantities. A certain complement of genes occurring in a certain type of environment together produces phenotypic variation:

$$\text{phenotypic variation} = \text{genes} + \text{environment}.$$

When the genetic contribution is trying to be understood but cannot be measured directly, that is, on a molecular basis, the equality is rearranged:

$$\text{phenotypic variation} - \text{environment} = \text{genes}.$$

The genetic contribution, which is what is trying to be understood, is isolated on one side and the environmental component subtracted from phenotypic variation. This is part of the process used in epidemiology to give some quantitative measure of the contribution of genes in relation to environment.

As a technical process, this is also intrinsically flawed. Neither the tools nor the statistical methods to do this effectively are available. Objections similar to ones raised previously with other analytic strategies also can be raised here:

1) Clearly, not all of the environmental factors can be identified and measured.
2) Many of them can be measured only imprecisely.
3) Perhaps more importantly, these factors are not all additive.

It is not simply a matter of having A+B, but having an interaction in the form of A×B. That is to say, genes in a particular environment have a different outcome. Therein lies the central conceptual limitation of race as a biologic construct for the study of disease causes: the logic of genetic explanations of disease risk (ie, genetic susceptibility) leads us astray since it tempts use to accept essentialist causes. This acceptance may arguably be even less tenable in the context of polygenic disorders, of which prostate cancer may be an example.[17]

Expression of genetic material is context-dependent. Therefore, when trying to determine the presence or absence of genetic effects, it is important to measure both the environmental and genetic contributions and account for potential interactions. Unfortunately, gene–environment interactions are extremely difficult to measure, and quantifying them is probably well over the horizon of our current technical capabilities. However, there is now a revolution in biology that allows us to make genetic measurements rather than talk about these as philosophical concepts.[17] This is cause for judicious optimism.

Conclusion

Serious technical and conceptual obstacles limit the use of race in the study of disease causes; racial comparisons to test genetic susceptibility hypotheses are particularly weak. That said, there is, at least theoretically, the potential to use race or ethnicity to advance our understanding of the cause(s) of racially variable diseases such as prostate cancer. However, much needed work remains, and numerous issues must be resolved in order to move forward. These include a more comprehensive understanding of the factors that mediate the apparent effect of race, valid measures of those factors, and creative strategies that help overcome the technical and interpretive limitations of statistical adjustment.

Finally, the "grand" theories of race-based genetic susceptibility should be renounced and rigorous criteria established to determine when a trait can be ascribed to some genetic origin. At minimum, these criteria should include: 1) evidence that the gene confers susceptibility in each of the groups being compared, 2) definition of the functional mutations or highly specific haplotypes, and 3) differences in the frequencies of the at-risk alleles between the groups. With the ability to make actual observations, that should be put forward as the only useful information: to talk about genetic effects should be to talk about genes. That is the challenge of the molecular revolution. Therefore, let us find the genes, find out how they work, identify the functional relations, and see if the frequency of mutations varies between groups. Genetic explanations, which are actually what the biologic concept of race is all about, should be about genes and not about vague notions that people are different and have different rates of disease, and that since genes cause disease, the differences between the two must be due to genetics.

Literature Cited

1. Centers for Disease Control and Prevention. *Chronic Disease in Minority Populations*. Atlanta, GA: CDC; 1992.
2. Wagenknect LE, Roseman JM, Alexander WJ. Epidemiology of IDDM in black and white children in Jefferson County, Alabama, 1979–1985. *Diabetes*, 1989;38:629–633.
3. Moore ML, Michielutte R, Meis PJ, Ernest JM, Wells HB, Buescher PA. Etiology of low-birthweight birth: a population-based study. *Prev Med.* 1994;23:793–799.
4. Zahm SH, Fraumeni JF. Racial, ethnic, and gender variation in cancer risk: considerations for future epidemiologic research. *Environ Health Perspect.* 1995;103(suppl 8):283–286.
5. Whittmore AS, Wu AH, Kolonel LN, John EM, Gallagher RP, Howe GR. Family history and prostate cancer risk in black, white, and Asian men in the United States and Canada. *Am J Epidemiol.* 1995;141:732–740.
6. Baquet DR, Horm JW, Gibbs T, Greenwald P. Socioeconomic factors and cancer incidence among blacks and whites. *J Natl Cencer Inst.* 1991; 83:551–557.
7. Rothman KJ. *Modern Epidemiology*. Boston, MA: Little, Brown and Co; 1986.
8. Liberatos R, Link BG, Kelsey JL. The measurement of social class in epidemiology. *Epidemiol Rev.* 1988;10:87–121.
9. Kaufman JS, Cooper RS, McGee DL. Socioeconomic status and health in blacks and whites: the problem of residual confounding and the resiliency of race. *Epidemiology.* 1997;8: 621–628.
10. Klahr S. The kidney in hypertension: villain and victim. *N Engl J Med.* 1989;320:731–733.
11. Law MR, Frost CD, Wald NJ. By how much does dietary sodium restriction lower blood pressure? III: analysis of data from trials of salt reduction. *BMJ.* 1991;302:819–824.
12. Brancati FL, Whittle JC, Whelton PK, Seidler AJ, Klang MJ. The excess incidence of diabetic end-stage renal disease among blacks: a population-based study of potential explanatory factors. *JAMA.* 1992;268:3079–3084.
13. Coughlin SS, Neaton JD, Sengupta A, Kuller LH. Predictors of mortality from idiopathic dilated cardiomyopathy in 356,222 men screened for the Multiple Risk Factor Intervention Trial. *Am J Epidemiol* 1994;139:166–172.
14. Wild S, McKeigue P. Cross-sectional analysis of mortality by county of birth in England and Wales, 1970–1992. *BMJ,* 1997;314:705–710.
15. Moul JW, Douglas TH, McCarthy WF, McLead DG. Black race is an adverse prognostic factor for prostate cancer recurrence following radical prostatectomy in an equal access health care setting. *J Urol.* 1996;155:1667–1673.

16. Huncharek M, Muscat J. Genetic characteristics of prostate cancer. *Cancer Epidemiol Biomarkers Prev.* 1995;4:681–687.
17. Schuler GD, Boguski MS, Stewart EA, et al. A map of the human genome. *Science.* 1996;274: 540–546.

Questions for Discussion

1. What diseases or health problems can you identify that are commonly also viewed in terms of moral failure? How are these conditions presumed to be caused or affected by immorality as opposed to medical considerations?
2. How can the members of the class or discussion group be stratified according to traditional epidemiologic variables? Do these classifications change when an individual assigns him or herself to these categories rather than being assigned by another person?
3. What kinds of personal medical information are most valuable for epidemiologic research on major health conditions? How fully do you think most people respond to their physician's requests for such information? How can the accuracy of personally reported medical information be improved?
4. What factors lead epidemiologists and medical researchers to conduct studies in developing countries? How should researchers conduct their work in countries that have no formal legal or ethical policies on the protection, rights, and responsibilities of participants in research?

Recommended Supplemental Reading

Council for International Organizations of Medical Sciences. *International Guidelines for Ethical Review of Epidemiological Studies.* Geneva: CIOMS; 1991; reprinted in *Law, Medicine, and Health Care.* 1991;19:247–258.

Coughlin SS. *Ethics in Epidemiology and Public Health Practice: Collected Works.* Columbus, GA: Quill Publications; 1997.

Coughlin SS, Beauchamp TL, eds. *Ethics and Epidemiology.* New York: Oxford University Press; 1996.

Mastroianni AC, Faden R, Federman DD, eds. Committee on the Ethical and Legal Issues Relating to the Inclusion of Women in Clinical Studies. *Women and Health Research: Ethical and Legal Issues of Including Women in Clinical Studies.* Vols. 1, 2. Washington, DC: National Academy Press; 1994.

Supercourse: Epidemiology, the Internet, and Global Health (Web-based lectures on multiple aspects of epidemiology). Available at http://www.pitt.edu/~super1

Tyler CW Jr, Last JM. Epidemiology. In: Wallace RB, ed. *Public Health and Preventive Medicine.* 14th ed. Stamford, CT: Appleton & Lange; 1998:5–32.

The Humane Care and Use of Animals in Research

The Humane Care and Use of Animals in Research

Elizabeth Heitman

The use of animals in biomedical research is undoubtedly one of the most contentious ethical issues in society today. Public attention to animal experimentation places researchers at the center of controversy over animal consciousness and pain, the meaning of suffering, and the role of animals in human life. While much of the academic debate rests on philosophical claims, policy related to the ethics of animal research has been shaped most directly by changing views about animals and practicing scientists' increasing awareness that the quality of animal studies ultimately depends on the welfare of animal subjects.

Most students in the life sciences take part in animal research during their education, and many will later find animal research central to their scientific careers. Researchers working with animals must be familiar with, and adhere to, the regulatory guidelines and procedures governing their work and understand the origins and purpose of these regulations. It is no longer enough for scientists to show that animal research benefits humanity. Moreover, they must be able to address the complex ethical and scientific questions that animal research involves. Even entry-level students must be able to justify their use of animals generally and the value of their specific animal work as they develop proficiency in the methods and techniques that a particular project requires.

The Scope of Contemporary Animal Research

The growth of biomedical science in the past 50 years has been accompanied by the use of animal models in almost all areas of research. Despite calls for a formal system to track the number and types of animals used in research,[1] the United States has no official accounting mechanism. A widely cited 1986 study by the U.S. Congress Office of Technology Assessment estimated that 17 to 22 million animals were used in research, education, and testing in 1983, of which less than 2% were cats, dogs, and nonhuman primates.[2] The Foundation for Biomedical Research (FBR) reports that in 1998 the U.S. Department of Agriculture (USDA), which is responsible for maintaining basic records under the Animal Welfare Act, registered some 1,213,000 research animals across the United States (available at http://www.fbresearch.org). However, FBR notes that USDA figures from the late 1990s are more than 40% lower than those recorded in 1968. Considering the explosive growth of research during that period, the FBR attributes this reduction to the impact of institutional concern for animal welfare and attention to cost-effective research methods.

Remarkably, the USDA's figures do not account for rats, mice, or birds, because before 2000 the Act did not classify these species as animals or subject their use to regulatory oversight. Rats, mice, and birds are typically thought to account for 90–95% of laboratory animals, suggesting that an additional 11 to 23 million animals were used in research in

1998. While these numbers are quite significant, they nonetheless pale in comparison to the hundreds of millions of animals killed annually in the United States for meat, leather, and assorted consumer products and the stray dogs and cats euthanized in pounds.

Scientists may readily complain that their work is unfairly targeted by animal rights activists – particularly in light of society's eagerness to exterminate wild rodents considered pests. However, as ethicist Arthur Caplan insists in an essay included in this section, it is important to assess whether *any* human use of animals is morally legitimate before judging the appropriateness of using animals in research.

Western Historical Views of Pain, Suffering, and Moral Status in Animals

The contradictions in social policy and practice regarding the place of animals in other areas of human life are highlighted by the debate over animal rights and welfare. The moral status of animals was not commonly a subject for analysis before the 1800s. The historical sources of Western moral thought – texts from ancient Judaism, ancient Greek philosophy, and early Christianity – consistently made a clear distinction between human life and animal life and highlighted the differences in the moral status granted to people and animals. Fundamental Jewish and Christian teachings hold that God gave dominion over animals to human beings. While Hebrew scripture on the treatment of meat animals and beasts of burden demonstrated concern for animals' welfare, animals were clearly intended to be used by humans for human benefit. And although the Pythagoreans (fourth–fifth century B.C.E.) insisted that animal life be treated with respect, in the ancient world moral concern for animals' welfare focused on its consequences for human activities and human well-being.

From the early Christian period through the nineteenth century, theologians and philosophers occasionally raised questions about animals in considering the special moral nature of human beings. They considered whether animals had souls, whether they were capable of rational thought, and whether they experienced pain and suffering, but such issues were typically discussed only to claim that humanity held a unique status in the eyes of God. Writers with a theological perspective interpreted animals' pain in terms of their perceived inability to reflect consciously and rationally on the experience – abilities typically associated with the human soul. Augustine (354–430) observed that animals experience pain but concluded that it was not morally comparable to human pain because animals had no soul; thus, he contended, the commandment "thou shalt not kill" did not apply to the killing of animals. Aquinas (1225–74) emphasized that human beings should have compassion for animals in pain but only for the sake of the moral benefit of the human being displaying compassion rather than for that of the animal.

Consideration of the use of animals in science began with the resurgence of anatomy and physiology in the sixteenth century. Across Europe, conflicting observations and scientific theories about animal pain and consciousness emerged from the practice of live dissection. From his own live dissections, French philosopher–scientist Rene Descartes (1596–1650) described animals' pain response as "mechanistic" rather than "conscious." Guided by contemporary theological views, Descartes held that animals do not suffer in the way that humans do because they cannot understand pain rationally. For Descartes the absence of rational ability left animals in a lower category than human beings.

In contrast, English philosopher–physician John Locke (1632–1704) concluded from his studies with animals that they do suffer when in pain and thus that killing animals or causing them pain is morally wrong. Scottish philosopher David Hume (1711–76) later argued that human minds and animal minds worked in analogous ways and thus that the human and animal experiences of pain were of equal moral significance. The moral meaning of suffering was redefined by English philosopher Jeremy Bentham (1748–1831), whose utilitarian theory claimed that it is not rationality but *sentience*, the ability to experience pleasure or pain, that determines moral standing. For Bentham and other utilitarians, animal and human pain and pleasure count equally.

The enormously influential German philosopher Immanuel Kant (1724–76), however, held that animals are not self-conscious and thus not rational. Because they are unable to reflect rationally on their pain, it had no moral significance for Kant. He argued that humans could ethically use animals as means to human ends in ways that human beings could not be used. His only caution was that causing pain to animals might make human beings indifferent to the suffering of other humans.

The real scientific challenge to a clear moral distinction between animals and human beings came from Charles Darwin's (1809–82) theory of evolution. In *The Descent of Man,* Darwin observed that the differences between humans and animals were a matter of degree, not of kind.[3] His work implied not only that animals do suffer, but that their suffering is morally significant.

Despite growing acceptance of Darwin's evidence, its moral connotations went unheeded. Animal research became an integral part of medical science in the late 1800s as a result of the revolutionary work of French physiologist and surgeon Claude Bernard (1813–78) and his extensive and highly instructive practice of vivisection. In *An Introduction to Experimental Medicine,*[4] Bernard argued that medical and surgical morality demands that human beings not be used in experiments that might be harmful to them. He maintained that even if animals experience pain in medical experiments, their use is morally legitimate because it permits the discovery of new knowledge and prevents the suffering of human beings in the painful experiments that such discovery requires.

Antivivisectionists and the Animal Welfare Movement

In many European countries, the growing use of animals in medical research coincided with growing public concern about animal welfare. As early as 1824, the English Society for the Prevention of Cruelty to Animals tried to prohibit animal blood sports and sought governmental protections for livestock and tamed wild animals. By the 1870s, the Society had counterparts in the United States and Germany with physician and scientist members actively working to end the practice of vivisection without the use of the recently developed anesthetics.

Antivivisectionists in England succeeded in establishing governmental regulation for animal research at the turn of the century, but dramatic advances in medicine attributed to animal research limited public criticism of laboratory animal use in the United States for over half a century. Moreover, by the 1950s, Bernard's claim that animal experimentation reduced the need for human research subjects was widely incorporated into governmental and professional standards for ethical medical research. Both the Nuremberg Code[5] and the World Medical Association's Declaration of Helsinki[6] called for animal studies before human experimentation to prevent unnecessary human harm.

The 1960s and 1970s saw a resurgence of public concern for laboratory animals in the United States and renewed philosophical discourse about the moral status of animals. In the mid-1960s, public fears that stolen family pets were being sold to laboratories as research animals led to the 1966 Laboratory Animal Welfare Act,[7] which regulated the sale of animals for laboratory use and set standards for their care. During the 1970s activist groups such as People for the Ethical Treatment of Animals (PETA) and the Animal Liberation Front (ALF) exposed the conditions and treatment of animals used in toxicology testing and trauma research and even broke into research and breeding facilities to free animals.[8] As philosophers and others in the new academic area of bioethics considered the ethics of medical research with human subjects and the nature of personhood, animal research also became a topic of academic ethical interest.

The most influential contemporary philosopher on the issue of animal experimentation is Australian Peter Singer, whose book *Animal Liberation* introduced the terms *animal rights* and *speciesism* – unjust discrimination on the basis of species – into public debate.[9] Singer built on the utilitarians' concept of sentience to argue that any animal capable of experiencing pain has both an interest in avoiding it and a right to be free from avoidable pain. For Singer, the claim that human benefit from animal research is more important than animals' interest in avoiding pain is *speciesist*, and any research that is not in the animals' own best interests violates the animal's rights.

Contemporary philosophers Martin Benjamin and Arthur Caplan reject Singer's emphasis on animals' equal rights but maintain that even if human beings have a higher moral status than animals, human beings should not use animals in ways that cause them pain, distress, or death except for vital human needs. Nevertheless, for Caplan, even the justifiable human use of animals is tragic. Both Benjamin and Caplan call on researchers to reduce their use of animals and to ensure that their studies are sufficiently well designed to eliminate wasting animal life.

Biomedical Scientists Reform Animal Research

Well before American philosophers called for a reduction in animal experimentation on moral grounds, scientists involved in the international animal welfare movement had offered strategies for limiting the use of animals in research in ways that were consistent with scientific method. The best-known proposal is the *3 Rs* (*refinement, reduction, and replacement*) of Russell and Burch.[10] They held that procedures for animal experimentation should be subject to continual refinement to eliminate physical or mental pain, distress, or injury, including the use of anesthetics and analgesics and appropriate monitoring. Using a clearly designed protocol based on a thorough knowledge of past work, they argued, researchers should reduce the number of experiments and the number of animals they use to the smallest number needed to test the research question in a statistically significant manner. Finally, researchers should replace animal research with nonanimal methods wherever possible and replace high-level animals with species lower in evolutionary complexity and consciousness to reduce the overall animal suffering related to the project.

Research into the nature of pain, its effects, and the physiology of the stress response has also made important contributions to the definition and protection of animal welfare.[11] Pain has been clearly described as a biological function that is not dependent upon consciousness, although its perception depends on central nervous system activity. In the 1980s, pain researchers made great strides in recognizing the effects of pain on physiologic functioning in all species. As the professional position papers included in this section indicate, veterinary pain specialists have argued for almost two decades that it is essential to minimize and control pain as a variable that affects research results. In 1998, the American College of Veterinary Anesthesiologists endorsed "a philosophy that promotes prevention and alleviation of animal pain and suffering as an important and tenable therapeutic goal."[12] In its position statement on pain and distress included in this section, the American Association for Laboratory Animal Science states that laboratory animal veterinarians now recognize a "legal and moral obligation to alleviate pain and distress in laboratory animals" irrespective of the moral debate about animals' ability to suffer.[13]

Similarly, research into environmentally induced stress has demonstrated that, as in humans, the physiologic effects of the neurochemical pain response can be affected by environmental factors. Housing and handling practices, including overcrowding and isolation, can lead to helplessness, boredom, and overall distress in research animals. Such phenomena have been linked to unhealthy neurobiological, endocrine, and immune responses that can skew research findings if they go undetected. In contrast, species-appropriate housing, exercise, socialization, and interaction with humans have been shown to improve the quality and reliability of research results by reducing animals' stress and its biological consequences. The AALAS statement reflects a growing international movement to prevent and manage stress and distress among laboratory animals through regulatory standards.

Regulation of Animal Experimentation

Since the 1970s, regulation of animal research has increased in scope and complexity worldwide. The first formal guidelines for animal research in the United States were published by the National Institutes of Health (NIH) in 1963 as the *Guide for Laboratory Animal Facilities and Care*.[1] The first U.S. regulations were issued in 1966 as the Animal Welfare Act (AWA), which required licensure of all institutions and individuals who bought or sold animals for laboratory use, mandated recordkeeping of all sales, and set standards for the care of laboratory animals in keeping with the *Guide*. The AWA has been amended five times since 1966. Today, all research facilities that use certain animal species in biomedical research must register with the U.S. Department of Agriculture (USDA) and comply with its standards and regulations on animal welfare, including standards for housing, handling, anesthesia and analgesia, and recordkeeping. These facilities are subject to yearly surprise inspection by the USDA as well as to annual reporting requirements on compliance with USDA standards. These standards are defined and regularly updated by the USDA's Animal and Plant Health Inspection Service (APHIS, http://www.aphis.udsa.gov).

A significant component of the AWA is the requirement that research facilities have an Institutional Animal Care and Use Committee (IACUC) to review animal research protocols for scientific merit and compliance with USDA standards (9 CFR 2.31). The facility's IACUC is also responsible for maintaining and regularly inspecting all animal study and housing areas, ensuring that investigators are properly trained and equipped to conduct approved research, reviewing complaints and reports of noncompliance with USDA standards, and, as necessary, suspending noncompliant animal research protocols. Every IACUC must have at least one veterinarian member as well as one member from outside the institution intended to represent community interests. Each IACUC is required to keep extensive records of its reviews and inspections as well as of the facility's sources of animals and housing and exercise plans.

In 1985, the Health Research Extension Act (P.L. 99–158) extended the requirement for IACUCs to all institutions that receive research funding from agencies of the Department of Health and Human Services (DHHS) (e.g., NIH, the Centers for Disease Control and Prevention [CDC], the Food and Drug Administration [FDA], and the Public Health Service [PHS]) irrespective of the species used in research. The PHS also requires its funded researchers to comply with its Policy on Humane Care and Use of Laboratory Animals and to follow the provisions of the most recent *Guide for the Care and Use of Laboratory Animals* updated in 1996.[14]

Since 1990, two lawsuits filed by animal welfare groups have also shaped U.S. regulation. Animal welfare organizations brought suit against the USDA, claiming that its standards on housing, exercise, and stimulus did not meet animals' needs. In early 1993, a federal court invalidated those standards on the grounds that they were too vague to be meaningful. While the USDA is still working to revise its standards to meet the court's practical demands, NIH policy continues to require compliance with the old USDA standards and adherence to the provisions of the *Guide*. In a potentially more far-reaching legal decision handed down in October 2000, a settlement was reached in a decade-old suit against the USDA that challenged the AWA's exclusion of rats, mice, and birds from the definition of research animal subject to its protections. However, almost immediately afterward, a U.S. Senate budget bill funding the USDA was amended to prohibit the use of federal monies to act on the settlement for at least a year.

Regulation of animal research internationally is highly variable. European countries, particularly the United Kingdom, regulate animal research quite stringently, while many developing nations offer little to no regulatory structure for animal use. In a 1983 conference, the Council of International Organizations of Medical Sciences (CIOMS) articulated international guiding principles on animal research with the expectation that the principles would serve as the basic professional standards in countries that have no regulations.[15] The principles emphasize the importance of animal work for the health and safety of humanity and animals but call for animals to be treated as sentient beings whose pain and suffering should be avoided or minimized. They stress the need for appropriate anesthesia and analgesia, appropriate housing for research animals, and veterinary supervision of research as well as the responsibility of each facility's director to ensure that researchers and staff are properly trained.

Additional Ethical Issues in Research with Animals

Training of Researchers in Humane Use and Care

While the housing and overall care of laboratory animals are provided by trained staff who follow specific federal guidelines, the researchers and research trainees who undertake animal work are subject to more general guidance from their individual IACUCs. Responsibility for establishing and maintaining expertise in the humane techniques necessary to perform high-quality research falls to the individual researcher, whatever his or her level of training, and to the principal investigator, who is charged with scientific and ethical oversight of the entire project. In principle, only researchers who are trained in a given procedure should use that procedure in research; for the purposes of training, the unskilled person should be appropriately supervised by someone already competent in the technique. Most IACUCs and their supervising veterinarians offer formal training in basic animal laboratory procedures and individualized training for less common techniques or new animal models. The development of new procedures should be undertaken only by persons with both the technical skills and theoretical preparation to maximize the potential for success, and even then consultation with a laboratory animal veterinarian may be warranted. Moreover, with new procedures and more common interventions, careful evaluation of mistakes and follow-up of animals with less positive outcomes may be as instructive as a traditionally defined success.

Choice of Species for Study

Choosing the appropriate animal model for a given research project is both a scientific and an ethical issue. The choice of species is determined by such practical factors as its physiological similarity to humans, suitability for housing and ease of care in laboratory facilities, purchase and upkeep costs, and the experience and preferences of the researcher, team, or institution. Ethically, the choice of species should maximize the applicability of research findings to humans in order to limit the need for intermediary animal models. The species chosen will also depend on the techniques to be used. Small animals such as mice may experience a greater physical burden from some procedures than a slightly larger animal such as a rat. However, when the animals are likely to experience significant unremediable pain or distress from a procedure, the ethical goal of using the least sentient animal models that can provide meaningful results may take precedence.

A major determinant of which species to use in research also appears to be the accepted "standard" role of certain species in human life apart from science. Dogs were once used frequently in research in many countries; today, however, they are much less common in the laboratory. In societies in which dogs are particularly valued as companion animals, their use in medical research is limited. Instead, researchers often use pigs, even though they are roughly as intelligent as dogs. Raising pigs for slaughter is already well accepted, and there seems to be little ethical distinction between medical experimentation and eating pork.

The apparent need for nonhuman primate models, such as chimpanzees and some types of monkeys, raises the issue of whether and how to use endangered species. In general, many believe that researchers should use endangered species only when no other animal can be used, and then only for research into serious threats to human life and health. Statistical analysis before the study begins should determine and clearly justify a specific number of animals needed to achieve valid results.

Source of Animals

The source of research animals depends largely on the need for healthy subjects. Thus, despite the public's fears, pound animals and wild animals, whose health may be difficult to assess, are seldom used in most types of studies. Researchers prefer animals raised by breeders whose known history limits the variables that may affect a study's outcome. However, animals raised by breeders may exhibit behavioral problems, such as high levels of stress or fear of handlers, which may be less prevalent among animals raised as pets. Proponents of using pound animals for certain studies note that doing so may save the life of two animals: the pet scheduled for euthanasia at the pound and the purpose-bred lab animal that will never be born.

Many parallels exist between raising animals to be used in research and raising animals for food or clothing and other consumer products. Typically, however, the regulation of breeding animals for consumption, environment before slaughter, and death is typically much less strict than the policies governing the breeding, use, and disposition of animals in research. Society's concern for animals in medical research appears to be greater than its interest in the welfare of animals whose products they use more directly. This concern is due in part to society's seemingly holding science and scientists to a higher level of ethical accountability than it does industry and consumers.

Creation of New Species for Research

One of the most scientifically remarkable and ethically controversial issues in genetic research is the development of genetically modified and transgenic animals. Transgenic animals are typically created to provide specialized models for the study of disease, but they are increasingly seen as a source of transplantable tissues. The creation and successful patenting of the Harvard oncomouse raised fundamental questions about property rights and the moral implication of creating new species. Before the genetic work is begun, researchers should consider how to meet the animals' need for care and stimulus as well as the possible consequences of their exposure to the natural population. Moreover, researchers should consider Caplan's contention that such animals are inherently tragic because they may be sentient but have no natural evolutionary place and no inherent purpose.

Disposition of Animals at the End of a Study

The disposition of experimental animals after they are no longer needed is an issue that the researcher or the IACUC must decide before the project begins. Regulatory standards prohibit researchers from subjecting an animal to more than one "major" surgical experiment from which it is allowed to recover, except when repeated procedures are required for scientific reasons. Such regulation presumes that the repeated use of a single animal is inhumane regardless of the methods used, and that repeated use is less ethical than the humane killing of multiple animals. Weighing the quality of life of an individual research animal against its death depends on an assessment of its likely experience of pain or distress from current and future use. The health of the animal after a procedure, together with the expected complications and stress, should provide an adequate predictive measure of the animal's future suffering. Where the suffering of one animal and several appears to be equal, the researcher and the IACUC should weigh the costs of caring for a single animal against the costs of obtaining its replacements.

   When governmental regulations do not prohibit the use of animals in more than one protocol, and when a previous protocol will not affect subsequent use, some animals may be transferred to other projects. Such a practice can reduce the number of animals sacrificed and potentially reduce economic costs. In many facilities, the adoption of research animals as pets is a common but seldom reported alternative to euthanasia. Adoption policies should consider whether the animal has medical needs that can be met outside the institution and whether it poses risk to other animals or to people. When a protocol requires the animal's death for scientific reasons, it should be killed as humanely as possible following procedures recommended by the American Veterinary Medical Association Panel on Euthanasia,[16] a portion of which is included in this section. Whenever possible, the organs and tissues of euthanized animals should be shared with researchers working with that animal model.

Conclusions

The integrity of animal research and the reputation of animal researchers depend on professional and institutional commitment to the welfare of laboratory animals. Biomedical scientists must take an active part in the public discussion and debate on animal research to ensure not only that they have a voice in related policy but also that their work is understood by critics and proponents alike. In light of the insights that pain research has provided on ethical and practical issues involved in animal research, animal researchers should be attentive to how their work may contribute to a fuller understanding of animal consciousness, purposefulness, and moral status. Animal researchers should also seek to develop alternative models wherever possible. In this complex and emotionally charged field, scientists, philosophers, and members of the lay public must ask questions and find answers together.

References

1. National Research Council, Institute of Medicine. *Use of Laboratory Animals in Biomedical and Behavioral Research.* Washington, DC: National Academy Press; 1988.
2. U.S. Congress Office of Technology Assessment, *Alternatives to Animal Use in Research, Testing, and Education.* Washington, DC: OTA; 1986.
3. Darwin C. *The Descent of Man.* London, John Murray; 1871.
4. Bernard C. *An Introduction to the Study of Experimental Medicine.* Greene H, trans. New York: Abelard–Schuman; 1867.
5. The Nuremberg Code. In: *Trials of War Criminals before Military Tribunals under Control Council Law No 10. vol 2.* Washington, DC: U.S. Government Printing Office; 1949: 181–182.
6. World Medical Association. The Declaration of Helsinki: Ethical Principles for Medical Research Involving Human Subjects. Geneva: WMA; 1964.
7. Animal Welfare Act, 1966, amended 1970, 1976, 1985, 1990, 2000; 7 U.S.C.2131–56.
8. Fraser C. Raid at Silver Spring: The case that launched the U.S. animal rights movement. *New Yorker.* 1993 (April 19):66–84.
9. Singer P. *Animal Liberation: A New Ethic for Our Treatment of Animals.* New York: Avon Books; 1975.
10. Russell WMS, Burch RL. *Principles of Humane Experimental Technique.* London: Metheun and Co. Ltd.; 1959.
11. Kitchell RL, Erickson HH, Carstens E, Davis LE, eds. *Animal Pain: Perception and Alleviation.* Bethesda, MD: American Physiological Society; 1983.
12. American College of Veterinary Anesthesiologists. Position paper on the treatment of pain in animals. *JAVMA* 1998;213:628–630.
13. American Association for Laboratory Animal Science. Position statement: Recognition and alleviation of pain and distress in laboratory animals. Memphis, TN: AALAS, 2000.
14. National Research Council, Institute of Medicine. *Guide for the Care and Use of Laboratory Animals.* Washington, DC: National Academy Press; 1996.
15. Howard-Jones N. A CIOMS Ethical Code for Animal Experimentation. *WHO Chronicle* 1985;39:51–56.
16. American Veterinary Medical Association Panel on Euthanasia. Report of the AVMA Panel on Euthanasia. *J Am Vet Assoc.* 2001;218:669–696.

Beastly Conduct

Ethical Issues in Animal Experimentation

Arthur L. Caplan

The Legitimacy of Means and the Legitimacy of Ends in Animal Experimentation

There has been a great deal of argument in recent years over the subject of animal experimentation. Few topics are able to elicit the degree of moral vehemence and passion that this topic does. Accusations of moral blindness fly back and forth between vivisectionists and antivivisectionists. Bills are submitted almost willy-nilly at both the federal and state level, lobbying efforts on both sides of the issue are best described as fierce, and the disputants seem to delight in holding meetings and conferences at which their opponents are persona non grata – on both sides opponents are rarely invited, and, if they somehow manage to appear, they are made the object of calumny usually reserved only for criminals or even politicians (12).

Despite the political and sociological vortex surrounding the issue of animal experimentation, it would be wrong for those on either side to underestimate the sincerity and thoughtfulness that can underlie much of the noise and rhetoric characteristic of current public debates over the issue. In recent years a rather rich philosophical literature (10,11) has developed on the subject of the moral responsibilities of human beings toward animals, and this literature surely must be reckoned with by all parties to the debate. Just as it is wrong to suppose that all vivisectionists are callous brutes, unconcerned about the effects of their work on their animal subjects, it is also wrong to assume that all antivivisectionists are misanthropic kooks who are too emotionally unstable to recognize the benefits that derive from research involving animals.

Before considering some of the moral questions that arise in the context of the practice of experimentation involving animals, it is important to make a distinction between two issues that are often conflated by parties on both sides of the issue. Oftentimes scientists go to great lengths to demonstrate to each other and the general public that they take every possible precaution to assure the humane treatment of any animals that may be used for experimental purposes. Scientists often note with pride that they have, through their own voluntary efforts, established clear codes of conduct about the care and handling

The author wishes to acknowledge De Anti-Vivisectie Stichting of The Netherlands for the opportunity to present some of the material in this paper in a series of lectures at the Universities of Leiden, Groningen, Wachningen, Nijmegen, and the Free University of Amsterdam; Corrie Smid, Eleanor Seiling, Janet Caplan, and Peter Singer for helpful conversations regarding many of the ideas presented in this paper; and the support of the Marilyn M. Simpson Charitable Income Trust in preparing this paper.

From *Annals of the New York Academy of Science*, 1983, 406, pp. 159–169. Reproduced with permission.

of laboratory animals. Moreover, most reputable scientists in America and other nations go to great lengths to minimize, through the use of anesthetics, anesthesia, and other means, the pain or suffering that animals endure as a result of the process of experimentation.

The many efforts now made to reduce animal suffering and to ensure the proper care and handling of animals used for research purposes are often brought forward in response to criticisms leveled by antivivisectionists concerning the enterprise of animal research. Unfortunately, persons who question the moral legitimacy of animal experimentation are not likely to be dissuaded from their view by demonstrations of the care and concern shown by those engaged in the practice.

There are really two issues involved in thinking about research involving animals and questions of humane care are pertinent only to one of them – (1) is it morally legitimate to conduct research upon animals?; (2) if it is morally permissible to utilize animals for research purposes, what moral responsibilities must be discharged by those engaged in such research? Questions on what conduct constitutes humane care, guidelines on the handling and transport of animal subjects, and efforts to teach students and professionals techniques that will minimize animal suffering and pain consequent to research interventions are all only relevant to the question of professional duty within the research context. However, before these issues can be usefully discussed, it is necessary to examine the prior question of whether it is morally justifiable to conduct any research on animals. For if the answer to this question is no, then no amount of guidelines, restraint, educational effort, or codified standards will suffice in response to criticisms of the activity.

The Major Areas of Contention Concerning the Moral Legitimacy of Animal Research

If one reviews the various public pronouncements (1,3,6,7,10,12) made about the issue of animal experimentation by parties on both sides of the issue, it quickly becomes evident that there exist three major areas of dispute. First, there is a good deal of disagreement about the need to conduct any research upon animals. Second, there is much disagreement about the moral value to be assigned to animals. Much of the attention to issues of animal sentience and consciousness in debates about the ethics of animal research are spin-offs from this issue since the more animals are felt to possess mental powers equivalent to or closely resembling those possessed by humans, the more various people feel disposed to assign moral worth to such creatures. Third, there is a good deal of tacit or between-the-lines argument about the moral priority that ought be accorded the whole issue of the ethics of animal experimentation. Many persons admit that the question of the legitimacy of animal experimentation is a vexing one, but there is no agreement over whether the topic is one that ought to command wide public attention and legislative concern. Other issues, such as human starvation, malnutrition, war, crime, poverty and the like are felt, oftentimes, to deserve precedence over the fates of animals in research laboratories (12).

It is interesting to compare and contrast the positions taken by the "pro" and "anti" vivisection camps on these three major issues. To some degree some of the stereotyping and caterwauling so characteristic of disputes over this issue can be defused by a little reflection over the stances adopted by the parties to the debate on the major question surrounding the legitimacy of the research enterprise.

The Provivisection Point of View

Need

Provivisectionists argue that it is ludicrous to talk at the present time about the complete replacement or elimination of animals from the context of experimentation. If human health and well-being are to be improved, if human safety is to be assured in both medical and non-medical contexts, and if human knowledge is to advance, then some amount of animal experimentation must be conducted. It is simply not possible, given our present knowledge, to utilize alternatives to animals and simultaneously maintain publicly acceptable levels of human health and well-being. In part, this is due to the fact that testing chemicals or pharmaceutical substances on cells or other limited organic systems fails to capture the complexities involved in the processing of such substances by whole organisms. The pursuit of such universally recognized human goods, as health, safety, and knowledge, requires that some animals be utilized in research contexts.

Moral Equality

Most provivisectionists do not accept the equation of animals and humans as entities deserving of equal moral consideration and concern. Some believe that animals do not suffer or feel pain in ways analogous to that experienced by human beings, and, thus, do not deserve the same sort of protections and considerations as human beings do in experimental settings. Others favoring vivisection simply see human beings and their goals and purposes as more worthy of moral respect than the goals and purposes of members of the animal kingdom. Thus, the general health of human beings or the welfare of any specific individual human being counts for far more, in their view, than the well-being or health of any single animal or groups of animals. This view is reflected in the fact that scientists will often comment to each other in private that they have actually heard some antivivisectionists say that they would rather one baby be used for experimental purposes than one thousand rats. Such statements are held up as exemplifying the moral blindness of those who would equate animal welfare with human welfare.

Priority

Many persons involved with or supportive of the use of animals in experimental studies find it hard to believe that so much energy, money, and time is devoted to this issue by opponents of such practices. They note that there is plenty of misery about in both the human and animal kingdoms and that antivivisectionists might better devote their frenetic energies to obviating the many other clear injustices that exist in the world. Why, it is sometimes asked, don't antivivisectionists attempt to stop such practices as pet abuse, hunting, or meat-eating rather than focus as they do on animal research? The numbers of animals who suffer at the hands of humans are surely greater in these other contexts, and these would therefore seem to be more appropriate places for political and legislative intervention by those concerned with animal welfare.

The Antivivisectionist Point of View

Need

Antivivisectionists believe that while it may be true that not all animal experimentation can be abolished (some believe that all could), it is nevertheless true that far more could be eliminated than is presently the case. They argue that there exist many techniques for replacing animals in experiments, including cellular studies, computer simulations, and careful field studies upon animals in natural settings. Moreover, they argue, even more could be done in the way of replacement and reduction in the number of animals used in scientific research but for the pernicious influence of the animal breeding industry, which has no obvious interest in seeing animal experimentation curbed or in developing suitable substitutes for whole live animals. Antivivisectionists see the continued and ongoing reliance of scientists upon animal studies as the natural outcome of an economic and political situation in which various parties have powerful vested interests in assuring the continuance of the status quo with regard to animal research.

It should also be noted that while most opponents of animal research do not challenge the legitimacy of such goals as the assurance of human health and safety or the advancement of human knowledge, they find defenses of animal research couched in terms of these broad social goals inadequate. First, they argue, it is not clear that human knowledge is likely to be advanced by the kinds of studies and experiments to which animals are currently put by scientists. There is simply too much waste, replication, and redundancy in scientific experimentation to justify the toll imposed on animals in the name of advancing scientific knowledge. Second, it is not clear that human health is always advanced by animal research since ultimately all drugs and procedures must be tried on humans anyway.

More importantly, they note, a good deal of animal experimentation is conducted in order to assure the American consumer a suitable range of cosmetics, toiletries, and other aesthetic paraphernalia. These are hardly indispensable aspects of human existence, and the antivivisectionists have been quick to note that safety with regard to perfumes and underarm deodorants is hardly an awe-inspiring moral imperative when assessing the legitimacy of the animal sacrifices involved in order to attain safety with regard to these frivolous ends.

Moral Equality

Sophisticated critics of the entire enterprise of animal research argue that science itself is in many ways responsible for skepticism about the acceptability of animal research. While there have existed strong traditions within both science and religion committed to the view that animals are nothing more than dumb brutes or automata, the fact is that scientific research has, over the years, revealed essential similarities between humans and animals with respect to many physical and mental properties. Surely, such critics note, we know enough about the physiology, neurology and behavioral capacities of higher vertebrates to make us realize that these creatures can feel pain, can suffer, and that they ought not be treated any differently than we would treat any human being endowed with such capacities and traits. There is an implicit demand for consistency behind much of the antivivisectionist opposition to research on animals – what we would not dream of doing to a child, a fetus, a newborn, a demented person, a retarded person, a senile person, a comatose person, or a dead person, we ought not dream of doing to a sentient animal.

The argument from consistency does not commit the antivivisectionist to the equation of animals and humans in terms of their moral worth. Rather, the view held by most antivivisectionists is that animals have the minimal properties capable of conferring moral standing upon an entity – sentience, consciousness, or the capacity to feel pain. These properties, or some one of them, seem sufficient for according moral status to animals. Animals and humans both possess, on this view, minimally sufficient attributes for becoming the objects of moral concern. Both kinds of organisms satisfy minimal requirements for being valued, and in this sense they ought be viewed as of equal moral worth.

Priority

While antivivisectionists argue that animals and humans are equal in terms of their both possessing capacities that qualify them for moral concern and respect, antivivisectionists give a higher priority to the need to attend to animal suffering than do many proponents of research. The primary reason that seems to motivate the view that animal suffering deserves our legislative and regulatory attention is that animals are not in a position to avoid the types of suffering they encounter in the laboratory. While it is true that animals cause each other harm in nature, the fact remains that the sorts of suffering they often encounter in research settings is entirely due to the activities of human beings. Human beings, thus, are responsible for inflicting an additional measure of pain and suffering upon creatures who are unable to protect themselves against these evils. While human beings can, assumedly, avoid at least some of the pain and misery they inflict on their fellows in various situations, animals in laboratories cannot and thus possess a special claim to human moral attention because they are so utterly dependent on humans for alleviating the suffering they encounter.

The Issue of Moral Equality

Having presented the basic outlines of the dispute about animal experimentation, the rest of this essay will focus on the thorny question of the moral worth of animals and humans. For, if it is true that at least some partisans on both sides of the issue are in basic agreement that human health, well-being, and safety are desirable goods and that the production of human knowledge that promotes these ends is also good, then it would seem that the real issue dividing "pro" and "anti" vivisectionists is the degree to which sacrifices and concessions have to be made with regard to these goods in order to promote animal well-being and decrease animal suffering. Both the level of priority accorded the enterprise of animal experimentation as a moral question and the zeal with which alternatives to animal use are pursued pivot around the degree to which animals are seen as worthy of moral concern. The moral equality of animals and humans is thus the crucial issue dividing the two sides in current disputes, and it is this question which merits close, critical scrutiny if any progress is to be made toward settling the issue.

Much of the basis for the belief that animals and humans have an equal claim to moral consideration arises from an awareness of recent history in the discipline of ethics (11). During the past two hundred years or so, many human beings have come to realize that differences in sex, race, ethnic group, or sexual preference are not relevant properties for excluding individuals from the moral realm. The recent popularity of the story of the

Elephant Man in the movies and on Broadway derives in part from the message conveyed by the leading character of the play, John Merrick, that despite his deformed and even ghastly appearance, he is still a person worthy of moral concern and respect. Physical form and appearance are not in themselves reasons for excluding someone or even something from the sphere of our moral concern. Thus, while animals are certainly different in their shape, form, and physical appearance from human beings, these differences are not in themselves sufficient for establishing a relevant moral difference between animals and humans any more than are the various shapes, colors, and sizes of human beings.

Some persons have turned to other criteria besides physical differences for distinguishing between the moral worth of animals and humans. Reason, language, intentionality, self-awareness, and a sense of personal identity have all been suggested as properties possessed by humans which distinguish them from animals with respect to their moral worth (2). But there are problems in using these properties as a basis for distinguishing animals from humans concerning moral worth. Many human beings lack some or all of the aforementioned properties. Certainly fetuses, comatose persons, and dead persons can be said to lack all of them. Yet, we do not feel free to do as we please with individuals who are in one of these categories of humanhood. It is also the case that the mental powers of many humans are, at various times, often severely impaired or entirely absent, i.e. when they are asleep, under the influence of drugs, etc., and yet we do not believe that the moral worth of such persons evaporates with the temporary disappearance of their mental powers.

Nor is it evident that animals lack the capacities and abilities to manifest some or all of the mental properties often held to distinguish man and beast. There is a voluminous literature in ethology and comparative psychology that indicates that at least some animals are capable of primitive forms of reasoning, intentionality, language, and self-awareness (1,3,5). Certainly enough evidence has accumulated in the behavioral and biological sciences to cast suspicions on claims for the complete absence of higher mental states and abilities in the animal world. Given the uncertainty surrounding the question of animal awareness, it seems reasonable, in light of what we know about other similarities and commonalities between humans and animals, to err in the direction of commonality when in doubt until definitive evidence can be produced – that what has proven true with regard to genetic, morphological, physiological, biochemical, and anatomical properties is not true with respect to mental properties.

Given the fact that not all humans always possess fully developed mental powers and the likely circumstance that at least some animals do, there would appear to be no basis for drawing a hard and fast line between animals and humans in terms of physical or mental properties. What is important about this claim is that the moral worth of entities does seem linked in important ways to abilities and capacities to suffer, feel pain, or have their goals and purposes frustrated. While it is evident that bodily form or physical appearance are unimportant in deciding whether one ought to be concerned about the welfare of another creature, it is true that certain properties must be presumed if talk about welfare is to make any sense. The ability to feel pain, to suffer anxiety or stress, and the capacity to have one's desires, purposes, or intentions frustrated, all seem to be grounds for speaking meaningfully about the welfare of something. If a creature can experience pain, then, other things being equal, it certainly seems wrong to inflict pain on that creature. Similarly, if an organism, be it human or animal, seeks to fulfill some purpose or end – to drink some water, return home, to rest – it seems wrong (again, other things being equal) to frustrate such desires or purposes.

Sentience and purposiveness seem to be the kinds of properties that confer moral worth on creatures. Any entity, human or non-human, terrestrial or nonterrestrial, that could reasonably be said to possess sentience or purpose seems to be the sort of thing to which it is reasonable to attribute moral worth (4,6). Unless some reason can be given for interfering with or hindering a creature so endowed, it seems inherently wrong to inflict pain on a sentient entity or to frustrate the purposes and goals of such a creature.

It is with respect to the properties of sentience or purposiveness that humans and animals can be said to be of equal moral worth. Most humans and many animals seem to possess some degree of sentience. They are alert to stimuli and will seek those they find pleasant and attempt to avoid those they find noxious. Many animals and most humans seem to harbor any number of desires, aspirations, intentions, and purposes as can be inferred from the efforts they will make to attain certain goals or to overcome certain obstacles that may stand between them and the objects of their desires. While the issue of sentience and purposiveness is in part a scientific question, at least with regard to the distribution and degree of such properties in the biological world, there would seem to be good reasons for thinking that these properties represent excellent candidates for conferring moral worth upon entities (4).

It should be noted that in arguing that sentience and purposiveness are sufficient properties for attributing moral worth to an entity, this does not mean that both or either property is necessary for having moral worth. Creatures may someday be found on this or other planets that lack these traits, but possess still others that might make them objects of our moral respect. Moreover, the fact that an entity possesses sentience or purposiveness only satisfies the minimal conditions requisite for having moral worth. It may be possible to distinguish further among various creatures as to which ones have more or higher degrees of these salient features. It would surely be a logical error to infer from the fact that animals meet minimal conditions for having moral worth that there are no relevant differences with respect to these properties that distinguish humans and animals – for example, few animals will modify their behavior toward other animals as a result of reading this paper, while it is possible that some human beings may do so.

If it is true that the existence of sentience and/or purposiveness are sufficient traits for imputing moral worth to someone/something, then it would seem there exists what philosophers term *prima facie* duties (2,9) that ought be exercised toward such creatures. Unless one can justify the behavior by an appeal to some higher moral reason or purpose, it would be wrong to harm or frustrate any creature, including an animal, for no reason. Perhaps the cruelest or meanest activity that humans can engage in is the harming or frustrating of others, human and animal, for no reason other than simple meanness of spirit. In some ways human beings are actually in a better position than minimally endowed animals to cope with the frustration and pain of being deceived, fooled, hindered, tricked, or duped since humans are at least bright enough to occasionally figure out what is going on and take steps to avoid or end their suffering. Animals, confronted with malevolent owners or mischievous children, are competent enough to serve as the objects of malevolent intentions (as the pet owners or children know all too well), but are not competent enough to avoid or evade their plight.

It is important to distinguish between an entity's having moral worth, a status I have argued derives from the properties of sentience and purposiveness, and an entity's being a moral agent. Or, in other words, to distinguish between being a moral object and a moral agent. It is true that many animals and some humans lack all of the properties of mentation we commonly associate with *Homo sapiens*. It would be ludicrous to think that we could hold all animals and humans morally responsible for their actions or that we should expect moral reciprocity from any creature capable of sentience and purpose. What is sufficient in terms of properties that concern moral worth or standing is hardly sufficient in terms of properties that confer moral agency and moral responsibility. We need not determine the nature of the properties that would be sufficient for establishing moral competence among creatures (although it is interesting to note that historically not a few animals have been punished by their owners and even by courts as liable for the untoward outcomes of their behavior!) in this paper. All that need be noted is that the class of moral agents is far smaller than the class of moral objects, and that arguments about the moral equality of animals and humans concern the latter status and not the former.

Sentience and Purposiveness as Criteria of Moral Worth

I have argued thus far that both sentience and purposiveness seem to me to be properties sufficient for conferring moral worth on entities who possess them. However, I have not faced the question of whether these properties must both be present, or whether either one of them is sufficient by itself for establishing moral worth. Since moral considerableness entails a number of responsibilities on human agents in terms of their not harming or interfering with creatures that have moral worth, it is important to look carefully at these two properties to see whether they are independent and individually adequate for conferring moral worth.

In recent arguments about the ethics of animal experimentation, some philosophers (10,11), notably and most vocally Peter Singer in his book *Animal Liberation*, have argued for the sufficiency of sentience as a property for conferring moral worth upon entities. Singer presents a four-part argument in this book that runs as follows: (1) Any creature that is sentient has an interest in not suffering and not feeling pain; (2) all interests must be taken into account in deciding how we ought to behave; (3) equal interests in not suffering or experiencing pain must be counted equally; (4) we should act to bring about the greatest amount of good and to minimize suffering and pain. Thus, if animals can suffer and feel pain as a result of being sentient, Singer argues we must treat them impartially in assessing the practice of animal experimentation. What counts is not only the degree to which human safety is assured and human health promoted, but the degree to which animal suffering is exacerbated by experimental procedures. We should not engage in any particular experiment where the degree of suffering or pain produced in sentient creatures is not outweighed by the amount of benefit to be produced for other sentient creatures, animal and human.

Singer's position is one of classical utilitarianism – the costs and benefits of every action must be computed as best as can be done and decisions about the acceptability or non-acceptability of any action or practice turn on the beliefs we have about the overall effects of the action or practice in terms of goods versus suffering produced. In most cases, Singer argues (11), animal experiments fail to be justifiable since, given animal sentience, the degree of suffering involved cannot, with certainty, be predicted to be outweighed by the goods to be obtained by engaging in any given case of animal experimentation. Since we should be impartial as to the source of suffering when it occurs, animals and humans being equally deserving of moral consideration when they are capable of suffering or feeling pain, we ought to modify our current experimental practices accordingly and drastically decrease the use of animals in research.

The difficulties confronting Singer's criterion of sentience and his four-part argument are many (9,10). For example, it is not clear that most scientists would disagree with the claim that human benefit ought outweigh animal suffering if animal experimentation is to be morally legitimated (12). Indeed, as critics of Singer's view point out, the issue of how much suffering is caused by animal experiments is an empirical question and it is not clear that the benefits do outweigh the harms in assessing most cases of animal research.

More seriously, Singer's argument against animal experiment founders on two other issues. First, his position would seem to permit experimentation on any creatures which cannot, for whatever reason, suffer or feel pain. Thus, if we can make animal experimentation, or human experimentation for that matter, pain-free, we would appear to be justified in conducting research that would produce benefits in terms of health, well-being, safety, or knowledge. Also, if we could produce vast benefits to animals or humans by utilizing only a few animals or humans in painful experiments, this practice would also escape moral condemnation since, on Singer's construction of the argument, it is only the net outcome of experimentation that legitimates the activity.

I suspect that sentience and the corresponding ability it confers upon animals to suffer or feel pain is a bit too lofty a standard to invoke in thinking about the question of moral worth. It seems wrong to treat humans or animals who are incapable of suffering or feeling pain as underserving of moral respect and consideration. For example, even if a human being were rendered unable to feel pain or to suffer by surgical intervention or through the use of drugs, I doubt whether members of our society would want to say that such persons could then be used in any way scientists deemed useful in the process of research.

It is interesting to note that Singer's view, while popular in antivivisectionist circles these days, does not lead to the view that all animal experimentation is wrong. Nor does it lead to the view that animals have rights – a concept that is antithetical to a utilitarian analysis of moral worth. However, if we look to purposiveness and intentionality rather than sentience and the ability to suffer as the standard of moral worth, I think we come closer to locating the kind of criterion that motivates much of the moral concern about animal experimentation.

If animals and humans are so organized as to be purposive creatures with various desires, drives, intentions, and aspirations, it seems wrong to cavalierly frustrate these purposes. It might be argued that if animals and humans are biologically constituted so as to pursue their own existence, which is a fact quite consistent with current thinking in evolutionary theory, then it is morally wrong to interfere with or deprive animals of the opportunity to fulfill this basic drive. In other words, animals and humans, endowed by nature with a will to survive, have a right to survive – rights being consequent upon the purposiveness and teleological orientation of living things (9). If all creatures who possess purposiveness have a right to be left alone to pursue their ends, then the basic moral repugnance felt by many people about animal experimentation can be easily understood – most experimentation deprives animals of the right to exist, or, at minimum, frustrates certain basic drives and intentions they manifest. While human beings are under no moral obligation to aid their fellows or animals in the pursuit of their basic purposes, they do appear to be under some constraint not to uncaringly interfere with other organisms.

I believe that purposiveness rather than sentience is a property that suffices for conferring moral worth upon entities. When organisms have sufficient organization to have basic drives, desires, and intentions, be they amoebas, bees, birds, or retarded humans, it is wrong to interfere with their efforts to fulfill these desires. It needs to be quickly added that such interference is wrong unless there exists some other reason or justification for doing so. The fact is that, as is the case with the abortion debate, most persons erroneously believe that once animal rights are established, the issue of animal experimentation is settled (2). If it is wrong to interfere with purposive creatures, then no animal research could ever be morally legitimate. But such a view confuses the question of how moral worth and moral rights arise with the question of what to do when rights conflict – a common, ordinary, and unavoidable consequence of the nature of the world we live in.

No animals or humans capable of purposiveness should be interfered with by others, other things being equal. But other things are rarely equal. If humans are to survive, they must eat, and animals may have to suffer the consequences. If human beings are to fulfill their desires to have medicines, then some creatures will have to suffer in the course of discovering whether different substances have therapeutic value. While it is true that we ought not interfere with or hinder the bringing to fruition of the desires and purposes of others, animals and humans, in a world of limited resources and conflicting purposes, some creatures will, of necessity, have their basic rights overridden.

The Legitimacy of Animal Experimentation Reconsidered

It should be evident from the preceding discussion that science has no one to blame but itself for the existence of worries about the ethics of animal experimentation. Science has shown the degree to which sentience and purposiveness permeate the animal kingdom, and thus has raised doubts about the validity of causing harm to or interfering with creatures who may not differ all that much from human beings in the properties that count from a moral point of view. If sentience or, minimally, purposiveness are sufficient for conferring moral worth on things, and if we are to be consistent in our moral practices and beliefs, then we may have to rethink our ordinary attitudes about the legitimacy of animal experimentation.

Perhaps the strongest caveat to emerge from an analysis of the morality of animal research is that the burden of proof always rests upon the experimenter to justify the use of animals in experimental contexts. The antivivisectionist has nothing to prove; many animals used in experiments are sentient and purposive, and thus have *prima facie* rights to live and be left alone. Those who would override or abrogate these rights must provide compelling reasons for doing so. Humility and sensitivity, not arrogance and hubris, must be the hallmarks of animal research since it is only out of ignorance and expediency that we put members of the animal kingdom to our purposes rather than theirs.

The other conclusion that follows from the analysis of the moral legitimacy of animal experimentation is that such activity is always morally tragic. No matter what goods are promoted by the process, some creatures who are unable to alter their circumstances will have their basic rights of life and fulfillment infringed. Since this is so, it would seem imperative that steps be taken to reduce waste and duplication in the use of animals for research purposes, put more funds toward the development of alternatives to animal testing, and make the public aware of the moral trade-offs that must be faced in deciding how best to achieve human well-being, health, safety, and knowledge at the expense of animal suffering. Ultimately, the public will have to decide what sorts of trade-offs are morally acceptable when animal and human interests conflict.

References

1. Bowd, A. D. 1980. Ethical reservations about psychological research with animals. Psychol. Rec. **30**(Spring): 201–210.
2. Caplan, A. L. 1978. Rights language and the ethical treatment of animals. *In* Implications of History and Ethics to Medicine – Veterinary and Human. L. McCullough & J. P. Morris, Eds.: 126–135. Texas A&M University Press. College Station, Tex.
3. Fox, M. S. 1981. Experimental psychology, animal rights, welfare and ethics. Psychopharm. Bull. **17**(2): 80–84.
4. Goodpaster, K. E. 1978. On being morally considerable. J. Phil. **76**(6): 308–324.
5. Griffin, D. R. 1976. The Question of Animal Awareness. Rockefeller University Press. New York.
6. Hoff, C. 1980. Immoral and moral uses of animals. N. Eng. J. Med. **302**(2): 115–118.
7. Morris, R. K. & M. W. Fox, Eds. 1978. On the Fifth Day: Animal Rights and Human Ethics. Acropolis Books. Washington, D. C.
8. Passmore, J. 1976. Man's Responsibility For Nature. Scribner's. New York.
9. Regan, T. 1980. Animal rights, human wrongs. Environ. Ethics **2**(2): 99–120.
10. Regan, T. & P. Singer, Eds. 1976. Animal Rights and Human Obligations. Prentice-Hall. Englewood Cliffs, N.J.
11. Singer, P. 1975. Animal Liberation. Avon Books. New York.
12. Visscher, M. B. 1979. Animal rights and alternative methods. The Pharos (Fall): 11–19.

Recognition and Alleviation of Pain and Distress in Laboratory Animals

American Association for Laboratory Animal Science

Background

The *Animal Welfare Act* mandates that Institutional Animal Care and Use Committees (IACUCs) oversee the care and use of animals covered by the *Act*. IACUCs are composed of scientists, veterinarians and at least one public member. They must assess warm-blooded animal research protocols to determine if (1) proposed animal use is essential for achieving relevant scientific goals, (2) the appropriate species have been selected, (3) the number of animals requested is properly justified, (4) the care of animals is appropriate, (5) provision for alleviating pain or distress is appropriate, and (6) alternatives to studies that might cause pain or distress have been sought.[1] The Public Health Service (PHS) *Policy on Humane Care and Use of Laboratory Animals* (which implements the *Health Research Extension Act* of 1985 and the *U.S. Government Principles for the Utilization and Care of Vertebrate Animals used in Testing, Research, and Training*) adopts a similar position that is applicable to all vertebrate animal research protocols.[2]

The *Animal Welfare Act* is administered by the U.S. Department of Agriculture (USDA), whereas the PHS *Policy* is administered and coordinated by the Office of Laboratory Animal Welfare (OLAW, formerly the Office for Protection from Research Risks).[3] These agencies, the laws and policies they administer, highly respected voluntary programs, such as the Association for Assessment and Accreditation of Laboratory Animal Care (AAALAC) International,[4] and local IACUCs provide effective, comprehensive assessment and monitoring to assure humane animal care and use.

A significant provision of the *Animal Welfare Act* requires that institutions provide an annual report indicating the number of covered species used in the following categories:[5]

Category C – animals in which procedures caused no pain or distress:

Category D – animals in which pain and distress during procedures was appropriately relieved by pain- or distress-relieving drugs;

Category E – animals involved in procedures which cause pain or distress that was not relieved by drugs for scientific reasons.

Animal use reported in Category E must be accompanied by an explanation and justification as to why drugs to relieve pain and distress were withheld. This information is readily accessible to the public through the *Freedom of Information Act*.[6]

The current USDA reporting categories have been in use for many years and would benefit from revision and expansion to improve their utility. Many IACUCs have recognized that the USDA system is outdated and have developed categories pertaining to the extent of pain and distress that are more accurate and informative. The USDA is currently reviewing policy pertaining to the annual report, which is a welcome initiative. However, it appears that potential revisions may not address the major limitation of the current categories: inadequate discrimination regarding the intensity or duration of pain or distress. In fact, they may further reduce the accuracy of reporting by increasing assignment to Category E of animals that experience mild or questionable pain or distress. It will be unfortunate if the policy revision misses the opportunity to improve reporting categories.

Issues

- The evaluation of potential pain or distress is complex because thresholds and manifestations of pain and distress vary among species and among individuals within a species.[7]
- The determination of what constitutes pain or distress in animals is further complicated by the fact that there are no universally agreed upon criteria for assessing for determining what is, or is not, painful or distressful to an animal.
- The alleviation of pain and distress is often a diverse task that may require drugs, adjustments to environmental enrichment, modifications in research protocols and other appropriate and humane strategies.[8]
- Pain and distress and the methods used to alleviate them, may interfere with research results.[9]
- The USDA categories for reporting pain and distress and measures to alleviate them are not optimally informative and potential policy changes may make them even less so.[10]

Positions

- Laboratory animal veterinarians and other animal caregivers have a legal *and* moral obligation to alleviate pain and distress in laboratory animals.[11]
- The complex nature of modern animal experimentation implies the need to report animal use accurately. Therefore, current USDA categories should be revised and expanded to facilitate more precise and informative reporting. Furthermore, annual reporting of animal use should be the responsibility of the IACUC in conjunction with assessment and monitoring by a qualified veterinarian.
- Alternatives to animal use in biomedical research should be sought. However, once a request to use animals has been made and approved, experiments should be performed as humanely as possible and with as few animals as possible.
- IACUCs must ensure that all personnel involved in the care and use of animals are adequately trained. Training should include concepts and methods to recognize pain and distress in laboratory animals and to alleviate them or seek assistance in doing so. This process will raise staff awareness regarding humane treatment and will improve the quality and documentation of monitoring.
- Qualified veterinarians should be involved in the design, monitoring and documentation of experiments that have the potential to cause more than momentary pain and distress to laboratory animals. The anticipated pain or distress level should be categorized and assigned during IACUC protocol review and monitored prospectively. The assignment

should be reviewed at appropriate intervals and changes may be recommended after additional observation and prior to submission of the USDA Annual Report.

- Conditioning and monitoring of research animals should be designed prospectively. The corresponding schedules should indicate the frequency of observation and responsibilities of monitoring and laboratory personnel. In addition, correct doses of appropriate anesthetics, analgesics and tranquilizers should be selected pre-emptively by the principal investigator in consultation with the veterinarian. Possible outcomes (endpoints) should be discussed among the veterinarian, the investigator, and other laboratory personnel listed in a given protocol.

- Potentially painful or distressful procedures should be closely monitored by the animal health care staff and appropriate treatment instituted. New or novel procedures that may be painful should initially be performed under veterinary surveillance or supervision. Analgesics should be administered pre-emptively for known potentially painful procedures.

- Death should be avoided as an endpoint for animal experiments. Alternatives such as behavioral changes, fluctuations in body temperature, body condition, and weight-loss patterns should be sought and implemented.[12]

- More research is needed on the assessment and alleviation of pain and distress to optimize the humane treatment of laboratory animals. The scientific and moral priorities inherent to animal research emphasize why such research is essential.

References

1. **Animal Welfare Act** (7 U.S.C. §§ 2131 et. seq.) *http://www.nal.usda.gov/awic/legislat/awa.htm*
   Code of Federal Regulations Title 9, Volume 1, Part 2, § 2.31 [Revised as of January 1, 2000] *http://www.access.gpo.gov/nara/cfr/waisidx 00/9cfrv1 00.html*
2. **Health Research Extension Act.** P.L 99–158. November 20. 1985 "Animals in Research" *http://grants.nih.gov/grants/olaw/references/hrea1985.htm*
   Interagency Research Animal Committee (IRAC). Federal Register; May 20, 1985. *http://grants.nih.gov/grants/olaw/references/phspol.htm # principle*
   Public Health Service Policy on Humane Care and Use of Laboratory Animals (Revised September, 1986, Reprinted March, 1996) *http://grants.nih.gov/grants/olaw/references/phspol.htm*
3. **USDA-APHIS Home page:** *http://www.aphis.usda.gov/reac/awainfo.html*
   OLAW Home page: *http://grants.nih.gov/grants/olaw/olaw.htm*
4. **AAALAC mission statement:** *http://www.aaalac.org/html/about.html*
5. **Code of Federal Regulations Title 9, Volume 1, Part 2, § 2.36** [Revised as of January 1, 2000] *http://www.access.gpo.gov/nara/cfr/waisidx 00/9cfrv1 00.html*
   US Department of Agriculture, APHIS, Animal Care Division. Policy #11 – Painful/Distressful Procedures – April 14, 1997. *http://www.aphis.usda.gov/ac/policy11.html*
6. **Animal and Plant Health Inspection Service Freedom of Information Act (FOIA) Home Page:** *https://foia.aphis.usda.gov/*
7. **Dennis SG and R Melzack.** 1983. Perspectives on phylogenetic evolution of pain expression. In Animal Pain: Perception and Alleviation. RL Kitchell and HH Erickson, eds. American Physiological Society. Bethesda, MD, pages 151–160.
   Hughes HC and CM Lang. 1983. Control of pain in dogs and cats. In Animal Pain: Perception and Alleviation. RL Kitchell and HH Erickson, eds. American Physiological Society. Bethesda, MD, pages 207–216.

Morton DB and HM Griffiths. 1985. Guidelines on the recognition of pain, distress and discomfort in experimental animals and a hypothesis for assessment. Vet Record 116(16):431–436.

Morton DB. 1986. Assessment of pain (Letter). Vet Record 119(17):435.

Spinelli JS and H Markowitz. 1987. Clinical recognition and anticipation of situations likely to induce suffering in animals. JAVMA 191(10):1216–1218.

National Research Council. 1992. Recognition and Alleviation of Pain and Distress in Laboratory Animals. Committee on pain and distress in laboratory animals. ILAR. National Academy Press. Washington, D.C., Chapter 4, pages 32–52.

FELASA Working Group on Pain and Distress. 1994. Pain and distress in laboratory rodents and lagomorphs. Laboratory Animals 28:97–112.

American College of Veterinary Anesthesiologists. 1998. Position paper on the treatment of pain in animals. JAVMA 213(5):55–57.

8. **Wolfle TL.** 1987. Control of stress using non-drug approaches. JAVMA 191(10):1219–1221.

Flecknell PA. 1996. Laboratory Animal Anesthesia: A Practical Introduction for Research Workers and Technicians. Academic Press; ISBN: 0122603613.

9. **Loew FM.** 1987. The challenge of balancing experimental variables: pain, distress, analgesia and anesthesia. JAVMA 191(10):1193–1194.

Benson GJ and JC Thurmon. 1987. Species differences as a consideration in alleviation of animal pain and distress. JAVMA 191(10):1227–1230.

10. **The Humane Society of the United States.** 2000. U.S. Humane Society challenges scientists to end research animal pain and distress by 2020. Press release 27 April.

11. **Morton DB.** 1985. Pain and Laboratory animals (Letter). Nature 317:106, 12 Sept.

Code of Federal Regulations Title 9, Volume 1, Part 2, § 2.31 d. [Revised as of January 1, 2000] *http://www.access.gpo.gov/nara/cfr/waisidx 00/9cfrv1 00.html*

National Research Council. Guide for the Care and Use of Laboratory Animals (Guide). ILAR. National Academy Press. Washington, D.C. 1996: Chapter 3, pages 64–65.

12. **Redgate ES; M Deutsch; SS Boggs.** 1991. Time of death of CNS tumor-bearing rats can be reliably predicted by body weight-loss patterns. Lab Anim Sci. 41(3):269–273.

Wong JP; Saravolac EG; Clement JG; Nagata LP. 1997. Development of a murine hypothermia model for study of respiratory tract influenza virus infection. Lab Anim Sci. 47(2):143–147 April.

Ullman-Cullere MH; CJ. Foltz. 1999. Body condition scoring: a rapid and accurate method for assessing health status in mice. Lab Anim Sci. 49(3):319–323.

Krarup A, P Chattopadhyay, AK Bhattacharjee, JR Burge and GR Ruble. 1999. Evaluation of surrogate markers of impending death in the galactosamine-sensitized murine model of bacterial endotoxemia. Lab Anim Science 49(5):545–550.

Vlach KD, JW Boles and BG Stiles. 2000. Telemetric evaluation of body temperature and physical activity as predictors of mortality in a murine model of staphylococcal enterotoxic shock. Comparative Medicine 50(2):160–166.

2000 Report of the AVMA Panel on Euthanasia

American Veterinary Medical Association Panel on Euthanasia

Preface

At the request of the AVMA Council on Research, the Executive Board of the AVMA convened a Panel on Euthanasia in 1999 to review and make necessary revisions to the fifth Panel Report, published in 1993.[1] In this newest version of the report, the panel has updated information on euthanasia of animals in research and animal care and control facilities; expanded information on ectothermic, aquatic, and fur-bearing animals; added information on horses and wildlife; and deleted methods or agents considered unacceptable. Because the panel's deliberations were based on currently available scientific information, some euthanasia methods and agents are not discussed.

Welfare issues are increasingly being identified in the management of free-ranging wildlife, and the need for humane euthanasia guidelines in this context is great. Collection of animals for scientific investigations, euthanasia of injured or diseased wildlife species, removal of animals causing damage to properly or threatening human safety, and euthanasia of animals in excess population are drawing more public attention. These issues are acknowledged in this report and special considerations are described for handling animals under free-ranging conditions, where their needs are far different from those of their domestic counterparts.

This report is intended for use by members of the veterinary profession who carry out or oversee the euthanasia of animals. Although the report may be interpreted and understood by a broad segment of the general population, a veterinarian should be consulted in the application of these recommendations. The practice of veterinary medicine is complex and involves diverse animal species. Whenever possible, a veterinarian experienced with the species in question should be consulted when selecting the method of euthanasia, particularly when little species-specific euthanasia research has been done. Although interpretation and use of this report cannot be limited, the panel's overriding commitment is to give veterinarians guidance in relieving pain and suffering of animals that are to be euthanatized. The recommendations in this report are intended to serve as guidelines for veterinarians who must then use professional judgment in applying them to the various settings where animals are to be euthanatized.

Excerpted from *J Am Vet Med Assoc*, 2001;218:669–696. Copyright © 2001 by the American Veterinary Medical Association. Reprinted by permission.

Introduction

The term euthanasia is derived from the Greek terms *eu* meaning good and *thanatos* meaning death.[2] A "good death" would be one that occurs with minimal pain and distress. In the context of this report, euthanasia is the act of inducing humane death in an animal. It is our responsibility as veterinarians and human beings to ensure that if an animal's life is to be taken, it is done with the highest degree of respect, and with an emphasis on making the death as painless and distress free as possible. Euthanasia techniques should result in rapid loss of consciousness followed by cardiac or respiratory arrest and the ultimate loss of brain function. In addition, the technique should minimize distress and anxiety experienced by the animal prior to loss of consciousness. The panel recognized that the absence of pain and distress cannot always be achieved. This report attempts to balance the ideal of minimal pain and distress with the reality of the many environments in which euthanasia is performed. A veterinarian with appropriate training and expertise for the species involved should be consulted to ensure that proper procedures are used.

Criteria for painless death can be established only after the mechanisms of pain are understood. Pain is that sensation (perception) that results from nerve impulses reaching the cerebral cortex via ascending neural pathways. Under normal circumstances, these pathways are relatively specific, but the nervous system is sufficiently plastic that activation of nociceptive pathways does not always result in pain and stimulation of other (non-nociceptive) peripheral and central neurons can give rise to pain. The term nociceptive is derived from the word *noci* meaning to injure and *ceptive* meaning to receive, and is used to describe neuronal input caused by noxious stimuli, which threaten to, or actually do, destroy tissue. These noxious stimuli initiate nerve impulses by acting at primary nociceptors and other sensory nerve endings that respond to noxious and non-noxious stimuli from mechanical, thermal, or chemical activity. Endogenous chemical substances such as hydrogen ions, potassium ions, ATP, serotonin, histamine, bradykinin, and prostaglandins, as well as electrical curents, are capable of generating nerve impulses in nociceptor nerve fibers. Activity in nociceptive pathways can also be triggered in normally silent receptors that become sensitized by chronic pain conditions.[3,4]

Nerve impulse activity generated by nociceptors is conducted via nociceptor primary afferent fibers to the spinal cord or the brainstem where it is transmitted to two general sets of neural networks. One set is related to nociceptive reflexes (eg, withdrawal and flexion reflexes) that are mediated at the spinal level, and the second set consists of ascending pathways to the reticular formation, hypothalamus, thalamus, and cerebral cortex (somatosensory cortex and limbic system) for sensory processing. It is important to understand that ascending nociceptive pathways are numerous, often redundant, and are capable of considerable plasticity under chronic conditions (pathology or injury). Moreover, even the transmission of nociceptive neural activity in a given pathway is highly variable. Under certain conditions, both the nociceptive reflexes and the ascending pathways may be suppressed, as, for example, in epidural anesthesia. Under another set of conditions, nociceptive reflex actions may occur, but activity in the ascending pathways is suppressed; thus, noxious stimuli are not perceived as pain. It is incorrect to use the term pain for stimuli, receptors, reflexes, or pathways because the term implies perception, whereas all the above may be active without consequential pain perception.[5,6]

Pain is divided into two broad categories: (1) sensory-discriminative, which indicates the site of origin and the stimulus giving rise to the pain; and (2) motivational-affective in which the severity of the stimulus is perceived and the animal's response is determined. Sensory-discriminative processing of nociceptive impulses is most likely to be accomplished by subcortical and cortical mechanisms similar to those used for processing other sensory-discriminative input that provides the individual with information about the intensity, duration, location, and quality of the stimulus. Motivational-affective processing involves the ascending reticular formation for behavioral and cortical arousal. It also involves thalamic input to the forebrain and the limbic system for perceptions such as discomfort, fear, anxiety, and depression. The motivational-affective neural networks also have strong inputs to the limbic system, hypothalamus and the autonomic nervous system for reflex activation of the cardiovascular, pulmonary, and pituitary-adrenal systems. Responses activated by these systems feed back to the forebrain and enhance perceptions derived via motivational-affective inputs. On the basis of neurosurgical experience in humans, it is possible to separate the sensory-discriminative components from the motivational-affective components of pain.[7]

For pain to be experienced, the cerebral cortex and subcortical structures must be functional. If the cerebral cortex is nonfunctional because of hypoxia, depression by drugs, electric shock, or concussion, pain is not experienced. Therefore, the choice of the euthanasia agent or method is less critical if it is to be used on an animal that is anesthetized or unconscious, provided that the animal does not regain consciousness prior to death.

An understanding of the continuum that represents stress and distress is essential for evaluating techniques that minimize any distress experienced by an animal being euthanatized. Stress has been defined as the effect of physical, physiologic, or emotional factors (stressors) that induce an alteration in an animal's homeostasis or adaptive state.[8] The response of an animal to stress represents the adaptive process that is necessary to restore the baseline mental and physiologic state. These responses may involve changes in an animal's neuroendocrinologic system, autonomic nervous system, and mental status that may result in overt behavioral changes. An animal's response varies according to its experience, age, species, breed, and current physiologic and psychologic state.[9]

Stress and the resulting responses have been divided into three phases.[10] Eustress results when harmless stimuli initiate adaptive responses that are beneficial to the animal. Neutral stress results when the animal's response to stimuli causes neither harmful nor beneficial effects to the animal. Distress results when an animal's response to stimuli interferes with its well-being and comfort.[11]

As with many other procedures involving animals, some methods of euthanasia require physical handling of the animal. The amount of control and kind of restraint required will be determined by the animal's species, breed, size, state of domestication, degree of taming, presence of painful injury or disease, degree of excitement, and method of euthanasia. Proper handling is vital to minimize pain and distress in animals, to ensure safety of the person performing euthanasia, and, often, to protect other people and animals.

An in-depth discussion of euthanasia procedures is beyond the scope of this report; however, personnel who perform euthanasia must have appropriate certification and training, experience with the techniques to be used, and experience in the humane restraint of the species of animal to be euthanatized, to ensure that animal pain and distress are minimized during euthanasia. Training and experience should include familiarity with the normal behavior of the species being euthanatized, an appreciation of how handling and restraint affects that behavior, and an understanding of the mechanism by which the selected technique induces loss of consciousness and death. Prior to being assigned full responsibility for performing euthanasia, all personnel must have demonstrated proficiency in the use of the technique in a closely supervised environment. References provided at the end of this document may be useful for training personnel.[12–21]

Selection of the most appropriate method of euthanasia in any given situation depends on the species of animal involved, available means of animal restraint, skill of personnel, number of animals, and other considerations. Available information focuses primarily on domestic animals, but the same general considerations should be applied to all species.

This report includes four appendices that summarize information from the text. Appendix 1 lists acceptable and conditionally acceptable methods of euthanasia, categorized by species. Appendices 2 and 3 provide summaries of characteristics for acceptable and conditionally acceptable methods of euthanasia. Appendix 4 provides a summary of some unacceptable euthanasia agents and methods. Criteria used for acceptable, conditionally acceptable, and unacceptable methods are as follows: acceptable methods are those that consistently produce a humane death when used as the sole means of euthanasia; conditionally acceptable methods are those techniques that by the nature of the technique or because of greater potential for operator error or safety hazards might not consistently produce humane death or are methods not well documented in the scientific literature; and unacceptable techniques are those methods deemed inhumane under any conditions or that the panel found posed a substantial risk to the human applying the technique. The report also includes discussion of several adjunctive methods, which are those methods that cannot be used as the sole method of euthanasia, but that can be used in conjunction with other methods to produce a humane death.

General Considerations

In evaluating methods of euthanasia, the panel used the following criteria: (1) ability to induce loss of consciousness and death without causing pain, distress, anxiety, or apprehension; (2) time required to induce loss of consciousness; (3) reliability; (4) safety of personnel; (5) irreversibility; (6) compatibility with requirement and purpose; (7) emotional effect on observers or operators; (8) compatibility with subsequent evaluation, examination, or use of tissue; (9) drug availability and human abuse potential; (10) compatibility with species, age, and health status; (11) ability to maintain equipment in proper working order; and (12) safety for predators/scavengers should the carcass be consumed.

The panel discussed the definition of euthanasia used in this report as it applies to circumstances when the degree of control over the animal makes it difficult to ensure death without pain and distress. Slaughter of animals for food, fur, or fiber may represent such situations. However, the same standards for euthanasia should be applied to the killing of animals for food, fur, or fiber, and wildlife or feral animals. Animals intended for food should be slaughtered humanely, taking into account any special requirements of the US Department of Agriculture.[22] Painless death can be achieved by properly stunning the animal, followed immediately by exsanguination. Handling of animals prior to slaughter should be as stress free as possible. Electric prods or other devices should not be used to encourage movement of animals and are not needed if chutes and ramps are properly designed to enable animals to be moved and restrained without undue stress.[23–27] Animals must not be restrained in a painful position before slaughter.

Ethical considerations that must be addressed when euthanatizing healthy and unwanted animals reflect professional and societal concerns.[28,29] These issues are complex and warrant thorough consideration by the profession and all those concerned with the welfare of animals. Whereas the panel recognizes the need for those responsible for the euthanasia of animals to be cognizant of these issues, it does not believe that this report is the appropriate forum for an indepth discussion of this topic.

It is the intent of the panel that euthanasia be performed in accordance with applicable federal, state, and local laws governing drug acquisition and storage, occupational safety, and methods used for euthanasia and disposal of animals. However, space does not permit a review of current federal, state, and local regulations.

The panel is aware that circumstances may arise that are not clearly covered by this report. Whenever such situations arise, a veterinarian experienced with the species should use professional judgment and knowledge of clinically acceptable techniques in selecting an appropriate euthanasia technique. Professional judgment in these circumstances will take into consideration the animal's size and its species-specific physiologic and behavioral characteristics. In all circumstances, the euthanasia method should be selected and used with the highest ethical standards and social conscience.

It is imperative that death be verified after euthanasia and before disposal of the animal. An animal in deep narcosis following administration of an injectable or inhalant agent may appear dead, but might eventually recover. Death must be confirmed by examining the animal for cessation of vital signs, and consideration given to the animal species and method of euthanasia when determining the criteria for confirming death.

Animal Behavioral Considerations

The need to minimize animal distress, including fear, anxiety, and apprehension, must be considered in determining the method of euthanasia. Gentle restraint (preferably in a familiar and safe environment), careful handling, and talking during euthanasia often have a calming effect on animals that are used to being handled. Sedation and/or anesthesia may assist in achieving the best conditions for euthanasia. It must be recognized that any sedatives or anesthetics given at this stage that change circulation may delay the onset of the euthanasia agent. Preparation of observers should also be taken into consideration.

Animals that are wild, feral, injured, or already distressed from disease pose another challenge. Methods of pre-euthanasia handling suitable for domestic animals may not be effective for them. Because handling may stress animals unaccustomed to human contact (eg, wildlife, zoo, and feral species), the degree of restraint required to perform any euthanasia procedure should be considered when evaluating various methods. When handling these animals, calming may be accomplished by minimizing visual, auditory, and tactile stimulation. When struggling during capture or restraint may cause pain, injury, or anxiety to the animal or danger to the operator, the use of tranquilizers, analgesics, and/or anesthetics may be necessary. A route of injection should be chosen that causes the least distress in the animal for which euthanasia must be performed. Various techniques for oral delivery of sedatives to dogs and cats have been described that may be useful under these circumstances.[30,31]

Facial expressions and body postures that indicate various emotional states of animals have been described for some species.[32–37] Behavioral and physiologic responses to noxious stimuli include distress vocalization, struggling, attempts to escape, defensive or redirected aggression, salivation, urination, defecation, evacuation of anal sacs, pupillary dilatation, tachycardia, sweating, and reflex skeletal muscle contractions causing shivering, tremors, or other muscular spasms. Unconscious as well as conscious animals are capable of some of these responses. Fear can cause immobility or "playing dead" in certain species, particularly rabbits and chickens. This immobility response should not be interpreted as loss of consciousness when the animal is, in fact, conscious. Distress vocalizations, fearful behavior, and release of certain odors or pheromones by a frightened animal may cause anxiety and apprehension in other animals. Therefore, for sensitive species, it is desirable that other animals not be present when individual animal euthanasia is performed.

Human Behavioral Considerations

When animals must be euthanatized, either as individuals or in larger groups, moral and ethical concerns dictate that humane practices be observed. Human psychologic responses to euthanasia of animals need to be considered, with grief at the loss of a life as the most common reaction.[38] There are six circumstances under which we are most aware of the effects of animal euthanasia on people.

The first of these is the veterinary clinical setting where owners have to make decisions about whether and when to euthanatize. Although many owners rely heavily on their veterinarian's judgment, others may have misgivings about making their own decision. This is particularly likely if an owner feels responsible for allowing an animal's medical or behavioral problem to go unattended so that euthanasia becomes necessary. When owners choose to be present during euthanasia, they should be prepared for what will happen. What drugs are being used and how the animal could respond should be discussed. Behaviors such as vocalization, muscle twitches, failure of the eyelids to close, urination, or defecation can be distressing. Counseling services for grieving owners are now available in some communities[39] and telephone counseling is available through some veterinary schools.[40,41] Owners are not the only people affected by euthanasia of animals. Veterinarians and their staffs may also become attached to patients they have known and treated for many years and may continue to struggle with the ethical implications of ending an animal's life.

The second is animal care and control facilities where unwanted, homeless, diseased, and injured animals must be euthanatized in large numbers. Distress may develop among personnel directly involved in performing euthanasia repeatedly. Emotional uneasiness, discomfort, or distress experienced by people involved with euthanasia of animals may be minimized. The person performing euthanasia must be technically proficient, use humane handling methods, understand the reasons for euthanasia, and be familiar with the method of euthanasia being employed (ie, what is going to happen to the animal). When the person is not knowledgeable about what to expect, he or she may mistakenly interpret any movement of animals as consciousness and a lack of movement as loss of consciousness. Methods that preclude movement of animals are more aesthetically acceptable to most technical staff even though lack of movement is not an adequate criterion for evaluating euthanasia techniques. Constant exposure to, or participation in, euthanasia procedures can cause a psychologic state characterized by a strong sense of work dissatisfaction or alienation, which may be expressed by absenteeism, belligerence, or careless and callous handling of animals.[42] This is one of the principal reasons for turnover of employees directly involved with repeated animal euthanasia. Management should be aware of potential personnel problems related to animal euthanasia and determine whether it is necessary to institute a program to prevent, decrease, or eliminate this problem. Specific coping strategies can make the task more tolerable. Some strategies include adequate training programs so that euthanasia is performed competently, peer support in the workplace, professional support as necessary, focusing on animals that are successfully adopted or returned to owners, devoting some work time to educational activities, and providing time off when workers feel stressed.

The third setting is the laboratory. Researchers, technicians, and students may become attached to animals that must be euthanatized.[43] The same considerations afforded pet owners or shelter employees should be provided to those working in laboratories.

The fourth situation is wildlife control. Wildlife biologists, wildlife managers, and wildlife health professionals are often responsible for euthanatizing animals that are injured, diseased, in excessive number, or that threaten property or human safety. Although relocation of some animals is appropriate and attempted, relocation is often only a temporary solution to a larger problem. People who must deal with these animals, especially under public pressure to save the animals rather than destroy them, can experience extreme distress and anxiety.

The fifth setting is livestock and poultry slaughter facilities. The large number of animals processed daily can take a heavy toll on employees physically and emotionally. Federal and state agricultural employees may also be involved in mass euthanasia of poultry and livestock in the face of disease outbreaks, bioterrorism, and natural disasters.

The last situation is public exposure. Because euthanasia of zoo animals, animals involved in road-side or racetrack accidents, stranded marine animals, nuisance or injured wildlife, and others can draw public attention, human attitudes and responses should be considered whenever animals are euthanatized. Natural disasters and foreign animal disease programs also present public challenges. These considerations, however, should not outweigh the primary responsibility of using the most rapid and painless euthanasia method possible under the circumstances possible under the circumstances.

***

References cited in this report do not represent a comprehensive bibliography on all methods of euthanasia. Persons interested in additional information on a particular aspect of animal euthanasia are encouraged to contact the Animal Welfare Information Center, National Agricultural Library, 10301 Baltimore Blvd, Beltsville, MD 20705.

The Panel on Euthanasia is fully committed to the concept that, whenever it becomes necessary to kill any animal for any reason whatsoever, death should be induced as painlessly and quickly as possible. It has been our charge to develop workable guidelines for veterinarians needing to address this problem, and it is our sincere desire that these guidelines be used conscientiously by all animal care providers. We consider this report to be a work in progress with new editions warranted as results of more scientific studies are published.

Acknowledgment: The panel acknowledges the assistance of Ms. Julie Horvath and Dr. David Granstrom in coordinating the preparation and circulation of various drafts of the report. The panel also acknowledges and thanks Dr. Laurence Roy, Dr. Leah Greer, and the many other individuals and organizations that provided valuable review, criticism, and input to the panel through the many drafts of the report. The research and humane communities were especially helpful in shaping important changes and additions to the report.

References

1. Andrews EJ, Bennet BT, Clark JD, et al. 1993 Report on the AVMA panel on euthanasia. *J Am Vet Med Assoc.* 1993;202:230–247.
2. *Webster's ninth new collegiate dictionary.* Springfield: Merriam-Webster Inc, 1990.

3. Wall PD. Defining pain in animals. In: Short CE, Poznak AV, eds. *Animal pain.* New York: Churchill-Livingstone Inc, 1992;63–79.

4. Vierck CJ, Cooper BY, Ritz LA, et al. Inference of pain sensitivity from complex behaviors of laboratory animals. In: Chapman CR, Loeser JD, eds. *Issues in pain measurement.* New York: Raven Press, 1989;93–115.

5. Breazile JE, Kitchell RL. Euthanasia for laboratory animals. *Fed Proc.* 1969;28:1577–1579.

6. Zimmerman M. Neurobiological concepts of pain, its assessment and therapy. In: Bromm B, ed. *Pain measurement in man: neurophysiological correlates of pain.* Amsterdam: Elsevier Publishing Co, 1984;15–35.

7. Kitchell RL, Erickson NH, Carstens E, et al, eds. *Animal pain: perception and alleviation.* Bethesda: American Physiological Society, 1983.

8. Kitchen N, Aronson AL, Bittle JL, et al. Panel report on the colloquium on recognition and alleviation of animal pain and distress. *J Am Vet Med Assoc.* 1987;191:1186–1191.

9. National Research Council. *Recognition and alleviation of pain and distress in laboratory animals.* Washington, DC: National Academy Press, 1992.

10. Breazile JE. Physiologic basis and consequences of distress in animals. *J Am Vet Med Assoc.* 1987;191:1212–1215.

11. McMillan FD. Comfort as the primary goal in veterinary medical practice. *J Am Vet Med Assoc.* 1998;212:1370–1374.

12. Grier RL, Clovin TL. *Euthanasia guide (for animal shelters).* Ames, Iowa: Moss Creek Publications, 1990.

13. Cooper JE, Ewbank R, Platt C, et al. *Euthanasia of amphibians and reptiles.* London: UFAW/WSPA, 1989.

14. Greyhavens T. *Handbook of pentobarbital euthanasia.* Salem, Ore: Humane Society of Willamette Valley, 1989;1–126.

15. *Operational guide for animal care and control agencies.* Denver: American Humane Association, 1988.

16. Fowler ME, Miller RE, eds. *Zoo and wild animal medicine: current therapy 4.* Philadelphia: WB Saunders Co, 1999;1–747.

17. Clark R, Jessup DA. *Wildlife restraint series.* Salinas, Calif: International Wildlife Veterinary Services Inc, 1992.

18. Kreeger T. *Handbook of wildlife chemical immobilization.* Laramie, Wyo: Wildlife Veterinary Services Inc, 1996.

19. Nielsen L. *Chemical immobilization of wild and exotic animals.* Ames, Iowa: Iowa State University Press, 1999.

20. McKenzie A, ed. *The capture and care manual.* South Africa: Wildlife Decision Support Services/The South African Veterinary Foundation, 1993.

21. Amass K, Neilsen L, Brunson D. *Chemical immobilization of animals.* Mount Horeb, Wis: Safe-Capture International Inc, 1999.

22. Humane slaughter regulations. *Fed Reg.* 1979;44: 68809–68817.

23. Grandin T. Observations of cattle behavior applied to design of cattle-handling facilities. *Appl Anim Ethol.* 1980;6:19–31.

24. Grandin T. Pig behavior studies applied to slaughter-plant design. *Appl Anim Ethol.* 1982;9:141–151.

25. Grandin T. Farm animal welfare during handling, transport, and slaughter. *J Am Vet Med Assoc.* 1994;204:372–377.

26. Grandin T. Objective scoring of animal handling and stunning practices at slaughter plants. *J Am Vet Med Assoc.* 1998;212:36–39.

27. Grandin T. Effect of animal welfare audits of slaughter plants by a major fast food company on cattle handling and slaughter practices. *J Am Vet Med Assoc.* 2000;216:848–851.

28. Tannenbaum J. Issues in companion animal practice. In: *Veterinary ethics.* Baltimore: The Williams & Wilkins Co, 1989;208–225.

29. Rollin BE. Ethical question of the month. *Can Vet J.* 1992;33:7–8.

30. Ramsey EC, Wetzel RW. Comparison of five regimens for oral administration of medication to induce sedation in dogs prior to euthanasia. *J Am Vet Med Assoc.* 1998;213:240–242.

31. Wetzel RW, Ramsay EC. Comparison of four regimens for oral administration of medication to induce sedation in cats prior to euthanasia. *J Am Vet Med Assoc.* 1998;213:243–245.

32. Beaver BV. *Feline behavior: a guide for veterinarians.* Philadelphia: WB Saunders Co, 1992; 1–276.

33. Houpt KA. *Domestic animal behavior for veterinarians and animal scientists.* 3rd ed. Ames, Iowa: Iowa State University Press, 1998;1–495.

34. Hart BL. *The behavior of domestic animals.* New York: WH Freeman & Co, 1985;1–390.

35. Beaver BV. *Canine behavior: a guide for veterinarians.* Philadelphia: WB Saunders Co, 1999; 1–355.

36. Beaver BV. *The veterinarian's encyclopedia of animal behavior.* Ames, Iowa: Iowa State University Press, 1994;1–307.

37. Schafer M. *The language of the horse: habits and forms of expression.* New York: Arco Publishing Co, 1975;1–187.

38. Hart LA, Hart BL, Mader B. Humane euthanasia and companion animal death: caring for the animal, the client, and the veterinarian. *J Am Vet Med Assoc.* 1990;197:1292–1299.

39. Neiburg HA, Fischer A. *Pet loss, a thoughtful guide for adults and children.* New York: Harper & Row, 1982.

40. Hart LA, Mader B. Pet loss support hotline: the veterinary students' perspective. *Calif Vet.* 1992; Jan-Feb:19–22.

41. Pet loss support hotlines (grief counseling). *J Am Vet Med Assoc.* 1999;215:1804.

42. Arluke A. Coping with euthanasia: a case study of shelter culture. *J Am Vet Med Assoc.* 1991;198:1176–1180.

43. Wolfle TL. Laboratory animal technicians: their role in stress reduction and human-companion animal bonding. *Vet Clin North Am Small Anim Pract.* 1985;15:449–454.

Members of the AVMA Panel

Bonnie V. Beaver, DVM, MS, DACVB, (Chair) Department of Small Animal Medicine and Surgery, College of Veterinary Medicine, Texas A&M University, 4474 TAMU, College Station, TX 77843-4474, representing the AVMA Executive Board.

Willie Reed, DVM, PhD, DACVP, DACPV, Animal Health Diagnostic Laboratory, College of Veterinary Medicine, Michigan State University, B646 W. Fee Hall-AHDL, East Lansing, MI 48824-1316, representing the AVMA Council on Research.

Steven Leary, DVM, DACLAM, Division of Comparative Medicine, Washington University, Box 8061, St Louis, MO 63110, representing the AVMA Animal Welfare Committee.

Brendan McKiernan, DVM, DACVIM, Denver Veterinary Specialists, 3695 Kipling St, Wheat Ridge, CO 80033, representing the American Animal Hospital Association.

Fairfield Bain, DVM, DACVIM, DACVP, DACVECC, Hagyard-Davidson-McGee Associates PSC, 4250 Iron Works Pike, Lexington, KY 40511-8412, representing the American Association of Equine Practitioners.

Roy Schultz, DVM, MS, DABVP, 1114 N Frost Ave, Avoca, IA 51521, representing the American Board of Veterinary Practitioners.

B. Taylor Bennett, DVM, PhD, DACLAM, Biologic Resources Laboratory (MC533), University of Illinois at Chicago, 1840 W Taylor St, Chicago, IL 60612-7348, representing the American College of Laboratory Animal Medicine.

Peter Pascoe, BVSc, DVA, DACVA, DECVA, Department of Surgical and Radiological Sciences, School of Veterinary Medicine, University of California, Davis, CA 95616-8745, representing the American College of Veterinary Anesthesiologists.

Elizabeth Shull, DVM, DACVB, DACVIM (Neurology), Veterinary Specialty Consultation Services, 1505 Bob Kirby Rd, Knoxville, TN 37931, representing the American College of Veterinary Behaviorists.

Linda C. Cork, DVM, PhD, DACVP, Department of Comparative Medicine, School of Medicine, Stanford University, MSOB Building, Room X347, Stanford, CA 94305-5415, representing the American College of Veterinary Pathologists.

Ruth Francis-Floyd, DVM, MS, DACZM, Department of Large Animal Clinical Sciences, College of Veterinary Medicine, University of Florida, Box 100136, Gainesville, FL 32510-0136, representing the International Association of Aquatic Animal Medicine.

Keith D. Amass, DVM, Safe-Capture International Inc, PO Box 206, Mount Horeb, WI 53572, representing wildlife regulatory/conservation agencies.

Richard Johnson, PhD, Department of Physiological Sciences, College of Veterinary Medicine, University of Florida, Box 100144, Gainesville, FL 32610-0144, representing the Society for Neuroscience.

Robert H. Schmidt, MS, PhD, Department of Fisheries and Wildlife, Utah State University, Logan UT 84322-5210, representing the wildlife damage management profession.

Wendy Underwood, DVM, MS, DACVIM, Lilly Corporate Center, Eli Lilly and Co, Indianapolis, IN 46285, representing the National Institute for Animal Agriculture Euthanasia Task Force.

Gus W. Thornton, DVM, DACVIM, Massachusetts Society for the Prevention of Cruelty to Animals (MSPCA), American Humane Education Society (AHES), 350 S Huntington Ave, Boston, MA 02130, representing an animal protection agency.

Barbara Kohn, DVM, USDA/APHIS/Animal Care, 4700 River Road, Unit 84, Riverdale, MD 20737-1234, representing the USDA/APHIS.

Questions for Discussion

1. How does interaction with domesticated animals (dogs, cats, horses, hamsters) as children and adults shape researchers' experience of animals in research settings?
2. Are there any animal research techniques that all or most students in the basic sciences need to learn as part of their theoretical education or laboratory training? Do students have a right to refuse to participate in animal research considered essential to their specific program?
3. How is the role of the Institutional Animal Care and Use Committee (IACUC) similar to that of the Institutional Review Board that oversees human research? Do the protective functions of the IACUC center more on scientific or ethical issues?
4. How should researchers who use animals respond to the challenges raised by the wide range of animal rights groups and members of the lay public?

Recommended Supplemental Reading

American College of Veterinary Anesthesiologists. Position paper on the treatment of pain in animals. *JAVMA*. 1998;213:628–630.

Ballis M. Why is it proving to be so difficult to replace animal tests? *Lab Animal*. 1998; 27(5): 44–47.

Bulger RE. Use of animals in experimental research: A scientist's perspective. *Anatomical Record*. 1987;219:215–220.

Festing MFW, et al. Reducing the use of laboratory animals in biomedical research: Problems and possible solutions – the report and recommendations of ECVAM Workshop 29, *ATLA* 1998;26: 283–301.

Gaertner DJ, Riley LK, Martin DG. Reflections on future needs in research with animals. *ILARJ*. 1998;39:306–310.

Hill RN, Stokes WS. Validation and regulatory acceptance of alternatives. *Cambridge Qtrly Healthcare Ethics*. 1999;8:73–79.

National Association for Biomedical Research. http://www.fbresearch.org

Orlans FB. *In the Name of Science: Issues in Responsible Animal Experimentation*. New York: Oxford University Press; 1993.

U.S. Department of Agriculture. *Consideration of Alternatives to Painful/Distressful Procedures* – Policy #12. June 21, 2000. Available at: http://www.nal.usda.gov

Management of and Access to Scientific Data

Ethical Issues in Data Acquisition, Access, and Management

Ruth Ellen Bulger

Science is driven by data. Scientists not only need to be honest in all of their experimental work, they need to be as objective as possible about the data that they generate as well. They must use good practices in the recording, retention, and analysis of their data. Because science is often a group endeavor, a clear understanding of who owns, maintains, controls, and has access to data is required. Fabrication or falsification of data clearly constitute scientific misconduct. However, without clear policies about data access, disputes over data that are actually data access and management issues have frequently turned into charges of scientific misconduct. This chapter addresses the issues of objectivity in the collection of data, data management, and data policies.

Objectivity in Data Collection

For data to be useful in modern scientific experiments, researchers should use the most up-to-date methods that are likely to provide data that will be significant in answering the questions being tested. The data collected need to be analyzed using appropriate statistical methods. It is wasteful to use more subjects than necessary to get meaningful results, yet it is equally wasteful to use too few subjects because the results will not have proper significance. And no matter how elegantly a study is done, the experiment is meaningless if the results are never published.

In their discussion of self-deception included earlier in Section II, Broad and Wade[1] clearly demonstrate how scientists who are gullible about their experimental results, or who deceive themselves about the data they have collected, have historically been plagued with unsubstantiated conclusions. Over time, scientists have developed a variety of ways to help ensure that they remain objective in their research. In addition to testing the identified experimental factor, scientists routinely use a variety of control experiments to test possible confounding variables. In conjunction with control experiments, various methods are used that blind the scientist to whether a given result is from the experimental group or from a control situation. Experiments are also repeated several times, and several independent investigators are frequently used to observe and assess results to ensure their own objectivity and the reliability of the data. The use of quantitative data measurements makes this process more open to independent evaluation.

Another way that researchers can guard against self-deception is to examine any personal *bias* that might affect the way in which they view or interpret their results. Researchers need to recognize and thoroughly evaluate both their *financial and intellectual conflicts of interest* or, better yet, avoid them, so that subconscious factors do not color their analysis. Strict rules are necessary about the circumstances under which experiments are to be stopped and data excluded from analysis. Without such a policy, it is too easy to justify retrospectively why data that do not fit the theory are not "normal" and can be discarded. Retrospectively explaining away an unexpected experimental result often leads to selection bias. Moreover, by dismissing such results, one may miss a crucial opportunity to profit from them by generating a new hypothesis to explain the unexpected findings. True scientific advance can be made by rethinking old hypotheses in the light of unexpected results.

Responsibilities of the Principal Investigator

The principal investigator (PI) is responsible for the validity and quality of all data and manuscripts generated by the laboratory. This includes understanding and following the federal, state, and local regulations relating to human research volunteers, animal subjects, radioactive substances, recombinant DNA, blood-borne pathogens, and hazardous chemicals. The guidelines from the Brain Tumor Research Center at the University of California at San Francisco, included in this section, are an excellent compilation of the roles and responsibilities of the PI concerning how data are to be handled at that institution.[2] This selection should be useful to laboratory directors as they establish procedures for their own facilities to follow.

The PI must ensure that research data are adequately collected, recorded, and maintained. How this is to be done will vary with the kind of data being collected, but each laboratory needs to develop well-articulated procedures. Educating all of the individuals who work in the laboratory – technicians, students, postdoctoral fellows, and all others who are involved with obtaining data – about the policies is equally important. The PI must supervise the research, which entails ensuring that these standards are followed.

An open atmosphere in which researchers can easily admit mistakes and then correct them without fear of recrimination is critically important in any laboratory. It is a cardinal idea that the only bad mistakes are those that are not admitted because those errors cannot be corrected and can taint all of the data from an experiment.

To ensure that experimental data are collected and maintained appropriately, at least two kinds of laboratory notebooks are routinely used: one for laboratory methods and at least one for experimental data. In addition, a system must be developed and followed to maintain other types of primary data, such as electron micrographs, audio and video recordings, negatives, gels, and cell lines.

The Methodology Notebook

A methodology notebook (or backed-up computer file) containing all of the standard procedures (with references) used in the laboratory is indispensable. Such a record ensures that each person is following the same procedures. This notebook can be a three-ring, loose-leaf type (with plastic sleeves to protect the instruction sheet because it is used frequently and is likely to get soiled). The methods notebook should be placed in a prominent area of the laboratory. This notebook normally contains a table of contents, descriptions of all standard procedures being used, and the inclusive dates for their use. Copies of original published articles are also useful for detailed reference. When the laboratory updates any procedure, the new procedure should be added to the notebook with the date that it was instituted, but the earlier procedure should remain in an archive section of the book. Such notebooks are indispensable in training new laboratory personnel and are invariably duplicated when laboratory personnel relocate.

The Experimental Data Notebook

Experimental data notebooks are crucial records of research progress. They should be kept in the laboratory at all times (except when removed briefly for duplicating). Bound notebooks with sequentially numbered pages are still the norm in most laboratories; however, some researchers, such as those doing field research, sometimes use the more flexible three-ring notebooks. (The use of computers for data storage will be addressed later.) Some bound notebooks have a second yellow sheet that is a copy that can be torn out and stored elsewhere. Experience with this type of notebook is that these second pages are often hard to read, and periodic duplication of a standard notebook is preferable. Because the laboratory notebook is so crucial for research, the data notebook should be duplicated at monthly intervals and copies kept in a separate location in case the original laboratory notebook might be lost or destroyed.

The data notebook generally begins with a table of contents listing the various studies that are included in the notebook. Research data from experiments are written directly into these notebooks in permanent ink. No erasures are used, and mistakes are indicated by a single line drawn through the incorrect material with the correct material written below, dated, and initialed by the investigator. All pages are used in chronological order.

Although the exact content will vary with the type of research, data notebooks usually follow a standard format determined for the laboratory. The book contains the date and name of the person doing each experiment, the title of the study and any background information, the objectives (why the study is being done, which is important to prove "first to invent"), the methods being used, and lists of important materials (such as the species, gender, and weight of experimental animals, type of anesthesia, etc.). Some laboratories use a different notebook for each investigator, but if several individuals are working on similar experiments, the primary notebook can document related experiments by any person. Separate books can be used for specific procedures such as renal clearances or for documenting lists of photographs taken of the experiments originally chronicled in the laboratory notebook.

It is important that each notebook be reviewed periodically by a second person involved with the work – usually the laboratory director. After review, the book should be signed by that person and dated. If it is anticipated that the data will be used for a patent application, it is wise to have an additional scientist who is not an investigator read, sign "as understood," and date the notebook also.

A properly documented experimental data notebook provides a record of intellectual property useful in resolving inventor and authorship disagreements. Notebooks must be available for review under appropriate circumstances by research funding agencies, institutional officials, institutional review boards (IRBs), or other auditors. Data notebooks serve to back up publications with easily located, identifiable data.

Data Kept on a Computer

As more and more data collection is undertaken using the computer, methods to store data on computers are being perfected. However, at present data can easily be lost or changed if kept only in that format. Keeping a detailed account of what is in each computer file and logs from each dataset has proved difficult for some people using electronic files.[3] Reconstruction of the data files after any period of time can be difficult without such detailed logs. The Collaborative Electronic Notebook Systems Association ((http://www.censa.org)

is currently developing "digital time stamps," "biometric signatures," and other kinds of certification of what was present at a certain date. But for the routine laboratory not using these techniques, data kept on a computer should also be kept in other formats. For example, the original worksheet may be kept on disk, but a back-up disk should routinely be made. A hard-copy printout is frequently pasted into a bound laboratory notebook and reviewed, signed, and dated as a handwritten notebook would be. In addition, a second hard copy can be printed to keep with the results, images, or other data if they are kept separately from the bound data notebook.

What Data Must Be Stored?

Data are generally divided into three categories: (1) primary, original, or raw data; (2) secondary or compiled data (in which the original data have been manipulated); and (3) tertiary or derived data (in which the derived data have been further changed, such as in graphics). There is general agreement that primary data should be retained. Retention of primary data confirms that the work was done. The availability of primary data is important in the replication of the experiments and in addressing questions of misconduct. Original data must be retained if they are derived from research under a government grant. The data must also be kept in conditions that are likely to preserve them. When data are generated in fulfilling a government contract instead of a grant, either the contract will specify the ownership of the data or the data will be regulated by the Federal Acquisition Regulations (FAR).[4]

The Environmental Protection Agency (40 CFR Part 742-EPA) and the Food and Drug Administration (FDA) (21 CFR Part 58-FDA) define primary (raw) data as "any laboratory worksheet, records, memoranda, notes or exact copies thereof that are the result(s) of original observations and activities of a study and are necessary for the reconstruction and evaluation of the report of that study. Raw data include photographs, microfilm and microfiche copies, computer printouts, magnetic media including dictated observations and recorded data from automated instruments." Data also include specimens developed in the course of the project. The Federal Acquisition Regulations define data as "recorded information, regardless of form of the media on which it was recorded."[4] The 1997 pamphlet, "Ownership and Retention of Data," provides an excellent in-depth report on this subject.[5]

Who Owns the Data Obtained Using External Funds?

Research data are widely recognized to belong to the institutions in which the research is carried out unless other contractual agreements are made in advance. Federal research funding creates institutional obligations regarding the resulting data. In September 1994, the Office of Research Integrity maintained that "research data generated under Public Health Service funding generally is owned by the grantee institution, not the principal investigator or the researcher producing the data. The institution is the grantee and assumes legal and financial accountability for the awarded funds (see 42 CFR 50.102 and 52.2(e)). . . . Therefore, a grantee institution has not only the right, but the obligation to require a researcher to produce accurate supporting data not only for funded programs but also for grant applications."[6] The *National Institutes of Health Guide* similarly states that "under the grant mechanism, recipient institutions have custody of and primary rights to data developed, subject to the Government's right to access."[7]

While many PIs would like to claim that they, not their institutions, own their research findings, Estelle Fishbein[8] points out that if the research was done in the course of employment, the data are owned by the institution "as a natural consequence of the conventional relationship between employer and employee, as it has developed under what is referred to in the law as 'common law agency doctrine'."

When funding comes from industrial sponsors, data ownership is usually negotiated between institutions, researchers, and sponsors. University policy can maintain that data must be available to be published and cannot be kept secret by any industrial sponsor. Original case report forms for clinical trials can either be given to the sponsors, or copies can be made for the sponsors, but the investigator should also retain these data. Again, the institutional policy should clarify this relationship. Medical records surveyed as part of approved human research using patients are always the property of the health care institution, and their data can be kept only with proper permission and IRB approval.

Ownership of the data by the grantee institution has decided advantages, for the institution can create a data policy tailored to its specific needs enumerating the responsibilities of those involved in generating, maintaining, and using research data and can serve as the arbitrator of disputes over data access among those who claim rights to data they were involved in obtaining. Institutions often remain silent on data *ownership* in data policies that they write. Institutions frequently assign to the PI the right to access and responsibility for the *custody and maintenance* of research data generated in the PI's laboratory. Institutions also generally give PIs the right to take data with them when they move to another institution as long as the PI promises to preserve the data for an appropriate period of time, make the data available to authorized users, leave copies as needed by others, and refrain from destroying data without permission.

How Long Must Original Research Data Be Retained?

A variety of factors dictate how long original research data must be retained and by whom. Most institutions have a general policy for how long scientific data must be kept unless the data fall into one of several categories for which specific regulations exist. In general, universities mandate that data be kept from 3 to 7 years with an average of 5 years. There are several exceptions to this generalization. Data obtained from research using federal funds must be kept for 3 years after the last expenditure report is submitted by the institution, which usually is due 90 days after the grant expires. The FDA requires that data from clinical trials of drugs are to be kept "for a period of 2 years following the date a marketing application is approved for the drug; or if no application is approved for the drug, until 2 years after shipment and delivery of the drug for investigational use is discontinued and FDA has been notified" (21 CFR 312).

Data that have been used to obtain patents at an institution should be kept for the life of the patent (20 years) to guard against interference or infringement of the patent. Original patent data should remain at the institution even if the investigator leaves, although the investigator can take copies of the data to the new institution.

Patient records are owned by the clinical care site and are not to be removed for research purposes. With the proper IRB approval and strict efforts to preserve patient confidentiality, certain data obtained from clinical care records for research may be maintained. The rights to, and responsibilities for maintaining, this type of data must be clearly defined by the IRB.

Contested data, such as data that have been questioned in a misconduct charge, must be retained until all litigation, claims, audit findings, and misconduct charges have been finally resolved. This time period may vary with the nature of the charges.

The Importance of an Institutional Policy on Data Management

A formal data management policy is of utmost importance for all research institutions.[5,9] First, a formal policy allows the institution to state its expectation that all data collected must be valid, of high quality, and appropriately recorded and maintained and that there is a responsibility to publish and disseminate data. A formal policy can likewise announce the institution's stance about researchers' rights to publish data freely from industrially funded research and the protection of funders' proprietary information.

Second, such a policy protects the intellectual property of the institution and its investigators and avoids unnecessary liability by defining researchers' responsibilities, deterring irresponsible conduct, and protecting the rights of all involved to use the data or products that have been produced. The policy should state to whom the data policy applies and who owns and who controls research data. It should notify investigators that data must be available to others under certain conditions such as IRB or FDA review. By notifying the investigators that data must be archived for an appropriate length of time depending on their type, a policy helps researchers comply with existing regulations.

Perhaps most important, a data policy can lay out how data are to be shared, by whom, and on what terms, preventing disputes whenever possible. If an investigator leaves the institution, a data policy outlines the procedures for taking data. The policy also needs to define a process to mediate any disagreements that do occur. Clear guidelines and processes for data sharing are of critical importance when professional relationships become problematic. When relationships are strained within a laboratory group, colleagues may be tempted to withhold research data and products from each other, prompting misconduct charges. A data management policy can provide a way to handle professional disputes fairly without raising the specter of scientific misconduct.

Data Sharing

Sharing research data outside the originating laboratory is an essential element of collaborative science. Barbara Mishkin[9] has observed that, "the public interest requires that data and materials developed with federal support be available to any scientist who wishes to extend the research after it has been published. When a collaborative team splits up, each member of the team should have continuing access to the data and biological materials with which he or she has been working, unless all parties agree to some other arrangements at the outset."

The Public Health Service Grants Policy Statement recognizes that investigators conducting biomedical research frequently develop unique research resources such as synthetic compounds, organisms, cell lines, and cell products.

The policy statement states that it is the policy of PHS to make available to the public the results and accomplishments of the activities that it funds. Restricted availability of unique resources upon which further studies are dependent can impede the advancement of research and the delivery of medical care. Therefore, when these resources are developed with PHS funds and the associated research findings have been published, or after they have been provided to the agencies under contract, it is important that they be made readily available for research purposes to qualified individuals within the scientific community. (PHS Grants Policy Statement; available at http://www.nih.gov/).

NIH similarly encourages the sharing of research resources in its recently published "Principles and Guidelines for Recipients of NIH Research Grants and Contracts on Obtaining and Disseminating Biomedical Research Resources" (http://grants.nih.gov/grants/policy/policy.htm/). According to NIH, the intent of these published principles and guidelines "is to help recipients ensure that the conditions they impose and accept on the transfer of research tools will facilitate further biomedical research consistent with the requirements of the Bayh–Dole Act and the NIH funding agreements." In addition, some journals have required that data used in publications be deposited in data registries.

Data can and should be shared in a variety of ways, especially data that have been produced using government funds. One primary way is the rapid publication of the experiments. A second way is for investigators to share research tools, including cell lines and molecules, with other qualified researchers. This exchange is frequently accomplished through a data or tumor registry. Cell lines can be placed in the American Tissue Type Culture (ATTC) for subsequent distribution. Research resources can be shared interinstitutionally through the use of material transfer agreements.

In the FY99 Health and Human Services Appropriation Bill (PL 105–277), Senator Richard Shelby placed an amendment that directed the Office of Management and Budget (OMB) to revise its Circular A110 to "ensure that all data produced under an award will be made available to the public through the Freedom of Information Act" (FOIA) to "allow the American people to review data for themselves to insure that the conclusions are solid."[10] There are nine exemptions to the FOIA, including data related to certain national security concerns, commercial and financial records, and personal and medical files. The OMB revised the circular (64 *Federal Register* 54926) in such a way that published data from federally supported research at universities, teaching hospitals, and nonprofit organizations could be obtained from the funding agency if the data were cited by a federal agency for actions with the force of law. Although this approach initially seemed to protect personal information obtained in medical research, the U.S. Chamber of Commerce has since used the FOIA to request personal and confidential research data from universities and hospitals. The OMB's rules now seem likely to provoke a lawsuit, and the appropriate openness of research data is likely to be established by the federal court.

References

1. Broad W, Wade N. Self-deception and gullibility. In: *Betrayers of the Truth*. New York: Simon & Schuster; 1982:107–125.
2. University of California at San Francisco Brain Tumor Research Center. *Guidelines on Research Data and Reports*. San Francisco, CA: UCSF; 2000.
3. Freedland KE, Carney RM. Data management and accountability in behavioral and biomedical research. *American Psychologist*. 1992;47:640–645.
4. Federal Acquisition Regulations, 45 CFR Subpart 27.401.
5. Stevens AR. Ownership and Retention of Data. The National Association of College and

University Attorneys, and the National Council of University Research Administrators; 1997. Available at http://www.nacua.org.

6. *Office of Research Integrity Newsletter.* Vol. 2, No. 4; 1–2, September 1994.

7. *National Institutes of Health Guide.* Vol. 24, No. 33; September 22, 1995.

8. Fishbein EA. Ownership of research data. *Acad Med.*1991;66:129–133.

9. Mishkin B. Urgently needed: Policies on access to data by erstwhile collaborators. *Science.* 1995;270:927–928.

10. Office of Management and Budget Circular A110, Retention and Custodial Requirements for Records, 45 CFR Part 74 Subpart D.

Sharing Research Data

Duncan Neuhauser

The National Research Council of the National Academy of Sciences has issued a report, *Sharing Research Data*[1] which has as its first recommendation, "Sharing data should be a regular practice." Other recommendations state that investigators should share their data by the time of publication of initial major results of analysis, except in compelling circumstances. Plans for data sharing should be an integral part of a research plan whenever data sharing is feasible. Investigators should keep data available for a reasonable period after publication of results. Subsequent analyses of data by others should explicitly acknowledge the contribution of the original investigators. These are exacting standards for medical care researchers to aspire to.

This report has four recommendations for editors of scientific journals:

1) "Journal editors should require authors to provide access to data during the peer review process." Although such a request would be extremely rare during the review process for *Medical Care* manuscripts, we believe that authors should, in principle, be willing to do so.

It is the expectation of the editors that the authors of papers published in *Medical Care* will allow access to their data. Keeping secret key parts of research reports in order to cash in on consulting and follow-up opportunities is inconsistent with full peer review. We have no objection to medical care researchers parleying their proprietary work into riches. In fact, if this happened, it might be good for the field. However, we are troubled by the thought that researchers might exploit the peer review process in spite of refusing to make their work available to peers, and thereby misrepresent their work as peer reviewed in the process of marketing it.

In the words of Donald Kennedy, President of Stanford,

Science relies very heavily on the capacity to replicate experiments; it is the only way at all to correct fraud. Although we referee journal articles, evaluate the logic of propositions, and check arithmetic, we cannot decide, merely from reading a report, that a result is right – only that it is not wrong in some obvious way. Accordingly, we require that scientific communications include enough detail about the way an experiment was done so that a competent investigator in the field can do it in exactly the same way. This is an exacting requirement; it compels the release of all relevant information about methods and techniques. Secret ingredients, magic sauces, and your own special glassware are fine in cookery or in product development, but in fundamental science they are out.[2]

A full description of most of the studies reported in this journal would take hundreds of pages to describe. Because this is not possible, we assume that detailed descriptions of method are available from the author on request.

From Duncan Neuhauser, Sharing Research Data, *Medical Care*, 1986, 24(10), pp. 879–880. Reprinted by permission.

2) "Journals should give more emphasis to reports of secondary analyses and to replications." We invite such submissions.

3) "Journals should require full credit and appropriate citations to original data collections in reports based on secondary analysis." We agree.

4) "Journals should strongly encourage authors to make detailed data accessible to other researchers." We assume that *Medical Care* authors accept this as a condition of submitting a paper to peer review and for publication.

The questions often raised about data sharing such as patient confidentiality, costs of reanalysis, requests by unqualified people, copyright laws, etc. are discussed in this National Research Council report, and those interested in these issues are urged to seek it out. In spite of potential problems with data sharing, the benefits of doing so greatly outweigh the risks and costs.

References

1. Committee on National Statistics, Commission on Behavioral and Social Sciences and Education, National Research Council. Sharing Research Data. Washington, DC: National Academy Press, 1985.
2. Kennedy D. The social sponsorship of innovation. In: Perpich J, ed. Biotechnology in Society. New York: Pergamon Press, 1986;26–27.

Retention of and Access to Research Data

*Henry M. Jackson Foundation for the Advancement
of Military Medicine*

A. Scope and Purpose of the Policy

Federal agencies and other sponsors of biomedical research have published requirements and guidelines on retaining scientific data obtained in biomedical research. The Henry M. Jackson Foundation for the Advancement of Military Medicine (Foundation) and investigators have a common interest in and a shared responsibility that research data be accurately recorded, retained for the required period of time, and available for review when appropriate. The Foundation is committed to the responsible maintenance and retention of and access to scientific data that is obtained during the conduct of research on projects that are managed by the Foundation. The Foundation's policy is in agreement with federal regulations on retaining scientific data and *embodies* the following:

- Compliance with federal regulations required by the acceptance of federal research awards or requirements of other sponsors related to data retention and access;
- Protection of the rights of investigators, the Foundation, government services, and the federal government with respect to scientific data;
- The confirmation or replication of published results;
- Protection of intellectual property rights of involved parties;
- Providing principal investigators, scientists, visiting scientists, graduate students, postdoctoral fellows, proper access to data they were involved with obtaining;
- Providing guidance for investigators who are moving to new research locations;
- Providing the means to effectively deal with problems that may arise if investigators disagree on possession of and/or access to data they were involved with producing;
- Facilitating proper access by the Foundation or federal agencies to address any questions regarding the propriety of scientific investigations; and
- Deterrence of irresponsible scientific behavior and to prevent unfounded allegations of scientific misconduct.

B. Definitions of Data

1. Data can be classified as original (primary or raw), compiled, or derived.
   a. The Good Laboratory Practice Standards of the EPA (40 CRF Part 742) and the FDA (21 CRF Part 58) define raw data as "Any laboratory worksheets, records, memoranda, notes or exact copies thereof, that are the result(s) of original observations and activities of a study and are necessary for the reconstruction and evaluation of the report of

that study. Raw data include photographs, microfilm or microfiche copies, computer print-outs, magnetic media, including detailed observations and recorded data from automated instruments." Other examples of raw data include specimens, slides, grids, embedded materials, gels, autoradiograms, Western blots, medical records, videos, sound recording, and other unique resources (cell lines) and methodologies (unless well established in the scientific literature).

   b. Compiled data are the original data subjected to some type of manipulation, such as statistical analyses.

   c. Derived data are the compiled data that is further transformed to facilitate the presentation to the scientific community such as in bar charts, tables, etc.

2. For contracts, the Federal Acquisitions Regulations (FAR) applies to data generated or developed from federal contract funds. The FAR classifies data as "recorded information, regardless of form or the media on which it may be recorded. The term includes technical data and computer software."

Technical data means "data other than computer software, which are of a scientific and technical nature."

C. Data to Be Retained

The Foundation agrees with the general consensus of universities, the federal government, professional societies (A.A.M.C.), and journal editors (American Federation of Clinical Research, J.A.M.A., N.E.J.M., American Journal of Public Health) that it is the original (primary, raw) data that must be retained. The data need to be maintained under conditions that are likely to preserve them safely. Original patient records are always the property of the medical institution not of the investigator.

D. To Whom the Policy Applies

This policy applies to all scientific investigators, including faculty, other scientists, visiting scientists, consultants, graduate students, and postdoctoral personnel supported by research funds awarded to and administered by the Foundation.

E. Control of and Responsibility for Data Retention

1. The person heading the research group (program director/head of the laboratory/principal investigator – whoever is in charge of the research) is responsible to retain original data and to make them accessible to the Foundation when needed for valid reasons for as long as this person remains at the research location. If the above person retires and no longer wants this responsibility, the person next in line for the responsibility of the research should keep the data. If there is no person involved in the research who wishes to keep the data, the department/program in which the research is done must assume the responsibility for the required time period (see E.2).

2. Scientific data (excluding patent data and clinical records) should be kept at least five years after the publication of the results. If no publication is involved, the data must still be kept for five years from completion of scientific work except for data from federally funded projects, which are to be kept three years past the last expenditure report. If any litigation, claim, negotiation, or audit is started before the expiration period, the

data records shall be retained until all litigations, claims, negotiations, or audit findings involving the records have been resolved or the end of the time period, which ever is later.

Patent data must be kept for the life of the patent (17 years) to guard against interference or infringement issues. The FDA requires records from clinical trials to be retained for at least two years following the date a marketing application is approved (21 CFR 312.62). Clinical records are owned by the clinical care site and are maintained indefinitely.

F. Access to Data

1. Access to the data will be controlled by the program director/head of the laboratory/ principal investigator. Co-investigators and pre or post doctoral trainees who were directly involved with obtaining of the data in question have rights to review the data. Extra costs for this review are the responsibility of the person seeking to review the data.
   If there is a dispute about data access among those directly involved in the data production, the Foundation President will appoint a committee of research peers to recommend a solution to the President. The President will make the ultimate decision.
2. The Foundation has the responsibility and accountability to produce the data that was obtained when supported by federal funds in situations of reasonable cause after providing adequate notice to the investigator. Confidential data shall be protected as appropriate.
3. In some situations private extramural sponsors may also have the right to review research data from experiments which they supported.
4. Access to proprietary, sensitive or confidential data and patient information, whether owned by the Foundation, or entrusted to the Foundation by a third party, is subject to additional controls over its use and dissemination. The specific program responsible for management of proprietary, sensitive or confidential data and patient information may, with the approval of the Foundation President, establish data access requirements and restrictions.
5. The Food and Drug Administration may require audit of clinical data relating to clinical trials.

G. Transfer of Data

The following are the provisions for transfer of data collected with Foundation administered funding from the institution at which the research was conducted by the departing investigator to a new institution.

1. In recognition of the rights of the faculty member who is changing the site of employment to continue with the ongoing research and the necessity for the Foundation to fulfill its contractual, ethical, and legal commitments, the head of a laboratory/principal investigator can arrange to transfer primary data when moving to a new research site by signing a transfer agreement with the Foundation (see attached draft of a transfer agreement). This transfer agreement assures that the principal investigator shall preserve the data for an adequate period of time and shall make the data available to authorized representatives of the Foundation, at the Foundation's request, for any lawful purpose. Consideration should be given to the division of non-reproducible raw data, and the

copying of reproducible data if some of the involved investigators remain at the original research site.

This form is to be used only where original data are to be kept by the investigator. In unusual cases, for example, data used for a patent application filed by the Foundation, it may be necessary for original data to be kept at the Foundation. In such a case, an individual written agreement shall be signed which preserves the investigator's right to access and copy (where practical) such data. Any dispute shall be resolved by the Foundation's President. Patient medical records shall remain at the Foundation and copying shall be only as permitted by law.

2. Original data that cannot be removed include patent data (unless the patent is assigned to the new institution) and clinical records.

3. Proprietary, sensitive, confidential data and patient information are subject to additional transfer controls. The specific program responsible for such data management may, with the approval of the Foundation President, establish data transfer requirements and restrictions applicable to proprietary, sensitive, confidential data, and patient information.

This policy was developed using the excellent materials presented by Anne R. Stevens, Ph.D., Emory University, at the NCURA Annual Meeting, November 1994.

References

1. "The Responsible Conduct of Research in the Health Sciences," a Report by a Committee on the Responsible Conduct of Research: Institute of Medicine, Division of Health Sciences Policy, National Academy Press, Washington, 1989.
2. Data Management in Biomedical Research: Report of Workshop, DHHS, US Public Health Service; OASH, Office of Health Planning and Evaluation, and OSIR, April, 1990.
3. Diane Morgan, "Battle Heats Up Over Who Owns Research Data," The Scientist, Volume 31, Page 7, May 28, 1990.
4. Estelle Fishbein, "Ownership of Research Data," Academic Medicine, Volume 66, page, 129, March, 1991.
5. Who Controls a Researcher's File? News and Comment: Science, Volume 256, Page 1620, June 1992.
6. Responsible Science, COSEPUP Report, National Academy Press, 1993.
7. Seminar on Ownership and Retention of Data, Anne R. Stevens, Ph.D., Emory University, NCURA Annual Meeting, Washington, DC, November, 1994
8. Code of Federal Regulations, Public Welfare, 45 (parts 1–199), Office of the Federal Register, National Archives and Records Administration, U.S. Government Printing Office, 1993.

Henry M. Jackson
Foundation for the Advancement of Military Medicine
Agreement on
Investigator Transfer of Research Data

In recognition of both the right of the undersigned research investigator, who is leaving the _____, but continuing the research, and the necessity for the Foundation to be able to fulfill its contractual and legal commitments, response to any allegations of research misconduct, and carry out its administrative, ethical, or moral duties, the _____ and the Foundation agree as follows:

1. Research data developed or generated by the investigator while employed by the above referenced institution shall be preserved for a period of not less than five (5) years (or such lesser period as designated below) from the later of: 1) the date on which the data were created or 2) the date of any publication utilizing such data.

Lesser period* (if applicable) _____ _____ _____
                                 Years   Investigator   Foundation
                                                Signature   Signature

2. The investigator shall have the right and responsibility to remove and preserve the data provided that the data shall be made available (including the right to copy) to authorized representatives of the Foundation, at the Foundation's request, for any lawful purpose including, but not limited to, the carrying out of a legal, contractual, administrative, ethical or moral duty. In case of dispute, the Foundation's President shall make the final decision after obtaining advice from a committee of the investigator's peers which shall be binding on both the Foundation and the investigator.

Dated this ____ day of _____. 19 __

_____ _____ _____
Research Investigator   Department Chair or Dean   Foundation President
                                  (if applicable)

* Please note that federal regulations require retention of records for a period of at least three (3) years after the final expenditure report. The FDA requires records of clinical trials to be retained for at least two (2) years following the date a marketing application is approved (21 Code of Federal Regulations 312.62).

This form is to be used only where original data are to be kept by the investigator. In the case of contracts, data handling will follow the terms specified in the contract. In unusual cases, for example, data used for a patent application filed by the Foundation, it may be necessary for original data to be kept at the Foundation. In such a case, an individual written agreement shall be signed which preserves the investigator's right to access and copy (where practical) such data. Any dispute shall be resolved by the Foundation's President. Patient medical records shall remain at the Foundation and copying shall be only as permitted by law.

Modified from the Emory University Transfer Agreement.

Guidelines on Research Data and Reports

University of California, San Francisco,
Brain Tumor Research Center

§1. Responsibilities of Principal Investigators

Principal investigators (PIs) have final responsibility for:

- the validity and quality of the data and reports generated from their laboratories or services.
- fulfilling the research, reporting, and publication standards, policies, and procedures of the Department of Neurological Surgery, the University of California, San Francisco<www.ucsf.edu/research>, and the USPHS, National Institutes of Health <www.nih.gov>, National Science Foundation <www.nsf.gov>, and Office of Research Integrity <http://ori.dhhs.gov>.
- formally orienting junior faculty, fellows, residents, and staff to those standards, policies, and procedures and, to the maximum extent possible, seeing to it that they are upheld.
- overseeing the work done by fellows, residents, and staff to assure that each has the knowledge, information, and skills necessary to meet the standards of the institution and scientific convention.

§2. Research Data

§2.1 Data Management and Review

In general, two primary forms of data records are maintained in a laboratory: the *methodology notebook* and the *experimental notebook*. Laboratories with several individual research projects also keep a *laboratory master log*. A *data selection file* containing data selected for publication and documents related to publication is kept for each paper resulting from a study. Standards for accurate collection and recording of data and for storing data are detailed in §3 of these guidelines.

§2.1.1 The PI has final responsibility for:

- the validity of the data.
- maintaining methodology notebooks and laboratory master logs relevant to the PI's

Excerpted from *BTRC Guidelines on Research Data and Manuscripts.* San Francisco: Brain Tumor Research Center, University of California, San Francisco, 1989 (revised 2000). Copyright © 2000 by the Brain Tumor Research Center and the University of California, San Francisco. Reprinted by permission.

laboratory and seeing to it that those books and all experimental notebooks, data selection files, and related data and records are kept and stored according to the standards set out in these guidelines.

- ensuring that data (*a*) are collected and recorded in the experimental notebook according to the standards described in these guidelines, and (*b*) are stored in a comprehensible way for others to have access to them.

§2.1.2 In some laboratories, a staff research associate designated by and responsible to the PI may maintain methodology notebooks, oversee experimental notebooks, have laboratory management responsibilities, and/or instruct new fellows and residents in laboratory techniques and protocols. In those laboratories, the PI meets with the staff research associate to review research progress and data at least once each month (*see* §2.1.4).

§2.1.3 The PI holds scientific meetings with junior investigators, fellows, and residents at least once each month, at which time the PI reviews the experimental notebooks and related data and records. For educational purposes, however, PIs are encouraged to meet with them more frequently, at least once a week, on a one-to-one basis (*see* §2.1.4).

§2.1.4 PIs are encouraged to initial and date the latest page of each experimental notebook reviewed in the event that documentation of these reviews is needed at a later date.

§2.2 Statistical Design and Analysis

Investigators are encouraged to consult a statistician during the earliest stage when designing a study, as well as when interpreting statistical data.

§2.3 Use of Pooled Data

An investigator wishing to base a study on pooled computerized data that was generated by anyone other than him/herself alone must discuss the project with the Director of the BTRC and the PI who derived the data *before work begins* to assure proper authorship, acknowledgment, and attribution of ideas and data.

§2.4 Ownership of Data

Methodology and experimental notebooks and related data and records are the property of the University of California. They may not be removed from the BTRC, although investigators may take a photocopy of all or part of them from the BTRC. [*Note*: When a PI resigns from the University, arrangements can generally be made to transfer ownership appropriately.]

§2.5 Storage of Data

PIs store all data notebooks and related data and records in their laboratory for 5 years after the date when funding for a study ends. They may then continue to store them in their laboratory or may make arrangements with the BTRC research administrator to have them moved to the University's storage facility; both the PI and the BTRC research administrator keep a record of the information necessary to retrieve the materials from the facility. Data notebooks and related data and records for any study may not be destroyed.

§3. Standards for Databooks

§*3.1 Data Notebooks*

§*3.1.1 Bound Notebooks with Consecutively Numbered Pages.*

These databooks, with a permanent (sewn) binding, are the hard copy of choice for data recording. Duplicate pages in the notebooks are intended for generating carbon copies.

§*3.1.2 Loose-Leaf Binders.*

These are used instead of bound data notebooks, at the PI's discretion, to log all or portions of experimental records or generated data. All pages of the loose-leaf binder should be numbered consecutively before the binder is used. Each page should be identifiable as consecutive and belonging to a specific experiment according to a system created and followed in the laboratory (*e.g.* an experiment-identification number followed by the sequential page number and the investigator's or technician's handwritten initials: 1.23.*MT*). The experiment-identification system used is clearly described on the first page of every binder in order to permit proper archiving and retrieval of data. When an experiment is completed, the consecutive pages of data and notes may be inserted into a plastic sleeve(s) for permanent storage in a binder for the one experiment, or in one binder including all experiments for the study.

§*3.1.3 Data and Relevant Material That Are Stored Separately*

(*e.g.* computerized data files, microscope slides): see §3.4.4–3.4.6.

§*3.2 Laboratory Master Log*

For studies involving several investigators, or for laboratories with several individual research projects, the PI(s) keep a master log that serves to catalog the experiments of the whole study or laboratory. This central log, a hardbound databook with consecutively numbered pages, should contain:

- the titles of the studies done by everyone in the laboratory,
- the investigators' names,
- the inclusive dates of the experiments, and
- the location of the experimental notebook and any raw data, computer files, or other relevant materials stored separately for each logged experiment.

§3.3 Methodology Notebook

§3.3.1 In each laboratory, certain techniques or protocols are used in common on a daily basis, such as specific cell-culturing techniques (*e.g.* cell transfers, dilutions, cell counting, media preparation), irradiation techniques, tumor implantation procedures, neurologic examinations, animal anesthesia, electrophoresis procedures, and others. Specific details about each of these commonly used methodologies (including the statistical) are documented and numbered or assigned reference notations that facilitate citation in experimental notebooks. Such documentation serves to standardize all experiments that generate data of the same form and is also instrumental in training new laboratory personnel.

- Notebooks have a section for each technique, and each section contains all versions of the technique, each dated for reference.
- A "table of contents" to the methodologies is kept at the front of the notebook.
- The specific entries in the methodology notebook are modified as improvements in the procedures are developed. Changes are noted precisely *and dated* in the methodology notebook.
- Outdated or discontinued methods remain in the methodology notebook with a notation of the precise date the modified or new method(s) went into effect (*e.g.* so that earlier methods can be readily retrieved for reference in writing a research report).

§3.3.2 The methodology notebook is the final and absolute arbitrating reference when questions of technique are raised in the context of the educational and training responsibilities of the BTRC.

§3.4 Experimental Notebook

§3.4.1 The experimental notebook is the vehicle by which the experiment is fully documented.

§3.4.2 The first several pages of the notebook are reserved for a "table of contents" in which are listed, as the study develops, the experiments and the pages on which the data are located.

§3.4.3 The following *minimum* information is entered for each experiment; PIs are encouraged to make up a "boilerplate" page that can simply be filled in with this information.

- Title of study
- PI's name
- Date the study starts; date it ends
- Associate investigator's name(s) (*i.e.* staff research associate/postdoctoral fellow/ resident/graduate student)
- Brief statement of hypothesis or study goals
- Cell line (passage no.)
  Animal strain and supplier
  Specific animal identification no. (large animals)
  Source of analyzed material
  Tumor type and passage no.

- Drug type (lot no. and/or source), dose(s), dilution(s)
  Radiation source and dose
  Special reagents (*e.g.* antibodies, probes)
  Cell culture batch/medium
  Serum batch/medium
- Experimental design
  ... *study-specific* treatment groups, projected number of subjects, and all other elements of the study design with reference to specific techniques or protocols from the methodology notebook [refer to each specific protocol or technique by its designation (e.g. number) in the methodology notebook].
  ... *statistical methodology* added to or deviating from that in the methodology notebook.
  ... *a "time line"* illustrating the sequence of study events (*e.g.* start – cells added – medium added –)
- Specific notes about special procedures or steps that differ from the techniques specified in the methodology notebook (*e.g.* changes in incubation time or temperature, concentration of trypsin, tumor cell inoculum, infusion rates, anesthetic procedure). *Any variance from the routine procedures recorded in the methodology notebook should be noted in detail* [refer to each specific routine protocol or technique by its designation (*e.g.,* number) in the methodology notebook].
- Raw data, or explicit instructions for locating the raw data or retrieving them from storage (*see* §3.4.4). *Of particular importance are notations about excluded data or animals with detailed information about why those data or animals were excluded.*
- A brief conclusion of the experiment, including a "value judgment" about the validity of the experiment, whether the study needs to be repeated to validate it, what can and cannot be definitively concluded from the data, and other observations. Simple concluding descriptions such as "bad study," or "data suspect," are not acceptable. It is essential to document why the study or data were considered suspect. Justifications for positive judgments should similarly be recorded.

§3.4.4 Raw Data

Whenever possible, raw data are stored together with the experimental notebook; *e.g.* they may be stapled on the duplicate page following the related databook entry or placed in a plastic sleeve(s) and inserted in the binder. Data too unwieldy to include is listed in the experimental notebook as it is collected, is described sufficiently for recognition, and is annotated with the name of investigator and explicitly where the data can be found (*e.g.,* location of the tape or disc and its identification number). Raw data include, but are not limited to:

- handwritten notes on, *e.g.* cell or colony counts, tumor dimensions, physiologic endpoints, daily observations on animals or other visually measured data (*e.g.* CT or NMR tapes) from which observations were made,
- photographs, photomicrographs, and negatives,
- spectra, EEG, evoked potential recordings
- films, scans, images

- slides (*e.g.* histologic sections)
- dated hard copy from computerized data files (*see* §3.4.5).

§3.4.5 Computerized Data Files

In the data notebook are included dated hard copy from these files or, if this is too unwieldy, dated summaries that describe the files sufficiently to find and recognize them, including the location of the data file and the particular computer disc(s) on which the data are stored.

§3.4.6 Blinded, Cooperative, or Multicenter Studies

Data for blinded or double-blind studies are kept in separate (perhaps smaller), bound notebooks by the respective investigators and are brought together with the experimental notebook(s) as a single unit for storage at the end of the study when the code is broken. Data management for cooperative or multicenter studies is in keeping with these guidelines to the greatest extent possible.

§3.4.7 Standards for Keeping Experimental Notebooks

§3.4.7.1 Each entry in the experimental notebook should be able to stand alone, to permit others to replicate the work at any time, whether immediately or even years after it is made.
§3.4.7.2 Experiments are logged in the notebook in chronological sequence.
§3.4.7.3 Data are recorded chronologically as they are collected on consecutive pages of the experimental notebook.
§3.4.7.4 Entries should be organized in such a way that someone not familiar with the specific experiment recorded can retrieve all the pertinent details of the study, from the hypothesis to the published article. Notes entered at the time of the experiment summarizing the goals, details, or problems can be invaluable during subsequent analysis or defense of the results and are therefore encouraged. Optimally, the experimental notebook is a journal of the study.
§3.4.7.5 *Databooks are kept only in ink and should contain no erasures or "whited-out" changes.* An entry made by mistake is deleted only by drawing a single line through it, preferably in ink of a different color. The deleted material should remain legible beneath the overstrike. Large blocks or a page to be disregarded are crossed over with an 'X' or diagonal line and marked, *e.g.* "OMIT." The page should remain legible.
  The corrected data are written beneath or beside the original entry. The explanation for the alteration is clearly written in close proximity to the alteration – preferably on the same page or on the facing page.
§3.4.7.6 If any changes are ever made in the experimental notebook – including a change in values, correction of a mistake, or like alterations – it is absolutely required that those changes be dated and initialed by the person making the alteration, and a clear explanation noted as to why the alteration was made.
§3.4.7.7 In permanently bound databooks containing duplicate (often perforated) numbered pages, only the original bound-in page is used to record data. The duplicate page is used only for a carbon copy or to paste in auxiliary material, *e.g.* photographs; it is otherwise simply left blank.

§3.4.7.8 Whether permanently bound or loose-leaf, only databooks with consecutively numbered pages should be used. Pages should never be torn from a databook.

§3.5 Data Selection File

Preparation of a research report involves the selection of specific experimental data from the experimental notebook. A data selection file, filed separately from the experimental notebook and clearly cross-referenced to it, is kept for each paper to be submitted for publication. *The data selection file consists of*

- Those data selected for reporting and their analyses (including, *e.g.* graphic presentations and statistical manipulations). These are photocopied from the original experimental notebook and cross-referenced to that notebook page by page (unless the cross-reference is evident on the photocopy).
- The rationale for selecting the specific data used in that particular paper recorded narratively ("I selected this datum on the basis of X, I excluded this datum on the basis of Y."), including justification for the selection of specific data to make a curve or other statistical representation.
- A document naming the coauthors and detailing their specific contribution(s) to the study.
- A document naming the persons cited in the acknowledgments as contributing to the paper and detailing their specific contribution(s) to the study.
- Any other material considered pertinent to selection of data, to authorship, or to any substantial related matter arising during the development of the paper.

At the completion of a research project, the data selection file for each paper developed from the project is archived in the PI's laboratory together with the experimental notebook(s) for the project and the photocopies of the relevant material from the methodology notebook(s).

***

Developed and written in 1989 by an Advisory Committee consisting of Susan Eastwood ELS(D) *(chair)*, Philip H Cogen MD PhD, John R Fike PhD, and Harold Rosegay PhD MD, with Michael Berens PhD. Adopted in consultation with BTRC Director (1968–1997) Charles B. Wilson MD, Associate Director Dennis F. Deen PhD, and the principal investigators of the BTRC. Revised in 1995. Revised and updated in 2000 by Susan Eastwood ELS(D), John Fike PhD, and Harold Rosegay PhD MD in consultation with BTRC Director Mitchel S. Berger MD and Associate Director Dennis F. Deen PhD.

***

The BTRC's *Guidelines on Research Data & Reports* is a working document produced to foster good research practice. Suggestions for additions or revisions are welcome.

Questions for Discussion

1. What claims can these participants in externally funded research rightfully make to "owning" the resulting data: the organization that funded the research, the institution to which the funds were granted, the principal investigator who wrote the research proposal, the person who collected the data, the person who analyzed the data? What are the strengths and weaknesses of their respective claims of ownership?
2. What is the difference between ownership of research data and access to research data?
3. Who should have custody of research data during a study? Who should have custody after a study is completed? What are some of the problems related to maintaining various kinds of research data?
4. Identify several situations in which maintaining research data may be difficult. How should anticipated difficulties in maintaining data affect the decision to do certain kinds of research?

Recommended Supplemental Reading

Fishbein EA. Ownership of research data. *Acad Med* 1991;66:129–133.

Freedland KE, Carney RM. Data management and accountability in behavioral and biomedical research. *Am Psychol.*1992;47:640–645.

Kanare HM. *Writing the Laboratory Notebook*. Washington, DC: American Chemical Society; 1985.

Stevens AR. *Ownership and Retention of Data*. The National Association of Colleges and University Attorneys and the National Council of University Research Administrators; 1997. Available at http://www.nacua.org.

The Work of the Academic Scientist

The Work of the Academic Scientist

Ruth Ellen Bulger

The academic scientist has traditionally been expected to undertake several roles at the same time, combining teaching, research, and service to society. The mechanisms used for combining these roles vary throughout academia according to the value or values that individual institutions or their faculty assign to the different functions. However, due to the complexity of modern research, the importance of excellence in teaching, and the changes in the funding of health care, it is becoming increasingly difficult to be a real "triple threat" faculty member, excelling at all three areas at once.

Pressures in Modern Biomedical Research

Doing research in the contemporary environment is becoming increasingly difficult. Research techniques used by academic scientists are rapidly becoming more complex and require up-to-date scientific equipment that is expensive to obtain and maintain. In addition, the emphasis on interdisciplinary research requires each scientist working on a project to spend more time in gaining a basic understanding of all the technologies being used and more time in communicating with collaborating colleagues from other disciplines. Economic pressures are requiring many universities to insist that investigators generate some of their salary support from clinical services, grants, or contracts. Another new pressure bearing upon the academic investigator is to patent discoveries and to work to translate them into marketable technologies.

Pressures in Teaching

As tuition for higher education continues to rise, the public is asking for more accountability concerning these increased educational costs. In return for the high costs, the public expects and deserves quality instruction for students. As biomedical science rapidly advances, the faculty must continue to stay abreast of changes in scientific content and present the new material in an understandable and interesting format. Institutions are faced with providing expensive computer facilities and the personnel to support their use. Developing new ways to deal with informatics and educational computer resources places still more pressure on institutions and the less technically oriented faculty who must learn to use the new technology. On the other hand, as the pressure from some quarters for enhanced teaching quality grows, there is all too often little financial reward or enhanced academic status to encourage high-quality teaching.

Pressures in Providing Health Care

Because academic health centers compete with managed care companies in the provision of health care services, they have had to discount the prices they charge for these services, and hence, clinicians have had to spend an increased amount of time providing medical care. This price discounting decreases not only the amount of money that the clinical faculty can provide for their own salaries and to subsidize research at the institution but also the amount of time they can spend in their own research endeavors.[1] As the clinical dollar shrinks, so does the cross-subsidy that the clinical enterprise has generated to support research in general within the institution.

Balancing the Roles

Shils[2] has stressed the dual roles of the university in both obtaining knowledge and passing it on. Although many, both inside and outside of academia, may think that teaching is the most fundamental responsibility of the university, academic scientists often believe that they are judged for promotion and tenure on the basis of their research and research funding. It appears to many faculty that universities value research as the most essential scholarly pursuit. In this view, the training of younger scientists and the application of knowledge have sometimes even been treated as functions related to the research itself. There is generally little instruction in how to become an effective teacher. The increasingly rapid translation of basic biological discovery to practical and marketable interventions has resulted in close interaction between the academic research university and commercial enterprises, thus raising the status of scientists whose discoveries are translatable into profit-making products. Fortunes may be made by perspicacious or lucky investigators, and this happens often enough to turn the heads of some faculty and to influence the culture in which science is now conducted.

In contradistinction, Boyer[3] has challenged the traditional perspective on academic life that favors research over other scholarly pursuits with a definition of scholarship that is more integrated than hierarchical. For Boyer, the scholarship of *discovery* [*sic*, research] must be complemented by the scholarship of *integration*, which interprets and gives contextual meaning to isolated findings; the scholarship of *application*, which offers new intellectual understanding of scientific findings in the act of using them; and the scholarship of *teaching*, which transmits, transforms, and extends knowledge into the future. Particularly as science becomes more specialized, such integration in academic life is essential in preserving the academic scientist's broader intellectual commitments. An excerpt from Boyer's writings is included in the readings in this chapter.

Boyer's ideas are being integrated into an increasing number of university appointment and promotion documents, which allows a broader definition of scholarship within our universities and a better appreciation of all aspects of university faculty responsibility. These changing values, which institutions express by the totality of their practices – including promotion and tenure, interdisciplinary collaboration and peer review, admissions, funding of student assistantships, grading, and advising – could shape a new self-image and social role of the academic scientists of the future.

Ethical Aspects of Collaborative Scientific Research

Most faculty have chosen careers in academic institutions not only because of their interest in the education of students but also because of a passion for, and commitment to, new scientific discoveries. Whether it is purely the intellectual joy of elucidating some new biological process or the desire to understand normal and abnormal biology and thereby to help in preventing or curing disease, the academic scientist understands that to succeed in a research-intensive university environment, research accomplishments are expected. The majority of the chapters in this book deal with ethical aspects of scientific research, and this material will not be repeated here. There is, however, one cross-cutting aspect of modern research that needs further emphasis: that of collaboration among scientists.

Both scientists and the funders of scientific research have recognized that a collaborative multidisciplinary approach is an excellent way to examine many aspects of complex research questions. No one scientist can be proficient in all research approaches that may facilitate the understanding of a complex research system. With the increased ability to communicate made possible by the Internet, such collaborations may easily involve scientists at local, national, or international sites.

That is the good news. However, along with these broad approaches in which several scientists contribute their expertise equally to solving the biological problem come several complex organizational issues that must be dealt with early in the planning of the multi-disciplinary research. What kind of a communications network will be established? How will the various scientists involved be able to ensure that each part of the work is done responsibly when they are not familiar with all of the techniques, or should publications clearly state who is responsible for which parts of the data? How are the data to be shared? Where will it be maintained? Who will be able to use the data independently? Who will have rights to any biologic products made during the joint work? How will money flow across the institutions? How will the conflicts of interest of individual scientists be shared with the other investigators?

These issues become even more important when one of the collaborating research partners is from industry. Then issues of secrecy of information and sharing of data and products need to be even more clearly defined.

Some institutions require that a formal Memorandum of Understanding or some similar document be written and accepted by each institution involved before any research is initiated. Investigators at each institution must follow the research regulations of their institution and coordinate with those of the other institutions. Written agreements may be helpful in establishing that the ground rules for collaboration are well understood.

Ethical Aspect of Teaching and Learning

Our institutions present several ethical concepts related to education to graduate students in the biomedical sciences. Bulger[4] identified three of these ethical aspects underlying ethics in teaching as *competence and communication, justice and caring,* and *creativity and freedom from control.* In demonstrating scholarly competence and communication, the teaching must accurately distinguish what is known about a topic from what is unknown or poorly understood. Knowledge of general educational principles is important, as is concentrating on a discipline's central intellectual principles and problems without giving excessively detailed information, thereby allowing adequate study time for the student. Irby[5] identifies essential factors outside of disciplinary competency that are essential to excellence in teaching: organization of material, clarity of presentation, enthusiasm, the ability to entertain questions openly, the ability to establish goals and evaluate progress, and the ability to transmit a sense of wonder and curiosity.

The principle of justice is demonstrated when the professor ensures equal access to materials, equal opportunity for instruction and remediation, and equitable grading standards; caring can be demonstrated in a variety of ways, including helping a student find a solution to academic problems and demonstrating a mutual respect for both faculty and students.

Teachers need to enhance the creative potential of their students. Teachers also need to examine their own motives so as not to exert undue pressure on students or to take advantage of their dependent position. Faculty members need to consider whether they are helping their students to obtain the degree in a reasonable amount of time or whether they are using their highly intelligent but low-paid students to further their own research advancement. It is crucial that faculty give proper credit to students for their work or ideas. It is equally important to be supportive of students and to look for positive aspects of their work so as not to impair their confidence by excessive criticism.

Reiser[6] focuses attention on ethical issues and relationships connected with the environment of both teaching and learning to help elaborate an ethics of education. He moves beyond the faculty-student relationship to examine the student's role with respect to the faculty and the responsibility for learning. In discussing the medical student's role with respect to future patients for which the student will care, Reiser believes that the faculty–student relationship will be mirrored in the student–patient relationship. The relationship of students to each other presages the future responsibility that the student will have in preventing harm to patients caused by other professionals. Finally, Reiser discusses the educational messages that the institutional administrator gives in making decisions about students, personnel, community, and society, which are not missed by those working within the institution. He concludes that the teaching and learning environment needs an ethical foundation to define the responsibilities and mission of teaching.

Being a Mentor

There is a growing understanding of the positive role that a mentor can have on the career of a young scientist. A wonderful book that discusses the many roles that faculty can play in the education of graduate students and other young scientists was recently published with the appropriate title *Advisor, Teacher, Role Model, Friend: On Being a Mentor to Students in Science and Engineering*.[7] It defines a mentor as "someone who takes a special interest in helping another person develop into a successful professional. . . . [An] effective mentoring relationship is characterized by mutual respect, trust, understanding, and empathy." In advising those who aspire to be mentors to others, the book gives good counsel: to listen patiently, giving the student time; to build a relationship by developing rapport; to refrain from abusing your authority by inappropriate requests; to nurture self-sufficiency and independent thinking by the student; to establish protected time together for the benefit of the student; to share your human side with the student; to provide introductions to your professional network; and to not be overbearing by dictating choices. Then the book advises that mentors find their own mentors to benefit themselves.

In most graduate programs, advisors or mentors are built into the educational process. If faculty take their designated roles seriously, the student can find the necessary support. It may come from several different people and not just from the thesis advisor. That is one reason why a graduate student has a committee of several people who can play differing roles in the student's education and research endeavors. Official mentoring roles are established less frequently for postdoctoral fellows. Some institutions do not even keep accurate lists of postdoctoral fellows working within the institution because they usually are hired under a variety of mechanisms and titles by an individual faculty member. Few specific institutional policies or educational activities are addressed directly to this group, and even those efforts can be resisted by the faculty member for whom the fellow is working, due to the time that such activities take from the research. Depending on the particular research advisor, a fellow may not get appropriate help to facilitate career development.

Finally, mentoring is rarely even broached when considering the needs of a new junior assistant professor. Yet the years as an assistant professor are some of the most difficult in an academic career. This is the period when the faculty member must establish an independent research program and writing grant applications to fund the research. It is also the time when new teaching assignments are given and lectures need to be prepared and presented. Finally, it is the time when many young faculty have responsibilities for bearing and caring for small children. Considering how an academic department can provide adequate mentoring for its younger faculty members can be a great help in establishing a successful career for such individuals.

Allowing and facilitating trainees to develop their own areas of scientific expertise and not just assigning them a part of a mentor's previously conceived of and written grant application are also key to adequate research training. The trainee needs to read the literature, propose a hypothesis that fills a gap in the present knowledge, and then test it under the tutelage of an experienced mentor. If new reagents or cell products are developed during the trainee's research experience, sharing them with the trainee as the person moves on to other research environments is also important to his or her continued career development.

Moving Beyond Compliance to a Culture of Social Responsibility

At present there are over 60 sets of compliance regulations that scientists must follow. The two sets of regulations most familiar to biomedical scientists regulate the humane care and use of animals and the protection of human subjects in research. The NIH now requires any research application for funding that will use human volunteers or human tissues in the research to describe the training for key personnel concerning human participant regulations. More recently, the Office of Research Integrity has proposed a rule describing additional areas in which each member of the research staff (those who have direct and substantive involvement in proposing, performing, reviewing, or reporting research or who receive research training supported by PHS funds) should receive training in the responsible conduct of research (http://ori.dhhs.gov/html/programs/finalpolicy.asp). If this policy is accepted, instruction in the responsible conduct of research would be similar to the training that NIH has required for all graduate and postgraduate trainees supported by National Research Service Award Institutional Training Grants since 1992.

How does one establish a culture in which all research participants understand and comply with these federal, state, and local regulations? One frequently used method is to provide required educational experiences for faculty, students, and research staff to ensure that they are cognizant of the regulations. The number of required educational experiences is increasing as societal concerns about how research is done have continued to surface. The humane use and care of animals, the use of radioactive substances in research, and in the handling of harmful chemicals or biological agents are examples of required courses already taught to potential investigators before they begin any research undertaking using these techniques. The recent NIH requirement that researchers receive training in the ethical treatment of human subjects in research before receiving funding of a grant that involves human research is just one example of additional required training.

Yet self-regulation, not required classes, would be more in keeping with what it means to be a member of a profession. It is important to consider how faculty and their institutions can establish a culture in which there is a basic desire to do research ethically and responsibly. Faculty play a key role in establishing such a culture by their individual actions and by the example they set for graduate students who work with them in the laboratory as well as for other young faculty. Pedagogy by example can be more effective than a rhetorical approach. Most universities have developed guidelines to help faculty recognize their responsibilities in such areas as supervision of trainees, data management, authorship, and research on human and animal subjects as well as procedures and requirements for promotion and tenure. The readings in this chapter include the NIH Intramural Guidelines for Scientists in their intramural program, which can serve as an example of the kinds of guidance that scientists can receive.

The Office of Management and Budget (OMB) has written several circulars (especially OMB Circular A110 and A21 or A122) enumerating the financial and scientific responsibilities that institutions and investigators have when they accept funding from a government agency. These documents are complex and generally never read by key research personnel on government-funded grants. Yet the scientists are bound by these regulations. To help make these responsibilities understandable to the scientists, I helped prepare a document entitled "Roles and Responsibilities of Principal Investigators for Research Projects" (see Appendix) that lists in a simple one-page format the responsibilities that each PI must read, sign, and agree to accept before having a grant submitted to a funding agency by the institution.

The Institutional Role in Establishing a Culture of Responsibility

The institution as well as the investigator must be involved in this process of establishing a culture of responsibility. Institutional administrators also need to manifest their ethical conduct in the way they treat all institutional employees by making administrative decisions that treat all students, faculty, and staff fairly and respectfully.

Mumford[8] has examined the nature and role of how an organization can influence scientific integrity. He investigated the role of individual and situational factors to integrity. In a recent abstract, he concluded that, at an individual level, lapses in integrity appear to be linked to overload, poor collegial support, a focus on extrinsic rewards, and a lack of involvement with the work. At a group level, it was poor leadership, lack of consensus, competitive pressure, and normlessness that were significant influences. At an organizational level, the operating environment – specifically its turbulence, munificence, interdependence, and climate with respect to its emphasis on trust, fairness, and openness – was related to integrity. It is therefore important that not only faculty but each institutional administrator examine the internal environment and work to make it conducive to the practice of integrity by all.

Reiser[9] believes that it is important for university administrators to recognize that they retain their basic role as teachers as they create and administer policy, and therefore that they need to think more critically about how to fulfill this responsibility. One way that he suggests is to hold regular open discussions with people in the institution about competing institutional pressures and policy alternatives. This could well be done within the framework of administrative case rounds in a manner similar to the very effective and often used clinical case rounds. Possible topics might include pressing issues involving institutional personnel, competing institutional expansion possibilities, or competing education or research opportunities.

Conclusions

Whatever the mechanisms used within an institution, the goal of the university should be to stimulate and reinforce the ethical conduct of faculty, administrators, and students in all aspects of their careers. Success in such an endeavor will invariably form an ethical institution. That is the proper work of the academic scientist.

Appendix   Roles and Responsibilities of Principal Investigators for Research Projects

When undertaking a research project, the Principal Investigator assumes numerous important responsibilities that include the preparation of the proposal, the compliance with appropriate assurances processes, the conduct and integrity of the scientific project and its close-out processes, and the subsequent dissemination of the research results.

The Principal Investigator is responsible for:

— the scientific soundness, accuracy, and completeness of the research proposal including
   Preparation of the technical research proposals or research fellowship applications;
   Submission of these proposal through the office of grants with the proper scientific, statistical, and departmental review and the verification of the adequacy of the resources to conduct the research; and
   Coordinating proper review of any off-site research activity.
— the scientific, ethical, and technical aspects of any resulting research project including
   Oversight of all activities in the laboratory and each study site involved;
   Training and education of all individuals working on the project in such areas as laboratory safety, scientific rigor, data collection and management, and scientific integrity including, but not limited to, issues such as authorship, conflict of interest and commitment, and humans and animal subjects issues; and
   Understanding that research conducted at this institution must satisfy not only the needs of the investigators but of the institution, society, and the funding agency.
— the proper budgetary management of awarded funds including
   Authorizing the allocation and verifying the appropriateness of research costs as legitimate, allowable, and correct; and
   Financial monitoring of accelerated expenditures, large unobligated balances and over-expenditures;
   Initiation and coordination of personnel actions for the research personnel;
   Re-budgeting in a timely and accurate way; and
   Ensuring that program income (if any) is returned to the grant.
— compliance with the specific terms of the award and statutes including
   Obtaining, maintaining, and adhering to all research assurances such as human subjects, animal care and welfare, radiation safety, hazardous chemical, recombinant DNA, and biological substances;

Compliance with terms including prior written approval for change in scope, foreign
travel, equipment purchases and disposition, hiring, contracting, and re-budgeting;
and

Submitting interim and final scientific reports and other required reports to the research
office before submission to the funding organization.

— protecting the University from legal liability related to the research project.

— following other Federal regulations such as those concerning proscriptions against lobbying, financial discussions with industry funding sponsors, and as specified in the
institution's Grant Terms and Conditions.

*Signed*_____ *Date*_____

(*From the Uniformed Services University of the Health Sciences, 1998*).

References

1. Weissman JS, Saglam D, Campbell N, Causino N, Blumenthal D. Market forces and unsponsored research in AHCs. *JAMA*. 2000; 281;1093–1098.
2. Shils E. The report of a study group of the International Council on the Future of the University. In *The Academic Ethic*. Chicago: University of Chicago Press; 1986.
3. Boyer EL. *Scholarship Reconsidered: Priorities of the Professorate.* Princeton, NJ: Carnegie Foundation; 1990.
4. Bulger RE. The need for an ethical code for teachers of the basic biomedical sciences. *J Med Educ.* 1988;63:131–133.
5. Irby DM. Evaluating teaching skills. *Diabetes Educator.* 1985;(suppl PPL)11:37–46.
6. Reiser SJ. The ethics of learning and teaching medicine. *Acad Med.* 1994;69:872–876.
7. National Academy of Sciences, National Academy of Engineering, Institute of Medicine. *Advisor, Teacher, Role Model, Friend. On Being a Mentor to Students in Science and Engineering.* Washington, DC: National Academy Press; 1997. Available at http://www.nap.edu/readingroom/books/mentor.
8. Mumford MD. Organizational influences on scientific integrity. *Procedings of the Office of Research Integrity Research Conference on Research Integrity*, Washington, DC;2000:13–14.
9. Reiser SJ. Administrative case rounds: Institutional policies and leaders cast in a different light. *JAMA.* 1991;266:2127–2128.

Enlarging the Perspective

Ernest L. Boyer

Since colonial times, the American professoriate has responded to mandates both from within the academy and beyond. First came teaching, then service, and finally, the challenge of research. In more recent years, faculty have been asked to blend these three traditions, but despite this idealized expectation, a wide gap now exists between the myth and the reality of academic life. Almost all colleges pay lip service to the trilogy of teaching, research, and service, but when it comes to making judgments about professional performance, the three rarely are assigned equal merit.

Today, when we speak of being "scholarly," it usually means having academic rank in a college or university and being engaged in research and publication. But we should remind ourselves just how recently the word "research" actually entered the vocabulary of higher education. The term was first used in England in the 1870s by reformers who wished to make Cambridge and Oxford "not only a place of teaching, but a place of learning," and it was later introduced to American higher education in 1906 by Daniel Coit Gilman.[1] But scholarship in earlier times referred to a variety of creative work carried on in a variety of places, and its integrity was measured by the ability to think, communicate, and learn.

What we now have is a more restricted view of scholarship, one that limits it to a hierarchy of functions. Basic research has come to be viewed as the first and most essential form of scholarly activity, with other functions flowing from it. Scholars are academics who conduct research, publish, and then perhaps convey their knowledge to students or apply what they have learned. The latter functions grow *out of* scholarship, they are not to be considered a part of it. But knowledge is not necessarily developed in such a linear manner. The arrow of causality can, and frequently does, point in *both* directions. Theory surely leads to practice. But practice also leads to theory. And teaching, at its best, shapes both research and practice. Viewed from this perspective, a more comprehensive, more dynamic understanding of scholarship can be considered, one in which the rigid categories of teaching, research, and service are broadened and more flexibly defined.

There is a readiness, we believe, to rethink what it means to be a scholar. Richard I. Miller, professor of higher education at Ohio University, recently surveyed academic vice presidents and deans at more than eight hundred colleges and universities to get their opinion about faculty functions. These administrators were asked if they thought it would be a good idea to view scholarship as more than research. The responses were overwhelmingly supportive of this proposition.[2] The need to reconsider scholarship surely goes beyond

From Ernest L. Boyer, *Scholarship Reconsidered: Priorities of the Professorate* (Princeton, NJ: Carnegie Foundation, 1990), pp. 15–25. © The Carnegie Foundation for the Advancement of Teaching. Reprinted with permission.

opinion polls, but campus debates, news stories, and the themes of national conventions suggest that administrative leaders are rethinking the definitions of academic life. Moreover, faculty, themselves, appear to be increasingly dissatisfied with conflicting priorities on the campus.

How then should we proceed? Is it possible to define the work of faculty in ways that reflect more realistically the full range of academic and civic mandates? We believe the time has come to move beyond the tired old "teaching versus research" debate and give the familiar and honorable term "scholarship" a broader, more capacious meaning, one that brings legitimacy to the full scope of academic work. Surely, scholarship means engaging in original research. But the work of the scholar also means stepping back from one's investigation, looking for connections, building bridges between theory and practice, and communicating one's knowledge effectively to students. Specifically, we conclude that the work of the professoriate might be thought of as having four separate, yet overlapping, functions. These are: the scholarship of *discovery;* the scholarship of *integration;* the scholarship of *application;* and the scholarship of *teaching.*

The first and most familiar element in our model, the *scholarship of discovery*, comes closest to what is meant when academics speak of "research." No tenets in the academy are held in higher regard than the commitment to knowledge for its own sake, to freedom of inquiry and to following, in a disciplined fashion, an investigation wherever it may lead. Research is central to the work of higher learning, but our study here, which inquires into the meaning of scholarship, is rooted in the conviction that disciplined, investigative efforts within the academy should be strengthened, not diminished.

The *scholarship of discovery,* at its best, contributes not only to the stock of human knowledge but also to the intellectual climate of a college or university. Not just the outcomes, but the process, and especially the passion, give meaning to the effort. The advancement of knowledge can generate an almost palpable excitement in the life of an educational institution. As William Bowen, former president of Princeton University, said, scholarly research "reflects our pressing, irrepressible need as human beings to confront the unknown and to seek understanding for its own sake. It is tied inextricably to the freedom to think freshly, to see propositions of every kind in ever-changing light. And it celebrates the special exhilaration that comes from a new idea."[3]

The list of distinguished researchers who have added luster to the nation's intellectual life would surely include heroic figures of earlier days – Yale chemist Benjamin Silliman; Harvard naturalist Louis Agassiz; astronomer William Cranch Bond; and Columbia anthropologist Franz Boas. It would also include giants of our time – James Watson, who helped unlock the genetic code; political philosopher Hannah Arendt; anthropologist Ruth Benedict; historian John Hope Franklin; geneticist Barbara McClintock; and Noam Chomsky, who transformed the field of linguistics; among others.

When the research records of higher learning are compared, the United States is the pacesetter. If we take as our measure of accomplishment the number of Nobel Prizes awarded since 1945, United States scientists received 56 percent of the awards in physics, 42 percent in chemistry, and 60 percent in medicine. Prior to the outbreak of the Second World War, American scientists, including those who fled Hitler's Europe, had received only 18 of the 129 prizes in these three areas.[4] With regard to physics, for example, a recent report by the National Research Council states: "Before World War II, physics was essentially a European activity, but by the war's end, the center of physics had moved to the United States."[5] The

Council goes on to review the advances in fields ranging from elementary particle physics to cosmology.

The research contribution of universities is particularly evident in medicine. Investigations in the late nineteenth century on bacteria and viruses paid off in the 1930s with the development of immunizations for diphtheria, tetanus, lobar pneumonia, and other bacterial infections. On the basis of painstaking research, a taxonomy of infectious diseases has emerged, making possible streptomycin and other antibiotics. In commenting on these breakthroughs, physician and medical writer Lewis Thomas observes: "It was basic science of a very high order, storing up a great mass of interesting knowledge for its own sake, creating, so to speak, a bank of information, ready for drawing on when the time for intelligent use arrived."[6]

Thus, the probing mind of the researcher is an incalculably vital asset to the academy and the world. Scholarly investigation, in all the disciplines, is at the very heart of academic life, and the pursuit of knowledge must be assiduously cultivated and defended. The intellectual excitement fueled by this quest enlivens faculty and invigorates higher learning institutions, and in our complicated, vulnerable world, the discovery of new knowledge is absolutely crucial.

The Scholarship of Integration

In proposing the *scholarship of integration,* we underscore the need for scholars who give meaning to isolated facts, putting them in perspective. By integration, we mean making connections across the disciplines, placing the specialties in larger context, illuminating data in a revealing way, often educating nonspecialists, too. In calling for a scholarship of integration, we do not suggest returning to the "gentleman scholar" of an earlier time, nor do we have in mind the dilettante. Rather, what we mean is serious, disciplined work that seeks to interpret, draw together, and bring new insight to bear on original research.

This more integrated view of knowledge was expressed eloquently by Mark Van Doren nearly thirty years ago when he wrote: "The connectedness of things is what the educator contemplates to the limit of his capacity. No human capacity is great enough to permit a vision of the world as simple, but if the educator does not aim at the vision no one else will, and the consequences are dire when no one does."[7] It is through "connectedness" that research ultimately is made authentic.

The scholarship of integration is, of course, closely related to discovery. It involves, first, doing research at the boundaries where fields converge, and it reveals itself in what philosopher-physicist Michael Polanyi calls "overlapping [academic] neighborhoods."[8] Such work is, in fact, increasingly important as traditional disciplinary categories prove confining, forcing new topologies of knowledge. Many of today's professors understand this. When we asked faculty to respond to the statement, "Multidisciplinary work is soft and should not be considered scholarship," only 8 percent agreed, 17 percent were neutral, while a striking 75 percent disagreed (see table). This pattern of opinion, with only slight variation, was true for professors in all disciplines and across all types of institutions.

The scholarship of integration also means interpretation, fitting one's own research – or the research of others – into larger intellectual patterns. Such efforts are increasingly essential since specialization, without broader perspective, risks pedantry. The distinction

*Multidisciplinary Work Is Soft and Should not
Be Considered Scholarship*

	Agree	Neutral	Disagree
All Respondents	8%	17%	75%
Research	7	9	84
Doctorate-granting	6	13	80
Comprehensive	8	14	78
Liberal Arts	8	16	77
Two-Year	9	27	63

Source: The Carnegie Foundation for the Advancement of Teaching, 1989 National Survey of Faculty.

we are drawing here between "discovery" and "integration" can be best understood, perhaps,
by the questions posed. Those engaged in discovery ask, "What is to be known, what is yet
to be found?" Those engaged in integration ask, "What do the findings *mean*? Is it possible to interpret what's been discovered in ways that provide a larger, more comprehensive
understanding?" Questions such as these call for the power of critical analysis and interpretation. They have a legitimacy of their own and if carefully pursued can lead the scholar
from information to knowledge and even, perhaps, to wisdom.

   Today, more than at any time in recent memory, researchers feel the need to move
beyond traditional disciplinary boundaries, communicate with colleagues in other fields,
and discover patterns that connect. Anthropologist Clifford Geertz, of the Institute for
Advanced Study in Princeton, has gone so far as to describe these shifts as a fundamental
"refiguration, . . . a phenomenon general enough and distinctive enough to suggest that what
we are seeing is not just another redrawing of the cultural map – the moving of a few disputed
borders, the marking of some more picturesque mountain lakes – but an alteration of the
principles of mapping. Something is happening," Geertz says, "to the way we think about
the way we think."[9]

   This is reflected, he observes, in:

. . . philosophical inquiries looking like literary criticism (think of Stanley Cavell on Beckett or
Thoreau, Sartre on Flaubert), scientific discussions looking like belles lettres *morceaux* (Lewis
Thomas, Loren Eiseley), baroque fantasies presented as deadpan empirical observations (Borges,
Barthelme), histories that consist of equations and tables or law court testimony (Fogel and
Engerman, Le Roi Ladurie), documentaries that read like true confessions (Mailer), parables posing
as ethnographies (Castañeda), theoretical treatises set out as travelogues (Lévi-Strauss), ideological
arguments cast as historiographical inquiries (Edward Said), epistemological studies constructed
like political tracts (Paul Feyerabend), methodological polemics got up as personal memoirs (James
Watson).[10]

   These examples illustrate a variety of scholarly trends – *interdisciplinary, interpretive,
integrative*. But we present them here as evidence that an intellectual sea change may be
occurring, one that is perhaps as momentous as the nineteenth-century shift in the hierarchy

of knowledge, when philosophy gave way more firmly to science. Today, interdisciplinary *and* integrative studies, long on the edges of academic life, are moving toward the center, responding both to new intellectual questions and to pressing human problems. As the boundaries of human knowledge are being dramatically reshaped, the academy surely must give increased attention to the *scholarship of integration*.

The Scholarship of Application

The first two kinds of scholarship – discovery and integration of knowledge – reflect the investigative and synthesizing traditions of academic life. The third element, the *application* of knowledge, moves toward engagement as the scholar asks, "How can knowledge be responsibly applied to consequential problems? How can it be helpful to individuals as well as institutions?" And further, "Can social problems *themselves* define an agenda for scholarly investigation?"

Reflecting the *Zeitgeist* of the nineteenth and early twentieth centuries, not only the land-grant colleges, but also institutions such as Rensselaer Polytechnic Institute and the University of Chicago were founded on the principle that higher education must serve the interests of the larger community. In 1906, an editor celebrating the leadership of William Rainey Harper at the new University of Chicago defined what he believed to be the essential character of the American scholar. Scholarship, he observed, was regarded by the British as "a means and measure of self-development," by the Germans as "an end in itself," but by Americans as "equipment for service."[11] Self-serving though it may have been, this analysis had more than a grain of truth.

Given this tradition, one is struck by the gap between values in the academy and the needs of the larger world. Service is routinely praised, but accorded little attention – even in programs where it is most appropriate. Christopher Jencks and David Riesman, for example, have pointed out that when free-standing professional schools affiliated with universities, they lessened their commitment to applied work even though the original purpose of such schools was to connect theory and practice. Professional schools, they concluded, have oddly enough fostered "a more academic and less practical view of what their students need to know."[12]

Colleges and universities have recently rejected service as serious scholarship, partly because its meaning is so vague and often disconnected from serious intellectual work. As used today, service in the academy covers an almost endless number of campus activities – sitting on committees, advising student clubs, or performing departmental chores. The definition blurs still more as activities beyond the campus are included – participation in town councils, youth clubs, and the like. It is not unusual for almost any worthy project to be dumped into the amorphous category called "service."

Clearly, a sharp distinction must be drawn between *citizenship* activities and projects that relate to scholarship itself. To be sure, there are meritorious social and civic functions to be performed, and faculty should be appropriately recognized for such work. But all too frequently, service means not doing scholarship but doing good. To be considered *scholarship*, service activities must be tied directly to one's special field of knowledge and relate to, and flow directly out of, this professional activity. Such service is serious, demanding work, requiring the rigor – and the accountability – traditionally associated with research activities.

The *scholarship of application*, as we define it here, is not a one-way street. Indeed, the term itself may be misleading if it suggests that knowledge is first "discovered" and then "applied." The process we have in mind is far more dynamic. New intellectual understandings can arise out of the very act of application – whether in medical diagnosis, serving clients in psychotherapy, shaping public policy, creating an architectural design, or working with the public schools. In activities such as these, theory and practice vitally interact, and one renews the other.

Such a view of scholarly service – one that both applies and contributes to human knowledge – is particularly needed in a world in which huge, almost intractable problems call for the skills and insights only the academy can provide. As Oscar Handlin observed, our troubled planet "can no longer afford the luxury of pursuits confined to an ivory tower.... [S]cholarship has to prove its worth not on its own terms but by service to the nation and the world."[13]

The Scholarship of Teaching

Finally, we come to the *scholarship of teaching*. The work of the professor becomes consequential only as it is understood by others. Yet, today, teaching is often viewed as a routine function, tacked on, something almost anyone can do. When defined as *scholarship*, however, teaching both educates and entices future scholars. Indeed, as Aristotle said, "Teaching is the highest form of understanding."

As a *scholarly* enterprise, teaching begins with what the teacher knows. Those who teach must, above all, be well informed, and steeped in the knowledge of their fields. Teaching can be well regarded only as professors are widely read and intellectually engaged. One reason legislators, trustees, and the general public often fail to understand why ten or twelve hours in the classroom each week can be a heavy load is their lack of awareness of the hard work and the serious study that undergirds good teaching.

Teaching is also a dynamic endeavor involving all the analogies, metaphors, and images that build bridges between the teacher's understanding and the student's learning. Pedagogical procedures must be carefully planned, continuously examined, and relate directly to the subject taught. Educator Parker Palmer strikes precisely the right note when he says knowing and learning are communal acts.[14] With this vision, great teachers create a common ground of intellectual commitment. They stimulate active, not passive, learning and encourage students to be critical, creative thinkers, with the capacity to go on learning after their college days are over.

Further, good teaching means that faculty, as scholars, are also learners. All too often, teachers transmit information that students are expected to memorize and then, perhaps, recall. While well-prepared lectures surely have a place, teaching, at its best, means not only transmitting knowledge, but *transforming* and *extending* it as well. Through reading, through classroom discussion, and surely through comments and questions posed by students, professors themselves will be pushed in creative new directions.

In the end, inspired teaching keeps the flame of scholarship alive. Almost all successful academics give credit to creative teachers – those mentors who defined their work so compellingly that it became, for them, a lifetime challenge. Without the teaching function, the continuity of knowledge will be broken and the store of human knowledge dangerously diminished.

Physicist Robert Oppenheimer, in a lecture at the 200th anniversary of Columbia University in 1954, spoke elegantly of the teacher as mentor and placed teaching at the very heart of the scholarly endeavor: "The specialization of science is an inevitable accompaniment of progress; yet it is full of dangers, and it is cruelly wasteful, since so much that is beautiful and enlightening is cut off from most of the world. Thus it is proper to the role of the scientist that he not merely find the truth and communicate it to his fellows, but that he teach, that he try to bring the most honest and most intelligible account of new knowledge to all who will try to learn."[15]

Here, then, is our conclusion. What we urgently need today is a more inclusive view of what it means to be a scholar – a recognition that knowledge is acquired through research, through synthesis, through practice, and through teaching.[16] We acknowledge that these four categories – the scholarship of discovery, of integration, of application, and of teaching – divide intellectual functions that are tied inseparably to each other. Still, there is value, we believe, in analyzing the various kinds of academic work, while also acknowledging that they dynamically interact, forming an interdependent whole. Such a vision of scholarship, one that recognizes the great diversity of talent within the professoriate, also may prove especially useful to faculty as they reflect on the meaning and direction of their professional lives.

Notes

1. Charles Wegener, *Liberal Education and the Modern University* (Chicago: The University of Chicago Press, 1978), 9–12; citing Daniel C. Gilman, *The Launching of a University and Other Papers* (New York: Dodd Mead & Co., 1906), 238–39 and 242–43.
2. Richard I. Miller, Hongyu Chen, Jerome B. Hart, and Clyde B. Killian, "New Approaches to Faculty Evaluation – A Survey, Initial Report" (Athens, Ohio; submitted to The Carnegie Foundation for the Advancement of Teaching by Richard I. Miller, Professor of Higher Education, Ohio University, 4 September 1990.)
3. William G. Bowen, *Ever the Teacher: William G. Bowen's Writings as President of Princeton* (Princeton, N.J.: Princeton University Press, 1987), 269.
4. Harriet Zuckerman, *Scientific Elite: Nobel Laureates in the United States* (New York: The Free Press, A Division of Macmillan, 1977), 282–88; citing *The World Book Encyclopedia*, vol. 14, 1975.
5. National Research Council, *Physics Through the 1990s* (Washington, D.C.: National Academy Press, 1986), 8.
6. Lewis Thomas, "Biomedical Science and Human Health: The Long-Range Prospect," *Daedalus* (Spring 1977), 164–69; in Bowen, *Ever the Teacher*, 241–42.
7. Mark Van Doren, *Liberal Education* (Boston: Beacon Press, 1959), 115.
8. Michael Polanyi, *The Tacit Dimension* (Garden City, N.Y.: Doubleday, 1967), 72; in Ernest L. Boyer, *College: The Undergraduate Experience in America* (New York: Harper & Row, 1987), 91.
9. Clifford Geertz, "Blurred Genres: The Refiguration of Social Thought," *The American Scholar* (Spring 1980), 165–66.
10. Ibid.
11. Lyman Abbott, "William Rainey Harper," *Outlook*, no. 82 (20 January 1906), 110–111; in Frederick Rudolph, *The American College and University: A History* (New York: Alfred A. Knopf, 1962), 356.
12. Christopher Jencks and David Riesman, *The Academic Revolution* (Garden City, N.Y.: Doubleday, 1968), 252.

13. Oscar Handlin, "Epilogue – Continuities," in Bernard Bailyn, Donald Fleming, Oscar Handlin, and Stephan Thernstrom, *Glimpses of the Harvard Past* (Cambridge, Mass.: Harvard University Press, 1986), 131; in Derek Bok, *Universities and the Future of America* (Durham, N.C., and London: Duke University Press, 1990), 103.

14. Parker J. Palmer, *To Know As We Are Known* (New York: Harper & Row, 1983).

15. *The New York Times*, 27 December 1954, D27.

16. Parker J. Palmer to Russell Edgerton, president of the American Association for Higher Education, 2 April 1990.

Obstacles to Collegiality in the Academic Health Center

Roger James Bulger and Ruth Ellen Bulger

> *"The unexamined life is not worth living"*
>
> Socrates, quoted by Plato, *The Apology*

In attempting to understand the obstacles to collegiality within a medical school, a full-blown academic health center with several health professional schools, or a university one cannot escape the need to understand societal and cultural elements that describe the particularly American experience from which our academic institutions have emerged. *Habits of the Heart*, by Robert Bellah and colleagues,[1] is to the America of the 1990s as *The Lonely Crowd*, by David Riesman, was to the America of the 1950s; that is, *Habits of the Heart* seeks to understand the particular searches for individual meanings characteristic of Americans in the postmodern age. The major thread that runs through Bellah and his coauthors' work is the American search for a sense of community, of connectedness, and of meaning for life. The authors point out that Americans need to reach common understandings about the appropriate sharing of economic resources based "on conceptions of a substantively just society,"[2] The authors look to our moral traditions for resources to think about these issues. They draw upon three major historical trends embedded in our nation's earliest years: the Biblical construction, exemplified by the search for a just and compassionate society to be shared with one's neighbors as personified by John Winthrop, first governor of Massachusetts; the utilitarian, individualistic, "God helps those who help themselves"[3] motif personified by Benjamin Franklin; and the Republican commitment "of a self-governing society of relative equals, in which all participate,"[4] best articulated by Thomas Jefferson. Alexis de Tocqueville, in 1835, worried for the fledgling nation about the naive individualism born of Benjamin Franklin but finding expression throughout the American frontier – an individualism that led people to believe that with their acres of land, their families and small sets of friends, and their guns, they had no need of any other human or social structure. If this tendency for isolation got the upper hand in America over the tendencies to community flowing out of the biblical and republican ideas, he felt that the great democratic experiment might break apart and fail.

In America, the scales of justice as expressed through equity and liberty, as well as through individual freedoms, are balanced differently than in most other Western democracies. In America we tilt inevitably more towards individual freedom than we do to equity. To a

Presented as part of a *Symposium on Academic Collegiality in American Medicine* held by the Foundation for Neurosurgical Research at Camp Topridge, New York, September 7–9, 1990.

From the *Bulletin of the New York Academy of Medicine*, 1991;68:304–307. Reprinted with permission of the Bulletin of the New York Academy of Medicine.

significant extent, our national meaning has been rooted in an expanding frontier, a limitless hope for improvement, a firm belief that each generation will be materially better than the last, and that our inventiveness and productivity are infinite. During recent decades, one after another of these self-conceptions, myths, and unifying ideas have been shattered or significantly discredited. Nuclear plant disasters, the Challenger tragedy, and our sense of loss of human control even over medically-related technologies have all contributed to our uncertainties. We are not first in the world in all ways; science has not brought us to Utopia; our children are not going to be better off than we are and they do not seem to want to propagate the race with much enthusiasm; and living longer is not a guaranteed good thing, especially when so many are frightened at the discomfort and expense with which they might die.

Our patriotism, our family structures and allegiances, our biblical language, and our unifying ideas have all been seriously weakened. As H. Tristam Engelhardt points out, we no longer have a canonical, content-full set of values to which we all subscribe, leading him to believe that consensus building and negotiation concerning pluralistic, competing values will be one of our most important communal tasks.[5]

Carol Gilligan's path-breaking book, *In a Different Voice: Psychological Theory and Women's Development*, shows how the two sexes have been conditioned toward different values and behaviors and how the dominant voice has created societal values that unfairly restrict a subset of our population.[6] How the new language of the different voices, based on responsibility and caring, will be integrated with the dominant voice's concern for rights and justice is yet to be played out. Our sensitivities have been similarly raised by the voices of various racial and ethnic minorities, soon to become majorities for large parts of our nation.

Grafted on to all these uncertainties, each with their own implications for collegiality when placed in academic health centers, are such university-specific factors as: physical and intellectual separation of the medical center from its parent university; incredible growth in power and influence of successful academic health centers due to their physical and fiscal size; the enormous post World War II investment in biomedical research via the National Institutes of Health, largely given to the medical schools in conformance with principles enunciated by Vannevar Bush;[7] the big dollars, big business fall-out of that research effort and the great increase in incomes from clinical practice; the enormous success of reductionist biology leading to specialized scientific fields that then have corresponding difficulties in interdisciplinary communication; specialized science that has led to specialized techniques that in turn have led to specialized practitioners who relate more to their specialty colleagues across the nation than to their medical center colleagues across the hall; the explosion in the availability of clinical dollars and research dollars reflected by the explosion of a seven-fold increase in full time medical school faculty members during the past few decades; and the role of our medical schools in technology transfer; the drive for patients, market share, and technology development, to be one of the economic winners rather than one of the losers. Each of these in turn may adversely affect the environment for open communication among scientists. The overall impact of this success can encourage insatiable greed to run amok, facilitated by the currently fashionable sociopolitical emphasis on entrepreneurial behavior and the drive to utilize medical centers as economic engines with which to positively affect local economies.

Add to all this the growing importance to the medical and health enterprise of the social sciences and nontraditional biomedical sciences (such as epidemiology and biostatistics) and the subsequent highlighting of the paradigm clash between the molecularly-oriented, reductionist, biomedical model and the population-based, epidemiologic model, and it is not hard to appreciate that collegiality at the medical school level, not to mention the health science center-wide level, is in for some tough sledding.

Complicating these considerations even further are the overwhelming time demands made upon our faculties. How do clinical faculty members balance the requirements of the modern highly competitive research laboratory with the demands of increased service for income production as well as service to the medically underserved, at the same time maintaining close personal relationships with our student colleagues? To the extent that the triple-threater is dead, faculty members seem to be becoming mostly researchers or mostly teachers or mostly clinicians, or significantly involved with administrative matters or external community service.

Faculty salaries have risen rapidly over the last decade. Such increases have been welcome but increase the pressure on those many faculty members supported partially or entirely by soft money that they must continually earn by medical practice or by obtaining research grants. In an increasingly competitive research environment, our colleagues become our competitors from whom we withhold our ideas and our hard-earned laboratory products. Greed replaces generosity and collegiality is diminished.

Tensions inhibiting collegiality have been known to develop at many levels in academic health centers: between basic science and clinical faculty concerns such as the size of salaries in each of their areas and the amount of time available to them for research pursuits; among the various members within medical school departments and across the departments themselves over turf considerations; among medical school and university faculty members over relative salary size, time required to be spent teaching students, and over differences in opinions on university values; and between basic scientists in basic science departments and basic scientists in clinical departments over such issues as tenured and nontenured positions, access to teaching responsibilities, salary and fringe benefits, and independence in choice of research topics.

The pace of our work life continues to accelerate; letters are whipped out of our computers, sent by fax or electronic mail, and the reply comes back almost instantaneously, eliminating the time we used to have for measured reflection. As we sit at our computers, we tend to use electronic mail even to reach the person just across the hall or next door, again decreasing collegiality.

The legal environment also impinges on our sense of colleagueship. As our actions are more frequently challenged by a litigious society, self evaluation among colleagues in activities such as clinical pathological conferences and morbidity/mortality conferences is increasingly abandoned. We react to questioning of our medical decisions with suspicion and fear. We are, in fact, being required by society to be more accountable for our actions not only with respect to medical liability but relating to honesty in our scientific laboratories as well as our use of animals in research. State legislatures and boards of trustees are playing a more active role in our day to day activities, constricting our spheres of influence, and limiting our control over our professional lives.

Who are these colleagues? Other faculty members are obviously colleagues, but how do we balance colleagueship with competition over teaching and service loads and for resources and attention? Are the students our colleagues? Surely they are. Hippocrates even spoke of the relationship of physicians and learners, using terms such as parents, sons, and family.[8] If they are our colleagues, how do our actions communicate colleagueship to them when they spend much of their first two years sitting in lecture halls as classes of 100–200 functioning as passive vessels responding to a parade of expert lecturers? Bulger proposed obligations in the area of faculty competence, communication skills, treating students with justice and caring, developing creativity and freedom from control.[9]

Finally, are our unknown neighbors our colleagues? It is easy to see our role with the patient in front of us, but what are our responsibilities to the faceless population, which in truth is composed of such individuals?

The core challenge to collegiality at both a professionwide and universitywide level becomes a challenge to develop the basis for and the mechanisms by which to bring about a meaningful sense of community, a discovery and iteration of shared core values, and a behavior change based upon a perception of the importance of living up to those shared values, while maintaining what we have attained and consolidating the progress already made. Meeting such a challenge may require us to consider how we might reapportion our time to achieve such goals. It will require courage to question and to change the basic assumptions on which so many of our daily activities are based.

References

1. Bellah, R., Madsen, R., Sullivan, W. M., et al.: *Habits of the Heart, Individualism and Commitment in American Life*. New York, Harper and Row, 1985.
2. Ibid., p. 26.
3. Ibid., p. 32.
4. Ibid., p. 30.
5. Engelhardt, H.T., Jr.: Integrity, Humaneness, and Institutions in Secular Pluralist Societies. In: *Integrity in Health Care Institutions*, Bulger, R. E. and Reiser, S. J., editors. Iowa City. University of Iowa Press. In press.
6. Gilligan, C. *In a Different Voice: Psychological Theory and Women's Development*. Cambridge, MA, Harvard University Press, 1982.
7. Bush, V. *Science, The Endless Frontier*, A Report to the President on a Program for Postwar Scientific Research. Washington, D.C., Office of Scientific Research and Development (Reprinted by the National Science Foundation), 1980.
8. Selections from the Hippocratic Corpus. In: *Ethics in Medicine. Historical Perspectives and Contemporary Concenrs*, Reiser, Stanley J., Kyke, A. J., and Curran, W. J., editors. Cambridge, MA, Massachusetts Institute of Technology Press, 1989, p. 5.
9. Bulger R. E.: The need for an ethical code for teachers of the basic biomedical sciences. *J. Med. Educ.* 63:131–33, 1988.

Integrity in the Education of Researchers

Terry Ann Krulwich and Paul J. Friedman

An aspect of research integrity that has received relatively little attention, despite the widespread concern that scientists learn how to conduct science responsibly in an increasingly complex environment, is the ethical development and treatment of research trainees. Great effort is currently being made to provide formal training in appropriate research practices, but there has been little public discussion about how trainees are treated, and how this treatment might affect the ethics that they absorb, possibly in contradistinction to the ethics they are taught.

There has always been an element of real or perceived exploitation of research trainees by their professors, a potential problem that is intrinsic to any apprenticeship system. The successful apprenticeship of the research trainee requires a delicate balance between development of the trainee's skills, general and specialized knowledge base, and potential for innovative independent work on the one hand, and the productive application of the trainee's developing abilities to a project of interest to the mentor on the other. The tension between the mutually sought productivity on a project that is fundamentally the intellectual property of the preceptor and the trainee's specific individual goals and needs has clearly increased with the hectic pace of contemporary biomedical sciences. This tension is exacerbated by our raised expectations with respect to the accomplishments of trainees and the generally increased time required to complete a doctoral degree or complete a useful postdoctoral period. There are corollary and additional issues that may reflect the increased competitiveness and anxiety of the research environment, the growing size of laboratories, and the increasing busyness of the faculty research supervisor.

A general statement of an increasing problem is: how often does the preceptor's interest in maximizing the trainee's progress on the research problem of mutual interest result in suboptimal or negligible support for both broad training to equip the trainee to move into new areas at some later time and sufficient theoretical rigor in the specific current area to serve as a model for mastery? For predoctoral trainees, coursework or tutorials, practice in presentation of research, understanding of unrelated work in other labs, and discussions in journal clubs are all part of the basis for a future independent career, but they are treated as noxious distractions by some preceptors. For postdoctoral trainees, some ongoing dialogue about future directions, possible paths of divergence that will provide an independent avenue for the new researcher, is seen by some as the obligation of the preceptor, by others as a problem for the trainee to handle "after hours." The behavior of preceptors concerning such

From *Academic Medicine*, 1993;68:S14–S18. Reprinted by permission.

issues, however, sends a very specific message to trainees with respect to how an individual is valued in the scientific enterprise.

Other such messages are communicated from the initial preceptor–trainee contact to the departure of the trainee from the training laboratory. Graduate schools need to be sensitive to the problem of how individual laboratory heads try to recruit students into their laboratories. For instance, it is woefully common for a would-be preceptor to woo a desirable PhD candidate by indicating or implying that the student is guaranteed the completion of a dissertation within some given number of years or is guaranteed a given number of publications within the first year or two. This practice is different from but no more ethical than the promise of what is essentially gift coauthorship to trainees at any level to reward them for joining a particular research group. Leadership should also recognize, however, that students often find negotiations with more than one interested preceptor difficult to manage; they should be offered guidance in how to handle such processes honestly and tactfully while assessing the opportunities in an appropriately self-interested manner. These issues arise again when the graduating student assesses postdoctoral positions, and such negotiations will recur throughout a trainee's career. There are skills to be taught with respect to maintaining rather than burning bridges when choosing one opportunity over others.

In the Laboratory or Research Setting

Once the trainee is in a laboratory or clinical research setting, the development of a project is the next challenge, and practices vary as much as do the research groups and their interests. Many trainees will have the opportunity to play a major role in the conceptual development of an idea within a range of ongoing effort. In many other instances, the trainee is encouraged to pursue one of several already well-conceived problems that have arisen from previous work. A balance must be sought between the sometimes naive but individual notions of the trainee and the clear-cut view that a preceptor often has of what should be done next. A balance must also be sought between the intrinsic sophistication of the project and the particular talents and training of the trainee and the feassibility of making productive headway on the project in a reasonable period of time.

At one extreme of trainee projects is the assignment of a routine task, of the kind that could be done by an experienced technician, that offers little opportunity for creativity or contribution by the trainee. This sort of assignment is sometimes appropriate for a rotation project or for getting a new trainee started and used to the laboratory but would hardly be appropriate for a thesis project or a postdoctoral experience. At the other extreme is the trainee working on a long shot, a "high-risk" project with a rather low probability of reaching a successful conclusion. This kind of task is tempting and justifiable when the idea is novel and the outcome is potentially exciting for both the field and the particular laboratory. Trainees often gravitate toward such projects. In such instances, the mentor has an obligation to help develop and maintain a back-up project, a more predictable study that is nevertheless interesting and worthy. The mentor also has the responsibility for remembering "to not kill the messenger" when the high-risk project fails to produce the mutually hoped-for results.

Once the trainee is launched on a project, it is commonplace in many research groups for a preceptor to make periodic requests for the trainee's "peripheral" or "temporary" participation in the development of an unrelated line of work that may have suddenly achieved a high priority in the laboratory. Such diversions from the main project can be among the most enjoyable and productive of a trainee's experiences, as he or she is invited to participate in the pursuit of the very latest thought and hottest opportunity, often with success for both trainee and preceptor. Nontheless, preceptors must initiate such requests with the honest understanding that they will not always be serving the professional interests of the trainee and that, if the new idea fails and the trainee has meanwhile lost momentum, the trainee may need additional support and, clearly, not the criticism that one occasionally witnesses. Also, if too frequently diverted on mini-forays, no matter how successful, a trainee may fail to learn the skills involved in the development of a particular line of research and the need to pursue research through periods of varying frustration and difficulty.

Although they are not the focus of this discussion, it is worth noting that clinically trained fellows who may be doing research for a short period, often with little prior training and less supervision than they might receive in a pure basic science setting, need especially carefully crafted projects. They also need designated junior mentors who will ensure that the needed technical and conceptual skills are developed in the trainee. All trainees, but less experienced ones in particular, must have explicit instruction on record keeping, radiation safety and biohazards, experimental design and data analysis, and the mores of the laboratory with respect to sharing of reagents and other materials. It is equally important that trainees learn their responsibilities with respect to the use of animals in research, and, where applicable, the ethics of human experimentation. Awareness of institutional and federal rules is essential.

In all research settings, preceptors must review data books and the status of primary materials and protocols from time to time to ensure that the research data are being properly maintained, but also to be sure that trainees are learning the subtleties involved in being able to reconstruct, go back and reinterpret, and otherwise optimally use the data derived from experimental research. Preceptors who fail to take a personal interest in how the trainee maintains data books are communicating a "paper towels are all right" ethos that will ill serve all parties.

A core issue for the training of researchers is the freedom with which trainees express their own opinions to their supervisor or mentor. Does the trainee have opportunity and encouragement to challenge the mentor's research hypothesis and experimental design either before or after data are generated? Can the trainee develop alternative hypotheses to explain the findings and to design new experimental approaches without derision or an automatically negative response? Are both preceptor and trainee appropriately cautious in handling data provided by a collaborating laboratory that may result from the application of techniques that the student-mentor pair cannot expertly evaluate? Trainees must be taught to question their own findings as well as to scrutinize those of others. They must not be consumed by the rush to publish, but they must be taught not to be pathologically afraid of error, not to be paralyzed when face to face with committing a piece of work to publishable paper. They must be taught that if they catch themselves in an error and correct it honestly and completely, they have safeguarded themselves and the laboratory better than they would have by failing to acknowledge a mistake or a misgiving.

Similarly, the preceptor is clearly best served and trainee best trained when the mentor invites critical evaluation and full participation by the trainee in how the trainee's data are to be presented at meetings and in print. It is shocking that preceptors may complete manuscripts that rely heavily on trainee data without the trainee's ever having seen the final compilation or discussion of those data. The preceptor who invites participation and critical comment is safeguarded against the inevitable biases formed by affection for a hypothesis, and the trainee is safeguarded against the natural desire to try to please the mentor by getting the results predicted by the hypothesis. The more competitive the research environment, the more crucial this self-critical and mutually critical dialogue becomes.

Laboratory meetings play a critical role in the development of the trainee and in the maintenance of the optimal atmosphere of the laboratory, so long as those meetings are not misused to intimidate or berate the trainees. Weekly presentations of research in progress to an entire group builds presentational, analytical, and critical skills. They also take the problems of a particular project out of the realm of a personal dialogue between one trainee and the mentor and bring them into the arena of shared concern and interest by all parties in the laboratory. Accordingly, many scientists regard these presentations as simply a part of doing research. They are by no means universal, however, and we are aware of researchers who do not provide this educational and quality-control activity.

Regular laboratory meetings also provide a semiformal opportunity for a modeling of behavior that should be part of research training. Such behavior includes the handling of delicate conflicts of interest, such as instances in which a preceptor may be asked to review the work of a colleague who is a competitor (and it is very important for preceptors to set an appropriate example in their handling of confidential material); the response to requests for probes or other materials by outside laboratories; and the resolution of complex issues of authorship, which are major sources of conflict, especially when trainees do not feel that there is openness. Laboratory meetings or informal discussions in the laboratory offer opportunities for transmission of basic information that trainees need to acquire about the life of the research laboratory.

What are the sources of research support and, in a general way, how does one wend one's way through the funding morass? Does the trainee understand the constraints involved in the very support mechanism that underwrites the training period? Have payback and rules about sources of supplemental funding, if any, been carefully reviewed? Do trainees recognize that they may generally not publish under the institutional name without some faculty review and approval albeit not necessarily coauthorship of the manuscript to be submitted? Does the research group agree on the criteria for authorship or for the order of authors?

Dilemmas of Commercialization

Recent trends toward increased commercialization of biomedical science have complicated the picture in several ways, while also enriching the apparent opportunities perceived by many trainees.[1] Competing laboratories have their eyes on more than achieving priority with new discoveries. They now look carefully at commercialization of their ideas and materials. This focus may incline them toward limiting the freedom of students in several ways. The limitation obviously includes what the trainee may be allowed to take away as part of future work, but problems arise even during the training period itself. If students take part in nondisclosure agreements, can they really execute a thesis project appropriately? Should graduate schools allow students to sign nondisclosure agreements? If students are asked to curtail their interactions with peers within and outside the institution in a particularly stringent manner, can they derive the needed interactive component of training?

There are no simple resolutions to some of these dilemmas; simply keeping students away from anything of commercial potential is not practical or really appropriate. On the other hand, as biomedical research moves into an era of more diverse funding, there are increasing opportunities for mentors to instruct trainees about the complexities of these relationships. Conflicts of interest should be pointed out and the institutionally approved means of dealing with them explained. All too often, explicit discussion and explanation are not pursued, but understanding conflicts of interest has become an important part of good laboratory technique. As in all matters of the ethics of research training, the interests of all will be best served by honest dialogue about the problems.

Issues of Completion and Separation

Other questions of great sensitivity are when is the trainee finished, and what may the trainee take away as part of developing an independent line of research? Students ask: is it just the greater complexity and apparent opportunities of research that have driven up the number of years to get a PhD, or is there an element of exploitation? What are the protective mechanisms for a student who is making inadequate progress or constantly being asked to take on side projects? Anecdotes of perceived abuses abound, in some institutions more than others.

On the other side of the picture, preceptors comment critically on the expectation of some trainees that when "they have put in their time" and learned how to do the experiments and gathered together a publishable aliquot of data, they should be allowed to move on. The trainees have this expectation despite their need to acquire the skills involved in putting data together, writing, and presenting, and to master doing a serious critical literature review and a prospectus on how the project might be extended to contribute further. In these arenas, there is an important role for advisory committees, program leadership, and ongoing discussions about the wider issues of training. The seeds sown by a mentor who has focused exclusively on the experimental progress of the trainee are sometimes reaped in the grudging reluctance of that student to participate fully in the work of writing up the results and finishing a promising coda to the main project. Even in nearly ideal student–preceptor relationships, however, the period of completion and separation is difficult. Faculty colleagues can give welcome and helpful perspective to both parties.

What may the trainee, especially the postdoctoral trainee who is about to establish an independent career, take from the laboratory as dowry? Clearly, both commercial interests and the ever-more-competitive funding climate have made this problem more complicated. It is more common than ever for a new junior faculty member to follow a line of investigation that is a direct offshoot of, and often quite close to, the investigation in which he or she became expert in the former mentor's laboratory. It is regrettable, in fact, that the difficulty of obtaining funds and the requirement for significant preliminary data and assurance of likely productivity discourage new investigators from putting forth ideas that depart markedly from familiar and successful work. When a trainee needs to write a proposal without the benefit of time to develop such an independent line of research, it is particularly important that the expectations of the preceptor be made clear in good time, and that complicating issues of commercialization be discussed.

Surprisingly, there is widespread ignorance among trainees even about technical but important matters such as the ownership of data notebooks. Few recognize that the research grantee owns the notebooks, and that is in almost all cases the institution, not the principal investigator, and certainly not the trainee. Yet, 35 percent of research trainees responding to a questionnaire thought that they had final authority in deciding what to do with their data.[2] About half recognized the authority of the principal investigator or mentor. Still, ethically, as opposed to legally, students are entitled to a share in the intellectual proceeds of their work. They are entitled to a fair and open discussion of expectations about later, independent activities.

If the mentor is reluctant to encourage the trainee to continue on a research endeavor that may ultimately place them in counterproductive competition, the resolution is best accomplished by the mentor's stimulating and allowing the trainee time and support to explore experimentally a truly separate research direction. Departing trainees are entitled to know whether they can expect coauthorship of later manuscripts that rely heavily on actual data that they have generated, or even on the methods or probes that they may have labored long to develop. In all instances in which a manuscript dependent on their work does emerge, they are entitled to review it before publication and to comment on the use of their data as well as on the credit that they have received.

Finally, it is worth reflecting upon the ever-present ethical aspects of recruiting research trainees in the absence of clear data on the job opportunities and the funding climate that will await them. Certainly these are issues that are discussed and debated, but it is beyond the scope of this paper to attempt to provide databased projections. Rather, like every other question in the realm of the ethics of research training, it is imperative for each training program and each would-be preceptor to monitor the opportunities that are in fact greeting the graduates of the program and the particular laboratory. These opportunities will bear varying relationships to the prospective goals with which those trainees entered, and those relationships should be carefully studied by the programs.

Can program trainees be made more competitive for the positions and types of career options that they most desire? Should recruitment efforts be focused on different skills in order to meet more closely the training goals of the entering trainees? Evaluation of the successes and the failures will be instructive in determining trainee numbers and structuring program features. As in other aspects of training, the trainees and applicants to the program and laboratories have the right to be provided with a candid and complete assessment of the accomplishments of program graduates and the institutional view of their training goals. Institutions and preceptors benefit highly from the work of trainees, but it should always be kept in mind that the training experience is primarily intended to benefit the trainee.

In an era of increasing research complexity, laboratory size, and public scrutiny, it is not enough to rely on the traditional approach of transmitting ethical as well as technically valid research practices "by example." Mentorship[3] now carries with it an obligation to inculcate these standards consciously and systematically; the first step is to ensure an ethical training experience.

References

1. Gluck, M. E., Blumenthal, D., and Stoto, M. A. University–Industry Relationships in the Life Sciences: Implications for Students and Post-doctoral Fellows. *Res. Policy* **16** (1987):327–336.

2. Kalichman, M. W., and Friedman, P. J. A Pilot of Biomedical Trainees' Perceptions Concerning Research Ethics. *Acad. Med.* **67**(1992):769–775.

3. Guston, D. H. Mentorship and the Research Training Experience. In *Responsible Science: Ensuring the Integrity of the Research Process*, vol. II, pp. 50–65. Panel on Scientific Responsibility and the Conduct of Research, National Academy of Sciences. Washington, D.C.: National Academy Press, 1993.

Administrative Case Rounds

Institutional Policies and Leaders Cast in a Different Light

Stanley Joel Reiser

Governing the institutions of health care provision is becoming increasingly difficult. This is largely caused by an accelerating pace of technological innovation that alters their financial status and internal structure, a growing number of constituencies in society that demand authority to influence institutional policies, and a widening gap between the professional and administrative staff of institutions concerning goals and purpose. To better cope with these issues, institutional leaders should recognize and learn to fulfill effectively the pedagogic role they take on for their staff and constitutents when they create and carry out policy. They also should consider holding regular discussions about institutional policy alternatives within the framework of one of the most significant and powerful means of teaching and research in medicine – the case round.

In reaching decisions, administrators who govern health care institutions, such as hospitals or health science centers, frequently separate the policies developed to guide institutional action from the formal teaching that goes on within them. However, the judgments that guide institutional choices and influence real-world decisions, such as the scope of offered services, speak volumes to staff as well as to patients, students, and society: they can be the most powerful lessons the institution is capable of giving. It is, accordingly, important that institutional leaders recognize their basic role as teachers and think more critically about how to exercise this responsibility.

Alongside the problem of how administrators as teachers should give their lessons is the difficulty of making policy decisions in modern health care institutions, given the conflict in values and opinions that exists among their multiple external and internal constituencies. Today health care institutions are buffeted by demands from constituencies such as government, business, private insurers, and patients, on the one hand, and professional and administrative groups within the institution on the other. They all have a significant stake increating effective institutional policies. But their diverse experiences, needs, and traditions often lead them to different views on what to do. Thus, a regular forum is needed in which these divergent perspectives can be aired and analyzed with the aim of integration into subsequent policies and through which the teaching function of administrators can be exercised. This situation is ideally suited for the introduction of the case round.

Reaching back to the writings of Hippocrates and his colleagues in the fifth century BC, and continuing through modern times, the case has been a key mode of capturing experience; analyzing through it the causes, effects, and significance of medical action; and using this learning to change practice. In the 20th century the case became a central

From *JAMA*, 1991;266(15):2127–2128. Copyrighted 1991, American Medical Association.

instrument in the teaching of clinical medicine to students and practitioners, challenging the dominion of the lecture. This idea emerged in 1900 when, as a student at Harvard Medical School, Walter Cannon drew on the example of C. C. Langdell at Harvard Law School, who used cases to teach law, to suggest that medicine take a similar step. The innovation achieved wide adoption. A decade later, the physicians Richard C. Cabot and James Homer Wright began a teaching conference at the Massachusetts General Hospital, Boston, in which a presented clinical case was analyzed by a physician unassociated with it. This was followed by the evaluation of a pathologist who commented and enlarged upon the clinical presentation. Thus the clinical-pathological conference was born; it continues to flourish.[1] Currently, cases serve to focus the attention of practitioners on new aspects of medicine from anthropological, social, and ethical factors to its economic aspects. As the number of case analyses grows, a body of experience is created that helps others learn lessons and gain knowledge from the daily actions taken in health care. Without such preservation as cases, these experiences vanish from view, remaining only in the memories of participants, changing and fading with time.

With the significance of institutions in health care decision making large and increasing, the need to capture and learn from the efforts to govern and formulate policy for them grows. Given the great help that case collection and analysis has been to physicians facing the complexities of clinical decisions, institutions and their administrators should consider recording their own experiences as cases and initiating regular administrative case rounds.

The choice of a subject for these cases is, of course, a critical step. The alternatives are as varied as the number of difficult issues administrators meet daily. However, particularly suitable for a case round are subjects that involve multiple constituencies that case discussion could bring together, or that have broad social importance, or that represent a recurrent or difficult institutional problem. Areas of interest include (*a*) personnel issues such as employee assessment and help programs for drug and alcohol use, providing day care for the children of students and employees, or mandating testing for the acquired immunodeficiency syndrome; (*b*) institution-building issues such as choices of expansion among research, learning, and patient care alternatives, or emphasizing outpatient vs inpatient development projects; (*c*) community issues such as deciding the level and type of services to offer the communities served by the institution, or responsibilities for their non-health care needs; (*d*) educational issues such as deciding which of the schools in a health science center should provide training programs for a given service, or student training requirements such as residency hours; and (*e*) research issues such as the inclusion of more women in clinical studies, or the relation of faculty with industry.

Decisions must be made whether to select cases that are past or ongoing. Analysis of cases whose outcome is known gives insight into how the institution deals with issues. Discussion of cases in progress provides opportunities to influence choices ahead. A mix of the two may be best at the outset, while examining how the case method works in the administrative venue.

The audience present for a case round can be any members of the institutional community wishing to attend – such as administrators, students, clinicians, and experts on subjects such as ethics and law. A mixed internal audience is wholly sufficient to conduct successful case rounds. However, where desired and feasible, as a regular or intermittent feature of the rounds, guests can be invited to introduce the views of experts not regularly present in the institution, or of external constituencies (eg, from government, business, or the community) whose opinions are relevant to the issue at hand.

Several formats are suited to the administrative case round, which is readily conducted in an hour. One, more expert driven, and adopted from the clinical-pathological conference, begins with the presentation of a case, is followed by analysis and commentary by designated participants, and ends with questions and discussion from the audience. A second, more audience based, and derived from my experience in ethics case rounds, also begins with a case presentation. A moderator then elicits from the audience key questions they discern in the case. The audience, with help from the moderator and experts present, discuss these questions and develop conclusions and suggestions for action.

No significant innovation is adopted without changes that, along with producing benefits, may create problems. In the instance of administrative case rounds, there are several understandable concerns that administrators reflecting on their use might have. Some may worry that the case discussion might create legal risks for the institution. That such a concern can arise in the context of an innovation to encourage the analysis of important health care issues reflects faults in the current liability system and the need for reform.[2] However, legal doubts about a case can be addressed by consultation with the institution's legal counsel in advance of the rounds to determine if problems exist. Where they do, particular aspects of the content of the case can be changed to allow its main aspects to be discussed. If such a revision is unsatisfactory, a different case should be chosen.

Others might be concerned that case discussion may cause unrest among the institution's constituencies and raise the level of argument. The adage "Let sleeping dogs lie" has much attraction for the harried administrator. The use of cases in clinical medicine provides reassurance here. In clinical-pathological conferences and other clinical forums, the presentation of controversy and error, and of cases ending in injury and death, has produced not unrest but enlightenment. The modern medical ethics movement, which began in the mid-1960s, depends fundamentally on case discussion. Its experience also offers comfort. Cases dealing with exceedingly difficult and controversial ethical issues such as truth-telling, abortion, and withdrawal of life-support systems now are regularly presented in all parts of hospitals and health science centers. These discussions have proved salutary, not discordant, to institutional functioning. In addition, organization literature supports the view that examination of policies and objectives among involved parties serves to advance, not thwart, organizational objectives.[3,4] This is particularly significant in health care institutions, where the professional and administrative sectors, driven by different values and viewpoints, often fail to come together adequately to discuss institutional policies and goals.[5] Their relationship would benefit by having a structured and regular forum for discourse provided through the case round.

An open discussion of ideas and experiences in health care to test knowledge, locate problems, and recommend change has been fundamental to the growth of its clinical, scientific, and ethical components. A hallmark of institutions of learning and patient care is to value reflection on actions contemplated and taken. Integrating the administrative and policy dimensions of health care into a framework of analysis within which its clinical and research constituencies thrive – the case method – would be a significant step forward. Like its use with these other constituencies, the administrative case can be transcribed to create permanent records that allow institutions to evaluate choices and pinpoint failings and transmitted to students and colleagues as relevant material to study and learn about health care. An effort to elaborate on the issues of institutional values and leadership, and to encourage the holding of administrative case rounds, is currently under way in the Association of Academic Health Centers.[6]

The case can be an important instrument in bridging the gap among the constituencies of health care institutions. Further, the benefits to institutions starting administrative case rounds can be shared by their leaders. By recognizing a basic responsibility for themselves as teachers, who fashion lessons through the policies they create, institutional leaders can more effectively meet the needs of those whom they serve and realize as well a new dimension of self.

References

1. Reiser SJ. The clinical record in medicine, part I: learning from cases. *Ann Intern Med.* 1991;114:902–907.
2. Huber PW, Litan RE. *The Liability Maze: The Impact of Liability Law on Safety and Innovation.* Washington, DC: The Brookings Institution; 1991.
3. Walton M. *Deming Management at Work.* New York, NY: GP Putnam's Sons; 1990.
4. Drucker PF. *Managing the Nonprofit Organization.* New York, NY: Harper Collins Publishers; 1990.
5. Bulger RE, Reiser SJ, eds. *Integrity in Health Care Institutions: Humane Environments for Teaching, Inquiry, and Healing.* Iowa City: University of Iowa Press; 1990.
6. Rich C, Barbato A, Griffith J, eds. *From Pragmatism to Vision: Leadership and Values in Academic Health Centers.* Washington, DC: Association of Academic Health Centers. In press.

Questions for Discussion

1. How do the multiple roles of the academic investigator create and affect collegial relationships among faculty and students (clinical versus basic science faculty, Ph.D.'s in basic science departments versus Ph.D.'s in clinical departments)?
2. How do your institution's policies on promotion and tenure reflect its commitments to teaching, research, and service to the community? Does your institution place special emphasis on any one aspect?
3. What are effective ways to teach good laboratory practices?
4. What factors should a graduate student or postdoctoral fellow consider when choosing a faculty mentor or advisor?
5. How does your institution encourage a culture of compliance with ethical principles?

Recommended Supplemental Reading

Ammons SW Jr, Kelly DE. Profile of the graduate student population in U.S. medical schools. *Acad Med.* 1997;72:819–830.

Callahan D, Bok C, eds. *Ethics Teaching in Higher Education.* New York, NY: Plenum Press; 1980.

Federation of American Societies for Experimental Biology. *Graduate Education: Consensus Conference Report.* Washington, DC: FASEB; 1997.

National Academy of Sciences, National Academy of Engineering, Institute of Medicine. *Reshaping the Graduate Education of Scientists and Engineers.* Washington, DC: National Academy Press; 1995.

The Scientist and Industry

The Scientist and Industry

Conflicts of Interest and Conflicts of Commitment

Ruth Ellen Bulger

In 1945, at the request of Franklin D. Roosevelt, presidential science adviser Vannevar Bush published a report entitled *Science – The Endless Frontier* proposing a peacetime science policy that could sustain the country's World War II investment in the funding of scientific research.[1] Since that time, there has been a continuing increase in government funding for biomedical research, which in 2001 exceeded \$20 billion. Many promising scientific findings have been made, and new information is being discovered at an ever-increasing pace. Today, life science research is thriving.

However, in the 1960s when this boom began, thoughtful observers noted that there seemed to be insufficient effort to convert health-related discoveries and patents into tangible products or useful tools to improve the health of the public. Because the federal agency that funded the research retained the patent on any new development, there was little incentive for the transfer of technology from the universities, where scientific discoveries were made, to industry, where they could be developed into useful products. The public did not seem to reap the expected benefits of research funding, for only about 5% of the 28,000 patents held by government agencies were being licensed for development.[2]

New patent contracts were needed to foster the efficient transfer of technology to public use. In 1968, the University of Wisconsin and the U.S. Department of Health and Human Services (DHHS, then the DHEW) negotiated the first "Institutional Patent Agreements" that gave the university title to the inventions of its faculty. In 1973 an additional agreement was created with the National Science Foundation (NSF).

The Wisconsin experience proved highly successful. Building on it, Congress passed a series of laws between 1980 and 1986 that have allowed universities, not-for-profit corporations, and small businesses to patent and commercialize federally funded inventions. The Stevenson–Wydler Technology Innovation Act of 1980 established offices in government to stimulate interactions with industry, allowing royalties to be shared with inventors. The 1980 Bayh–Dole Act (PL96–517) allowed federal contractors in small businesses and nonprofit organizations, including universities, that make patentable discoveries with federal funding to retain property rights to these inventions and any subsequent patents. The Bayh–Dole Act allowed the institution and researcher to share the resulting income, and the remaining funds to be used for scientific research or education. Implemented by the U.S. Department of Commerce in 1987 as 37 CFR 401, the Federal Technology Transfer Act of 1986 extended these incentives to inventions developed in government laboratories using cooperative research and development (R&D) agreements with nonprofits and nongovernmental profit organizations. Again the inventor could share in profits from the invention, and the remaining funds could be used by the company for the transfer of the technology into public use.

The government's actions of the 1980s have radically changed the relationships between universities and industry and have greatly restructured the goals and conduct of university researchers. By stimulating more interaction between universities, not-for-profit organizations, and government agencies and industry, governmental efforts to accelerate the transfer of technology have encouraged academic investigators to patent and further develop their research findings. Still, this changing relationship between academic scientists and for-profit companies poses new rewards and new threats to the academic mission of the university. This chapter considers the traditional role of the university and some of the changes and challenges that occur when closer relationships develop with industrial partners.

Intellectual Property

Intellectual property is a concept that addresses the ownership of things that a person or persons have created. It includes ideas; written works; inventions, and processes that are protectable using copyrights, trademarks, and trade secrets; and patents. (See reference 3 for an in-depth analysis of intellectual property). The property rights to such creations were granted to the creators in the U.S. Constitution in 1787 (U.S. Constitution, Article 1, Section 8).

A *copyright* protects ideas that exist in some tangible medium such as a book or journal, and now, original material placed on the Internet. Copyrights are used to grant exclusive rights for a limited time to those who write essays, books, musical or dramatic works, or make sound recordings. With a copyright, the owner can make, display, and distribute copies of the work or of derivative works. Officially, one can obtain a copyright by submitting the appropriate forms to the U.S. Copyright Office.

Trademarks include some representation by which the owner of a concept, service, or product identifies or distinguishes that service or product from one offered by others. Trademarks are issued by the U.S. Patent and Trademark Office (PTO). A trade secret includes information that has economic value when its contents are not generally known. It is protected by the process of secrecy.

A *patent* is a title to an invention granted to the inventors by a government in exchange for the inventor's disclosing relevant information about the invention to the public. In the United States, the patent is an official U.S. government document issued to the inventor granting the inventor certain rights. The rights include the ability to exclude others from making, using, or selling or offering for sale the patented invention within the country. The rights also include the freedom to transfer the patent to others and to sue others who infringe upon the patent. Patents are also granted by the PTO.

To encourage faculty to patent their discoveries, many universities have established offices to help investigators handle intellectual property and technology transfer actions efficiently. For a more complete description of the patent process, the Association of University Technology Managers Educational Series begins with a pamphlet entitled "An Inventor's Guide to Patents and Patenting."[4]

Several kinds of inventions can be patented, including: (1) processes, (2) machines, (3) composition of matter, (4) manufacturer's, and (5) new improvements of such inventions. However, several other kinds of inventions are not patentable, including an arrangement of printed matter, items that occur naturally, laws of nature, ideas without application, and a way of doing business.

To grant a patent, the PTO must find that the invention is *new* or *novel* (i.e., it has not been described previously in print anywhere in the world). There is a one-year grace period during which the inventor may have published some material on the patent without loss in patentable rights in the United States, but this grace period does not exist for obtaining a patent in other countries. Because, in general, an inventor wants to obtain worldwide patents, it is extremely important not to publish or give an oral description of a new invention before filing for a patent in the United States and other countries in which the invention might be developed and used.

Besides novelty, the invention is judged by its *utility*. The invention must have a function with some benefit and must do what the inventor claims it can.

Finally, to be patentable, at the time of the invention a discovery must be *nonobvious* to a person with ordinary skill in the "art" to which this patent pertains. Part of the application process is to ensure that no previous patent or publication describing the invention exists in the world (35 U.S.C. Section 103, 1995).

Exactly who qualifies as the inventor of a patented invention is a legal decision, and a patent can involve more than one inventor. Each inventor may have made a different kind of contribution or different amount of input to the invention. Yet each inventor has the right to "practice" the patent without the permission of the other inventors. Once granted, a patent can be licensed to another party for further development or use if the licensee and the inventor can agree on the legal terms of this use or development. New patents extend for 20 years from the filing date or 17 years from when the patent was granted, whichever is longer.

The University and Technology Transfer

The goal of technology transfer is to ensure that advances in basic research made at academic or nonprofit institutions move to the private sector, where they can be efficiently developed and made available rapidly and effectively as products for public use.

Much of the biomedical knowledge that underlies technical advances is attained at the universities or their health science centers through research funded by governmental grants. The role of the university includes the effective transmission of that knowledge to other scientists, students, and the public. Publication of the research findings produced within the institution in the peer-reviewed literature is one primary way to transmit this new knowledge. Developing patents is another.

Disciplined discovery of new biomedical knowledge happens effectively at a university because universities provide investigators with space and facilities in which to do research and individuals in many crucial ancillary roles to facilitate the research process. Perhaps even more important, the university has a proud tradition of maintaining an intellectually free and open environment in which scientists can not only choose their field of study but also determine the questions to be asked and answered by their research. The excellent reputation of the university is based on the previous good work of the faculty. The university then becomes the site of the generation of new knowledge and new ideas that lead to patentable inventions, and, most important, the production of well-educated graduates, both of which are valuable to the public as well as to industry.

Certain obligations result from the privilege of being employed by, and doing research within, a university. Both the institution and the faculty must work in such a way as to increase the good reputation of the institution and not to threaten the not-for-profit status or endowment of the institution. The university must maintain the necessary open environment for both students and faculty. The university must protect academic freedom, provide excellent instruction to students, offer a stimulating environment for the research, ensure information exchange among colleagues and students, and preserve the rights to its intellectual property by maintaining data ownership and allowing the free publication of research results. To accomplish this, the institution must decide on the appropriate types and amount of information transfer to be undertaken on both an inclusive and exclusive basis. It must undertake all research in full compliance with local, state, and federal laws and regulations.

Balancing these traditional university roles in the new more entrepreneurial environment generates new kinds of conflicts: *conflicts of interest* and *conflicts of commitment*. Bradley[5] defines a conflict of interest to exist "when an individual exploits, or appears to exploit, his or her position for personal gain or for the profit of a member of his or her immediate family of household ... [or] ... the undue use of a position or exercise of power to influence a decision for personal gain." Conflicts of interest can exist for both the individual or the institution. Conflicts of interest can be either financial (relating to money obtained) or intellectual (relating to how many of one's academic responsibilities are handled). Financial conflicts of interest are easier to understand and to regulate because they can be quantified, whereas intellectual conflicts of interest can be more subtle and complex to regulate.

Conflicts of commitment are concerned with time and effort – how much of an investigator's or teacher's time must be devoted to teaching, research, and service directly for the institution and how much time and effort are allowed for consulting with industry, starting an independent company, or other activities not directly related to the university's direct functions. It is possible that external activities can become so time-intensive that they interfere with one's primary responsibilities, which creates a conflict of commitment. Many schools have adopted a policy defining the maximum percentage of time external activities may consume. Often 20% of one's working time is allowed for these external activities, which include not only working with industry but providing advice to other institutions such as NIH.

All investigators have many *interests* that may lead to conflicts in how to act. Obtaining grants, promotions, loyalty to academic or industrial sponsors, expected financial gain, pleasing others, gaining increased fame or fortune, or strongly held social, intellectual, or religious convictions are all *interests* that investigators may have. Conflicts occur when an individual experiences opposing desires between private interests and official responsibilities. For example, whether an investigator should write one manuscript describing a complete study or break the material into several small, incomplete pieces to increase the number of publications in his or her bibliography can be a conflict between responsible conduct as a scientist and the wish to be promoted on the basis of the number of publications written. Whether one's actions serve the public interest by providing information openly or help a particular company succeed by giving it special information could be another conflict.

These conflicts can be destructive if they threaten one's scientific objectivity by increasing ones's tendency for self-deception and thereby intensifying the risk of scientific error. Conflicts can undermine public trust when they emerge into the public's view. Undermining of trust might change Congressional and public willingness to fund important scientific research. Other inappropriate conflicts can threaten the openness of members of the research community to each other. Scientists have reported using secrecy or withholding information from publication for prolonged periods beyond that necessary to submit a patent application.[6–8] Because conflicts of interest are part of our lives, it is important to recognize their existence and to learn to eliminate them or manage them fairly and effectively.

Various kinds of conflicts have been defined. The conflict is *potential* if it exists but no judgments have been made relating to it; the conflict is *actual* if a conflict exists and a judgment was made with respect to it. In the *appearance of a conflict of interest*, no real conflict exists, but others who view the situation are justified in concluding that a conflict of interest existed. One test frequently used to detect the appearance of a conflict of interest is to ask how the situation would look if you read about it in the headlines of the local newspaper.

How an institution manages conflicts of interest varies. Most institutions have published policies to regulate financial and, in some instances, intellectual conflicts of interest and conflicts of commitment. In July 1995, both the NSF and the Public Health Service (PHS) issued final regulations relating to financial conflicts of interest. The goal of these regulations is to protect government-sponsored research from bias that relates to the financial interests of the grantee investigator. Each regulation requires that institutions accepting funds from those agencies have a conflict of interest policy that is at least as restrictive as the regulations have established. For example, exceeding what the agency defines as a significant financial or equity interest is a conflict of interest that must be managed. For these agencies, when the salary, royalties, or other payments that, when aggregated for the investigator and the investigator's spouse and dependent children over 12 months, exceed $10,000 for any one related interest, a conflict of interest exits . For equity interest, a similar limit of $10,000 in value as determined by reasonable measures of fair market value, or more than 5% ownership in any single entity, is also defined as a conflict of interest. To meet the PHS policy, academic institutions must have a written enforced policy on financial conflict of interest, they must inform investigators of that policy, and they must report the existence of any conflicting interests to the awarding offices and ensure that the conflict has been managed, reduced, or eliminated in accordance with the regulations.[9] A similar policy exists for the NSF.[10] Since 1998, the FDA also has had regulations requiring clinical investigators to make financial disclosures.

The policies of academic institutions can regulate conflicts of interests in many ways, depending on the type and amount of the conflicts of interest. The one used most frequently is public disclosure of the interest. An increasing number of scientific journals require that all financial conflicts of interest be disclosed when an author submits a manuscript, and many journals publish these conflicts of interest with the article so that the reader can evaluate the conflict along with evaluating the publication. Krimsky et al.[11] have looked at the financial interests of authors in 14 scientific journals and found that 20% of authors serve on scientific advisory boards for industry; 7% are either officers, directors, or major shareholders in a biotechnology firm; and 22% are listed as an inventor of a related patent. Krimsky and Rotherberg[12] conclude that the scientific community and the public are best served by open publication of financial disclosures for readers and reviewers.

Other ways to manage conflicts of interest include either internal or external monitoring or review with modification of the research plan to eliminate investigator bias. Institutions also can require divestiture of significant financial interests, disqualification of conflicted investigators from participation in funded research, and, in severe cases, severance of relationships between the institution and the individual.

Relationships between Academics and Industries

The NSF reports that U.S. research and development (R&D) spending was at an estimated $220.6 billion in 1998.[13] However, industry is responsible for the largest part of the increase from $205.6 billion spent in 1997. Most of the industry R&D funds are used within the industry itself, but $1.8 billion was spent in academic institutions and another $1 billion in nonprofit organizations. Most of the industry R&D funds are spent for development.

Many types of relationships occur among scientists, their institutions, and industry.[14] Frequently the investigator receives research support given as a grant, contract, or gift by a company. Campbell et al.[15] surveyed 2,167 of 3,394 faculty (64% response rate) from research-intensive universities and found that 43% of respondents had received a research-related gift in the last 3 years that was independent of a grant or contract. Twenty-four percent had received biomaterials, 15% received discretionary funds, 11% received research equipment, 11% received funding for a scientific meeting, 9% received student support, and 3% got other research-related gifts. Recipients reported that donors expected a return for the gift: 63% wanted acknowledgment in the publications, 60% required that the gift not be passed on to others, 59% said it could only be used for the agreed-upon purposes, 32% said that donors wanted pre-publication review of publications resulting from the work, 30% wanted testing of their product, and 19% wanted ownership of all patentable results from the research in which the gift was used.

Another relationship with industry is formed when scientists consult directly with a company. This consultation is often associated with compensation and payment of expenses. In addition, companies also pay for scientists to give training lectures or courses to physicians or other possible users of the product. However, the FDA has established rules mandating that the agenda for such courses be planned by nonindustry individuals so that the information is not biased to a particular product.

As the number of patents held by university faculty increases, the licensing of the patent (or infrequently, the sale) to industry will allow further research or development for the subsequent use of the patent rights. This development could be carried out by the inventor in the university laboratory or within the industry laboratories. When the product is marketed, the institution and the inventor can share in the royalties generated by its sale.

A closer relationship between the investigator and the industrial sponsor includes the granting of equity in the company. Scientists or their institutions have also started companies to develop the inventions further independently of industry. This type of relationship can become problematic if the investigator in an academic role can act in a biased way to increase the value of the equity. Similar concerns relate to the institution's holding equity in an employee investigator's company because the institution might also act to favor the investigator or the company over other equally worthy investigators, or it may make an unwise institutional investment. An even closer relationship can occur if the investigator becomes an officer in the company, thereby having what can easily become conflicting loyalties.

The number of relationships between industry and academics is large and represents a substantial amount of research funding. Blumenthal et al.[7] surveyed 210 U.S. life science companies and found that 90% of those that conducted research had relationships with academia. Of these, 59% supported research at universities, providing $1.5 billion in 1994, which was 11.7% of the research funding received by those universities. Of those companies, over 60% received patents, products, or sales as a result of the money. However, many of the agreements included keeping the research results secret beyond the time needed to apply for a patent. The authors concluded that such relationships may pose a greater threat to the openness of scientific research than is generally acknowledged. In fact, in another study Blumenthal et al.[6] found that about 20% of life science faculty admitted withholding data from publication for more than 6 months to protect the commercial value. Thirty-four percent of faculty have been denied access to research results, and there is a significant correlation between withholding research results and a relationship with commercialization or with an industrial sponsor.[8]

Many obvious benefits can result from partnerships between academia and industry. Presumably, the main benefit is to ensure that the research results of the inventor are efficiently transferred to the public for the improvement of people's health. Developing products with the required testing to ensure safety and efficacy is expensive, and usually it is industry that foots the bill for the development and testing of an idea into a salable product.

Funds provided by the industrial sponsor can provide financial support to further the inventor's work in the laboratory or may be used by the institution. Interactions between the scientists at the company and the university have the potential to increase scientific and commercial productivity – even for the development of more patents. Finally, it is a stated government policy that scientific advances should fuel the economic position of the United States. That type of reasoning may partially explain the bipartisan support for increasing the biomedical research budget in the United States.

However, along with the benefits that can be derived from the advances, there are real risks to the academic research structure. Secrecy and the withholding of research results can slow the progress of science and disrupt the normal collegial relationships and discourse among scientists. Companies provide negative incentives that restrict the sharing of data and research reagents among scientists. Working with industry can shift the type of research that scientists do to support their research laboratories. If scientists are not careful to avoid conflicts of interest (or apparent conflicts of interest) and conflicts of commitment, both congressional and public support of research may diminish. The question has recently arisen whether financial conflicts of interests pose any threat to human research volunteers who are participating in clinical research, for there is no comprehensive approach to conflicts of interests in human research. How does the payment of a finder's fee to a physician sending a volunteer into the trial affect what is said by that physician to the volunteering patient about the trial? What is the effect on studies involving human subjects when the researcher will benefit financially if the company making the product to be tested does well? These are questions that need to be answered.

Scientists who have successful patents can earn substantial amounts of personal money while making real contributions to the public's health. That is laudable, but there is a school of thought that reminds scientists of the overall social value of science. Scientists must also remember that their efforts are important for many aspects of science as they relate to other societal needs. The stress on economic competitiveness in producing expensive products needs to be balanced by advances in areas that are not so richly rewarded via industrial relationships. George Brown, Jr., recently deceased Congressional representative from California and great supporter of the funding for scientific research, reminded scientists of this in a *Los Angeles Times* story called "It's Down to the Last Blank Check." He said, "Society needs to negotiate a new contract with the scientific community … rooted in the pursuit of explicit, long-term social goals, such as zero population growth, reduced generation of waste, reduced consumption of nonrenewable resources, less armed conflict, less dependence on material goods as a gauge of wealth or success, and greater opportunity for self-realization for all human beings."[16]

Insider Trading

Another industry-related conflict of interest relates to the rules that govern insider trading of stocks. When investigators are involved in clinical trials supported by for-profit companies, they must realize that it is illegal to trade in stocks (or inform other traders about these stocks) if, owing to their scientific work, they come into possession of information about the clinical trial that is not generally available to the public. Durso[17] describes a case in which the U.S. Securities and Exchange Commission (SEC) brought a charge of insider trading against an investigator working on a pharmaceutical drug research clinical trial. Although it is hard to know how prevalent the use of nonpublic scientific information is for the purchase or sale of stocks, investigators need to know and follow the SEC rules.

The Effect of For-Profit Relationships on Students' Research

As academic institutions become increasingly involved with industry research, the effect of these relationships on the education of students must be carefully considered. It is easy to list the advantages of students working in relationships with an industrial sponsor. They include the possible funding of stipends while doing the research, obtaining supplies and equipment needed in the research, cooperating with investigators in the industrial labs as well as those in the university environment, and learning about working in industry as a possible career goal.

However, if students are to work in conjunction with industry, either in the industry laboratory or in the university laboratory funded by an industrial sponsor, the academic institution must ensure that the student's efficient progress toward receiving his or her degree is not hampered by this type of relationship.

Students must be able to consult freely with any university faculty member about the techniques to be used or the results that have been obtained freely and openly as would any other graduate student who is supported by institutional funds. Scientific openness helps to ensure that quality research is being accomplished. The student must have the ability to publish or share the research results promptly. The student and the institution should share or retain an appropriate amount of the intellectual property that is being produced and should not be limited by secrecy and trade secrets or undue control of publications. Disclosure of ideas by graduate students at open scientific meetings should not be restricted.

The choice of the research topic to be studied should not be controlled by the company providing the stipends. Being able to review the literature, generate a hypothesis, and test it using the appropriate techniques are all part of the optimal graduate student experience. If the student is working in an industrial setting, clear mechanisms for including the student in the university learning community must be maintained.

How the academic institution will establish and monitor these interactions must be clearly understood before any project supported by industry is undertaken.

Conclusions

Various Congressional actions have provided incentives to encourage scientists to transfer their inventions into useful technology by allowing them to retain the intellectual property rights and to obtain financial rewards. These new technologies also fuel the economic development of the country. However, a quandary exists because, as scientists develop their inventions, they must also consider the negative side effects that these entrepreneurial activities have on the academic environment. These two sides must be carefully considered and balanced to prevent harm to the traditional roles of the university.

References

1. Bush V. *Science – The Endless Frontier: A Report to the President on a Program for Postwar Scientific Research.* Washington, DC: The National Science Foundation; 1990.
2. Massing, DE, ed. *Association of University Technology Managers Licensing Survey, FY1990–1995.* Norwalk, CT; Association of University Technology Managers, Inc: 1996.
3. Mays TD. Ownership of data and intellectual property. In: Macrina FL, ed.: *Scientific Integrity; An Introductory Text with Cases.* 2d ed. Washington, DC,: American Society of Microbiology Press; 2000.
4. von Bargen Mueller L. *An Inventor's Guide to Patents and Patenting.* Norwalk, CT; Association of University Technology Managers, Inc; 1995.
5. Bradley SG. Managing conflicting interests. In: Macrina FL, ed.: *Scientific Integrity: An Introductory Text with Cases.* 2d ed. Washington, DC: American Society of Microbiology Press; 2000.
6. Blumenthal D, Campbell EG, Causino N, Louis KS. Participation of life sciences faculty in research relationships with industry. *N Engl J Med.* 1966a;335:1734–1739.
7. Blumenthal D, Causino N, Campbell EG, Louis KS. Relationships between academic institutions and industry: an industry survey. *N Engl J Med.* 1966b;334:368–373.
8. Blumenthal D, Campbell EG, Anderson MS, Causino N, Louis KS. Withholding research results in academic life science: evidence from a national survey of faculty. *JAMA.* 1997;277:1224–1228.
9. Department of Health and Human Services, Public Health Service. Responsibility of applicants for promoting objectivity in research. 60 *Federal Register* 3132 (1995), 35810–9. Codified at 37 CFR §401. Available at: http://grants.nih.gov/grants/guide/notice-files/not95-179.html.
10. National Science Foundation. NSF investigator financial disclosure policy, with changes and clarifications published in the *Federal Register.* Vol. 60 (132);July 11, 1995.
11. Krimsky S, Rotherberg LS, Scott P, Kyle G. Financial interests of authors in scientific journals: A Pilot study of 14 publications. *Sci Eng Ethics.* 1996;2:395–410.
12. Krimsky S, Rotherberg LS. Financial interest and its disclosure in scientific publications. *JAMA.* 1998;280:225–226.
13. Payson S. *National Patterns of R&D Resources:1998.* Washington, DC: NSF Division of Science Resources Studies, NSF; 1999. Available at http://www.nsf.gov/sbe/srs/nsf99335/start.htm.
14. Blumenthal D. Academic–industry relationships in the life sciences: Extent, consequences, and management. *JAMA.* 1992;268:3344–3349.
15. Campbell EG, Louis KS, Blumenthal D. Looking a gift horse in the mouth: corporate gifts supporting life sciences research. *JAMA.* 1998;279;995–999.
16. Brown G, Jr. It's down to the last blank check. *Los Angeles Times.* September 8, 1992.
17. Durso TW. Insider-trading case poses concerns for researchers. *The Scientist.* 1997;11:1.

Patenting Life

Summary, Policy Issues, and Options for Congressional Action

U.S. Congress, Office of Technology Assessment

Intellectual Property

Rooted in the Constitution, intellectual property law provides a personal property interest in the work of the mind. Modern intellectual property law consists of several areas of law: patent, copyright, trademark, trade secret, and breeders' rights.

Patents

A patent is a grant issued by the U.S. Government giving the patent owner the right to exclude all others from making, using, or selling the invention within the United States, and its territories and possessions, during the term of the patent (35 U.S.C. 154). A patent may be granted to whoever invents or discovers any new, useful, and nonobvious process, machine, manufacture, composition of matter, or any new and useful improvement of these items (35 U.S.C. 101). A patent may also be granted on any distinct and new variety of asexually reproduced plant (35 U.S.C. 161) or on any new, original, and ornamental design for an article of manufacture (35 U.S.C. 171).

The first patent act was enacted by Congress in 1790, providing protection for "any new and useful art, machine, manufacture, or composition of matter, or any new and useful improvement [thereof]." Subsequent patent statutes were enacted in 1793, 1836, 1870, and 1874, which employed the same broad language as the 1790 Act. The Patent Act of 1952 replaced "art" with "process" as patentable subject matter (35 U.S.C. 101). The Committee Reports accompanying the 1952 Act demonstrate that Congress intended patentable subject matter to include "anything under the sun that is made by man." However, the Supreme Court has held that laws of nature, physical phenomena, and abstract ideas are not patentable.

Patents have many of the attributes of personal property (35 U.S.C. 261). Property is generally viewed as a bundle of legally protected interests, including the right to possess and to use, to transfer by sale and gift, and to exclude others from possession. Patents are designed to encourage inventiveness by granting to inventors and assignees a limited property right – the right to exclude others from practicing the invention for a period of 17 years. In return for this limited property right, the inventor is required to file a written patent application describing the invention in full, clear, concise, and exact terms, setting forth the best mode contemplated by the inventor, so as to enable any person skilled in the art of the invention to make and use it. **Although a patent excludes others from making,**

From U.S. Congress, Office of Technology Assessment, *New Developments in Biotechnology: Patenting Life* (Washington, DC: U.S. Government Printing Office, 1988), pp. 4–5, 7–9, 12–18.

using, or selling the invention, it does not give the patent owner any affirmative rights to do likewise. As with other forms of property, the right to make, use, or sell a patented invention may be regulated by Federal, State, or local law.

Patents are more difficult to obtain than other forms of intellectual property protection. All applications are examined by the Patent and Trademark Office (PTO), which is responsible for issuing patents if all legal requirements are met. Once obtained, the enforceability of a utility patent is maintained by the payment of periodic maintenance fees.

***

Patenting of Micro-organisms and Cells

Patents on biotechnological processes date from the early days of the United States. Louis Pasteur received a patent for a process of fermenting beer. Acetic acid fermentation and other food patents date from the early 1800s, while therapeutic patents in biotechnology were issued as early as 1895.

The development of recombinant DNA technology (rDNA) – the controlled joining of DNA from different organisms – has resulted in greatly increased understanding of the genetic and molecular basis of life. Following the first successful directed insertion of recombinant DNA into a host micro-organism in 1973, scientific researchers began to recognize the potential for directing the cellular machinery to develop new and improved products and processes in a wide variety of industrial sectors. Many of these products were micro-organisms (microscopic living entities) or cells (the smallest component of life capable of carrying on all essential life processes). With the development of recombinant DNA technology, the potential of patenting the living organism resulting from the technology arose.

Prior to 1980, PTO would not grant patents for such inventions, deeming them to be "products of nature" and not statutory subject matter as defined by 35 U.S.C. 101. Although patent applications were rejected if directed to living organisms per se, patent protection was granted for many compositions containing living things (e.g., sterility test devices containing living microbial spores, food yeast compositions, vaccines containing attenuated bacteria, milky spore insecticides, and various dairy products). In the absence of congressional action, it took a catalytic court decision to clarify the issue of patentability of living subject matter.

The Chakrabarty Case

The Supreme Court's single foray into biotechnology occurred in 1980 with its ruling in the patent law case of *Diamond v. Chakrabarty*. Chakrabarty had developed a genetically modified bacterium capable of breaking down multiple components of crude oil. Because this property was not possessed by any naturally occurring bacteria, Chakrabarty's invention was thought to have significant value for cleaning up oil spills.

Chakrabarty's claims to the bacteria were rejected by PTO on two grounds:

- micro-organisms are "products of nature;" and
- as living things, micro-organisms are not patentable subject matter under 35 U.S.C. 101.*

---

* Section 101. Inventions Patentable. Whoever invents or discovers any new and useful process, machine, manufacture, or composition of matter, or any new and useful improvement thereof, may obtain a patent therefor, subject to the conditions and requirements of this title.

Following two levels of appeals, the case was heard by the U.S. Supreme Court, which in a 5–4 ruling, held that **a live, human-made micro-organism is patentable subject matter under Section 101 as a "manufacture" or "composition of matter."** The court reached several conclusions in analyzing whether the bacteria could be considered patentable subject matter within the meaning of the statute:

- The plain meaning of the statutory language indicated Congress' intent that the patent laws be given wide scope. The terms "manufacture" and "composition of matter" are broad terms, modified by the expansive term "any."
- The legislative history of the patent statute supported a broad construction that Congress intended patent protection to include "anything under the sun made by man."
- Although laws of nature, physical phenomena, and abstract ideas are not patentable, Chakrabarty's micro-organism was a product of human ingenuity having a distinct name, character, and use.
- The passage of the 1930 Plant Patent Act (affording patent protection for certain asexually reproduced plants) and the 1970 Plant Variety Protection Act (providing protection for certain sexually reproduced plants) does not evidence congressional understanding that the terms "manufacture" or "composition of matter" do not include living things.
- The fact that genetic technology was unforeseen when Congress enacted Section 101 does not require the conclusion that micro-organisms cannot qualify as patentable subject matter until Congress expressly authorizes such protection.
- Arguments against patentability based on potential hazards that may be generated by genetic research should be addressed to Congress and the executive branch for regulation or control, not to the judiciary.

Post-Chakrabarty Events and Trends

The *Chakrabarty* decision and subsequent actions by Congress and the executive branch provided great economic stimulus to patenting of micro-organisms and cells, which in turn provided stimulus to the growth of the biotechnology industry in the 1980s. In addition to the *Chakrabarty* decision, revisions in Federal patent policy promoted increased patenting of inventions in general, including living organisms and related processes. The Patent and Trademark Amendments of 1980 (Public Law 96–517) as amended in 1984 (Public Law 98–620) encourage the patenting and commercialization of government-funded inventions by permitting small businesses and non-profit organizations to retain ownership of inventions developed in the course of federally funded research.

These policies, which gave statutory preference to small businesses and nonprofit organizations, were extended to larger businesses by Executive order in 1983. The Technology Transfer Act of 1986 (Public Law 99–502) granted Federal authority to form consortia with private concerns. An Executive order issued in 1987 further encouraged technology transfer programs, including the transfer of patent rights to government grantees.

Increased patenting of biotechnology inventions has led to litigation, primarily related to patent infringement issues. Already, patent battles are being fought over interleukin–2, tissue plasminogen activator, human growth hormone, alpha interferon, factor VIII, and use of dual monoclonal antibody sandwich immunoassays in diagnostic test kits. It is likely that patent litigation relating to biotechnology will increase given the complex web of partially overlapping patent claims, the high value of products, the problem of prior publication, and the fact that many companies are pursuing the same products.

One negative trend arising from the increase in patent applications is the inability of PTO to process biotechnology applications in a timely manner. The number of these applications has severely challenged the process and examination capabilities of PTO. In March 1988, PTO reorganized its biotechnology effort into a separate patent examining group. As of July 1988, 5,850 biotechnology applications had not yet been acted on. **Currently, approximately 15 months lapse, on average, before examination of a biotechnology application initiates, and an average of 27 months passes before the examination process is completed by grant of the patent or abandonment of the application.** Turnover among patent examiners, lured to the private sector by higher pay, is cited as a significant reason for the delay in reviewing patents.

***

Patenting of Animals

In April 1987, the Board of Patent Appeals and Interferences ruled that polyploid oysters were patentable subject matter. Subsequently, PTO announced that it would henceforth consider nonnaturally occurring nonhuman multicellular living organisms, including animals, to be patentable subject matter under general patent law. This statement initiated broad debate and the introduction of legislation concerning the patenting of animals.

The first animal patent was issued in April 1988 to Harvard University for mammals genetically engineered to contain a cancer-causing gene (U.S. 4,736,866). Exclusive license to practice the patent went to E.I. du Pont de Nemours & Co., which was the major sponsor of the research. The patented mouse was genetically engineered to be unusually susceptible to cancer, thus facilitating the testing of carcinogens and of cancer therapies. Specifically, the patent covers "a transgenic nonhuman eukaryotic animal (preferably a rodent such as a mouse) whose germ cells and somatic cells contain an activated oncogene sequence introduced into the animal . . . which increases the probability of the development of neoplasms (particularly malignant tumors) in the animal." In November 1988, du Pont announced its intention to begin sales of the patented "oncomouse" in early 1989. The 1987 PTO policy and the 1988 issuance of the first patent on a transgenic animal spurred public debate on scientific, regulatory, economic, and ethical issues.

Producing Transgenic Animals

Most potentially patentable animals are likely to be transgenic animals produced via recombinant DNA techniques or genetic engineering. Transgenic animals are those whose DNA, or hereditary material, has been augmented by adding DNA from a source other than parental germplasm, usually from different animals or from humans.

Laboratories around the world are conducting research that involves inserting genes from vertebrates (including humans, mammals, or other higher organisms) into bacteria, yeast, insect viruses, or mammalian cells in culture. A variety of techniques, most developed from early bacterial research, can now be used to insert genes from one animal into another. These techniques are known by a number of exotic names: microinjection, cell fusion, electroporation, retroviral transformation, and others. **Of the currently available scientific**

techniques, microinjection is the method most commonly used and most likely to lead to practical applications in mammals in the near future. Other methods of gene insertion may become more widely used in the future as techniques are refined and improved. If protocols for human gene therapy, now being developed in animal models, or laboratory cultures of mammalian cells prove successful and broadly adaptable to other mammals, other gene insertion techniques could supplant microinjection.

Although the number of laboratories working with transgenic animals remains small (no more than a few hundred, worldwide), and researchers with the required skill and experience are not common, the number of research programs using these techniques has grown steadily in recent years. For reasons of convenience, much research involving transgenic mammals continues to be done using mice, although programs using several larger mammals have made significant progress. **It is anticipated that some animals of research utility or substantial economic importance will become more common as subjects of transgenic modifications in the near future (within 5 to 10 years). Beyond mice, the major research efforts involving transgenic modifications focus on cattle, swine, goats, sheep, poultry, and fish.**

Producing transgenic animals by microinjection, although tedious, labor intensive, and inefficient (only a small fraction of injected eggs develop into transgenic animals), compares favorably in at least three respects with traditional breeding techniques:

- The rapidity with which a specific gene can be inserted into a desired host means that **the time it takes to establish a line of animals carrying the desired trait is much reduced.**
- The specific gene of interest can be transferred with great confidence, if not efficiency, and if proper purification protocols are followed, **without any accompanying, unwanted genetic material.**
- With proper preparation, **genes from almost any organism can be inserted into the desired host,** whether it is a mouse or some other animal. Historically, genetic material exchanged by classical hybridization (crossbreeding) could only be transferred between closely related species or different strains within a species.

If there is a fundamental difference arising from the new techniques, it is that breeders have greatly augmented ability to move genes between organisms that are not close genetic relatives (e.g., human and mouse, or human and bacterium). Most transgenic animal research in the near future will likely focus on traits involving a single gene. Manipulation of complex traits influenced by more than one gene, however, such as the amount of growth possible on a limited food regimen, or behavioral characteristics, will develop more slowly (perhaps within 10 to 30 years) because of greater technical difficulty and the current lack of understanding of how such traits are controlled by genes.

Species Barriers and Species Integrity

Some concern has been raised over negative impacts transgenic animals might have on their own species, based on the assertion that transferring genes between species transgresses natural barriers between species, and thus violates their "integrity" or identity.

Modern biologists generally think of species as reproductive communities or populations. They are distinguished by their collective manifestation of ranges of variation with respect to many different characteristics or qualities simultaneously. The parameters that limit these ranges of variation are fluid and variable themselves: different species may have substantially different genetic population structures, and a given species may look significantly different in one part of its range than it does in another while still demonstrably belonging to the same gene pool or reproductive community. Although research into the nature of species continues to be vigorous, marked by much discussion and disagreement among specialists, general agreement among biologists exists on at least one point: **nature makes it clear that there is no universal or absolute rule that all species are discretely bounded in any generally consistent manner.**

The issue of species integrity is more complex and subtle than that of species barriers. If a species can be thought of as having integrity as a biological unit, that integrity must, because of the nature of species, be rooted in the identity of the genetic material carried by the species. Precisely how a species might be defined genetically is not yet apparent.

Any genetic definition of species, grounded in the perception of a species as a dynamic population, rather than a unit, cannot be simple; it must be statistical and complex. Therefore, **to violate the "integrity" of a species it is not sufficient to find a particular gene, once widespread throughout the species, now entirely replaced by a different gene.** Such changes occur repeatedly throughout the evolutionary history of a lineage and are described as microevolutionary. These changes are usually insufficient to alter a species in any fundamental way or to threaten any perceived genetic integrity.

If it is possible to challenge the integrity of a species, it would have to be by changing or disrupting something fundamental in its genetic architecture, organization, or function. Mammals like mice, cattle, or humans may contain from 50,000 to 100,000 or more genes. Whatever it is in the organization and coordination of activity between these genes that is fundamental to their identity as species, it is not likely to be disrupted by the simple insertion or manipulation of the small number of genes (fewer than 20) that transgenic animal research will involve for the foreseeable future.

The right of a species to exist as a separate, identifiable creature has no known foundation in biology. Species exist in nature as reproductive communities, not as separate creatures. The history of systematics and taxonomy (the disciplines of naming and describing species) demonstrates that species' existence has often been independent of scientists' shifting understanding or abilities to discern this existence. Furthermore, most of the domestic animals that are now the subjects of transgenic research (with the possible exception of some fish), and are likely to be for the foreseeable future, are already the products of centuries, and in many cases millennia, of human manipulation.

Federal Regulation and Animal Patents

To gain an understanding of the potential use and regulation of genetically altered animals that might be patented, OTA asked selected Federal agencies the following questions:

- How are genetically altered animals currently used in research, product development, and mission-oriented activities conducted or funded by your agency?
- What are the potential uses of such animals during the next 5 years?
- How does (or would) your agency regulate such animal use? What statutes, regulations, guidelines, or policy statements are relevant?

Several agencies currently use transgenic animals. The National Institutes of Health is currently the largest user of such animals for biomedical research projects. USDA has conducted research on the genetics of animals for many years. USDA's Agricultural Research Service reported projects involving the use of growth hormone in sheep and swine, and chickens engineered by recombinant DNA technology to be resistant to avian leukosis virus. USDA's Cooperative Research Service is in the early stages of supporting extramural research projects involving genetically engineered animals. The National Science Foundation (NSF) currently funds research involving transgenic animals in a range of experiments, all involving laboratory animals. With the use of transgenic animals becoming central to whole lines of investigation, NSF expects that work with such animals will increase. The Agency for International Development (AID) funds research involving conventional and transgenic animals at international research centers that are only partially funded by the United States. Accordingly, AID has minimal control over such research activities.

Several Federal agencies regulate experimental use or commercial development of genetically altered animals. Because current statutes regulate various uses and protections for animals, no single Federal policy governs all uses of genetically altered animals. In the absence of a single policy, Federal agencies will rely on existing statutes, regulations, and guidelines to regulate transgenic animal research and product development. **Current federally funded research efforts could lead to patents on animals. The patentability of an animal, however, does not affect the manner in which the animal would be regulated by any Federal agency.**

Economic Considerations

Economic considerations will influence the order in which different transgenic animals are produced for commerce. Transgenic animals used for biomedical research are likely to be developed first, primarily due to extensive research in this area. Transgenic agricultural animals are also likely to be produced, although large-scale commercial production of such livestock and poultry is unlikely in the near future (5 to 10 years).

The largest economic sectors likely to be influenced by animal patents are the different markets for agricultural livestock and some sectors of the pharmaceutical industry. The principal agricultural markets involve poultry, dairy, and red meat. These markets are organized quite differently, and are subject to different degrees of economic concentration. Poultry is most concentrated (though still diffuse by the standards of other industries, such as automobiles) and the dairy and red meat sectors much more diffuse. Different economic forces are important in markets as well: Federal price supports are of major importance in the dairy market, while the market for poultry is more open and competitive.

It is difficult to predict the manifold consequences of any particular approach to protecting intellectual property, especially across so wide a range of economic activity as that spanned by patentable animals. This range embraces diverse sectors of the agricultural livestock markets, pharmaceutical and other chemical production, as well as academic research or industrial testing. The economics of patenting and the effect on inventors and consumers will be determined by the potential use of the animal, its market, its reproduction rate, and its relative value.

The existence of animal patents and the degree to which they are employed in the different markets may introduce some new economic relationships. It is not now clear that these are likely to have any substantially adverse effects on the major markets or existing market forces. **The same types of pressures that have driven economic choices in the past are likely to continue to dictate them in the future. If an innovation increases costs (e.g., if a patented animal costs more than the unpatented alternative) it is unlikely to be adopted unless it commensurately increases outputs or product values.** It therefore seems that although cost savings can be anticipated to follow from animal patenting in some areas (e.g., pharmaceutical production or drug testing), innovations attributable to patented animals are likely to advance more slowly in low margin operations such as raising beef cattle.

In some cases, efficient alternatives to protection of intellectual property via patents are feasible. Trade secrets or contractual arrangements might serve well where the animals involved have a high intrinsic value and are limited in number (e.g., animals used for pharmaceutical production). When faced with the complexity of the markets for pork or beef production, however, such alternatives are clearly less practical, although the same complexity complicates any scheme for enforcement or royalty collection associated with patenting animals per se.

Ethical Considerations

A number of ethical issues have been raised in regards to patenting animals. Many of these arguments focus on the consequences that could occur subsequent to the patenting of animals. Other arguments focus on religious, philosophical, spiritual, or metaphysical grounds. These arguments have been used to support and oppose the concept of animal patenting.

Many arguments relating to the consequences of animal patenting are difficult to evaluate since they are speculative, relying on factual assertions that have yet to occur or be proven. Arguments based largely on theological, philosophical, spiritual, or metaphysical considerations are likewise difficult to resolve, since they usually require the assumption of certain presuppositions that may not be shared by other persons. Thus, such arguments are not likely to be reconciled with those persons holding opposing and often strongly held beliefs.

Most arguments that have been raised both for and against the patenting of animals concern issues that would be materially unchanged whether patents are permitted or not. Most arguments center on issues that existed prior to the current patenting debate (e.g., animal rights, the effect of high technology on American agriculture, the distribution of wealth, international competitiveness, the release of novel organisms into the environment). It is unclear that patenting per se would substantially redirect the way society uses or relates to animals.

Many concerns about the consequences of patenting can be addressed by appropriate regulations or statutes, rather than by amendments to patent law. Other arguments, particularly those of theological, philosophical, spiritual, or metaphysical origin, need to be debated more fully and articulated more clearly.

Looking a Gift Horse in the Mouth

Corporate Gifts Supporting Life Sciences Research

Eric G. Campbell, Karen Seashore Louis, and David Blumenthal

Throughout the last decade there have been a number of studies of academic-industry research relationships (AIRRs) that have focused on corporate support of research in the form of grants or contracts.[1-5] However, these studies have not examined a less formal method of resource exchange between companies and academic scientists – research-related gifts. These gifts can be in the form of discretionary funds, biomaterials, support for students, research equipment, or trips to professional meetings.[6-8]

Unlike other AIRRs, gifts are rarely subjected to significant oversight by the university. This is partly because gifts are given to individuals without an institutionally negotiated research grant or contract. In addition, because gifts are believed to be given with innocuous restrictions, many recipients assume they do not require significant university oversight.

Nevertheless, anecdotal evidence suggests that research-related gifts may come with problematic restrictions and expectations that may justify more active university management of these relationships. For example, accepting gifts may obligate recipients to keep results of their research confidential or provide donors with prepublication review that may significantly delay publication. In other cases donors may expect recipients to turn over all ownership rights of patentable results that arise from use of a gift.[7,9]

Because no systematic data have been collected to address this issue, the extent, characteristics, and implications of these exchanges have been difficult to judge. In this article we begin to explore these issues by examining the following questions: (1) How prevalent in major universities are research-related gifts? (2) How important are these gifts to faculty members' research? (3) What characteristics exemplify faculty who are likely to receive research-related gifts? (4) What, if anything, do donors expect in return for a research gift?

Answers to these questions will inform university policymakers regarding the extent and potential consequences of gift relationships for faculty and their institutions.

Methods

Sample

The data used in this study were derived from a survey of a stratified, random sample of 4000 life science faculty conducted between October 1994 and April 1995. This sample was selected by identifying the 50 universities that received the most research funding from the National Institutes of Health in 1993. Then, using medical school catalogs and *Peterson's Guide to Graduate Programs in the Biological and Agricultural Sciences,*[10] we identified all life science departments and graduate programs at these institutions. Departments were classified as "clinical" or "nonclinical" depending on whether their names referred to a clinical discipline (eg, anesthesiology, medicine, or surgery) or a nonclinical discipline (eg, biochemistry, molecular biology, genetics, or chemistry). From each institution, we randomly selected 1 department of medicine (internal medicine or other medicine subspecialties), 1 additional clinical department (eg, surgery, anesthesiology, or pathology), and 2 nonclinical departments. Departments of medicine, internal medicine, and medicine subspecialties were oversampled with respect to the nonmedicine specialties (surgery, pathology, etc) because they often receive the majority of extramural research funds at academic health centers.[11]

After identifying members of the selected departments, we constructed our mailing sample so that half was drawn from clinical departments and half from nonclinical departments. To avoid including individuals who were not truly functioning as faculty (eg, pure clinicians, residents, fellows, and hospital staff), we included only those clinical faculty who had published at least 1 article listed in the National Library of Medicine's MEDLINE database in the 5 years preceding the study. We also included all faculty who were identified by the National Center for Human Genome Research as recipients of funding from the Human Genome Project (HGP).[1] This process yielded a final sample of 1871 clinical faculty, 1871 nonclinical faculty, and 258 HGP recipients.

Survey Design and Administration

The survey instrument was a modified version of a questionnaire administered in 1985 to 1238 faculty concerning their relationships with industry.[2] The survey was conducted by mail and administered by the Center for Survey Research at the University of Massachusetts, Boston. Of the 4000 faculty in our mailing sample, 606 were ineligible because they were duplicate listings, were deceased or retired, held no faculty appointment at the sampled university, or could not be located. To determine how respondents differed from nonrespondents, the survey firm conducted a brief follow-up telephone survey of 124 nonrespondents. We asked nonrespondents about their academic rank and whether they had any extramural research funding. Nonrespondents were significantly more likely to have nontenure track or junior appointments (eg, lecturer, instructor), and they were significantly less likely to have any extramural research support. Of the remaining eligible 3394 faculty, 927 (63%) of the clinical faculty, 1125 (67%) of the nonclinical faculty, and 115 (51%) of the recipients of HGP funding returned completed questionnaires, yielding a total of 2167 completed surveys and an overall response rate of 64% after 3 survey mailings.

Important Variables

Gift Variables

In order to measure the frequency and importance of research-related gifts we asked faculty, "In the last 3 years have you received any of the following gifts (independent of a research grant or contract) from industry to support your research? (Check all that apply.)" The response categories were "equipment," "biomaterials (reagents, clones, antibodies, tissues, cell lines, etc.)," "discretionary funds," "support for students," "trips to professional meetings," "other (please describe)," and "none of the above." We then asked, "How important were these gifts to the progress of your research?" The response categories were "essential," "very important," "important," "not very important," and "not at all important."

To measure the extent and nature of restrictions and expectations of return associated with gifts we asked, "Do you think the company (or companies) expected any of the following in return for the gift(s)? (Check yes or no for each.)" The follow-up statements were as follows: "use only for the agreed-on purposes," "acknowledgment in publications," "prepublication review of articles or reports," "coauthorship on papers," "the gift not be used for commercial applications," "the gift not be used for applications that compete with company products," "the gift not be passed on to third parties," "ownership of all patentable results of the gift," "a future consulting relationship between you and the company," "general access to faculty and graduate students," "recruitment of graduate students," "evaluation testing of company products," "training of company employees," and "other (please explain)." It is important to note that this item measured what recipients *thought* companies expected in return for a gift, not necessarily what requirements they actually experienced.

Classifying Faculty by Research Type

Since membership in a clinical or nonclinical department may not fully predict whether faculty conduct clinical or nonclinical research, we classified faculty based on their responses to 2 survey items: "In the last 3 years, has any of your university research consisted of clinical trials of drugs, devices, or other diagnostic or therapeutic technologies?" and "In the last 3 years, has any of your university research, other than clinical trials, required approval of a human subjects committee?" Those faculty who responded affirmatively to either question were classified as clinical researchers. Faculty who indicated that they did not conduct any of these types of research within the last 3 years were classified as preclinical researchers.

Analysis

In addition to tabulating responses, we used simple and multiple regression analysis to test differences in means. Differences in simple proportions were tested using χ^2 analysis. Differences in proportions involving multiple variables were tested using logistic regression analysis.

We conducted several analyses to distinguish the effects of receiving gifts of different types. For clarity, these analyses involve only faculty who received a single type of gift (eg, biomaterials alone), since it would be impossible to relate a restriction or expectation of return to a particular class of gift where faculty received more than one type.

Results

Table 1 shows that in the last 3 years, 43% of respondents (920 faculty) received a gift from industry (independent of a grant or contract) to support their research. The most frequently received type of gift was biomaterials (24% of respondents), followed by discretionary funds (15%), equipment and trips to professional meetings (11% each), support for students (9%), and other (3%).

Among the 920 gift recipients, 459 (49.9%) received a single type of gift and 461 (51.1%) received more than 1 type of gift. Of those who received a single type of gift, 64 (14%) received only equipment, 252 (55%) received only biomaterials, 77 (17%) received only

Table 1. *Frequency of Research-Related Gifts From Industry**

Type of Gift	Faculty Who Received a Gift, No. (%)
Equipment	235 (11)
Biomaterials (reagents, clones, antibodies tissues. cell lines, etc.)	502 (24)
Discretionary funds	315 (15)
Support for students	186 (9)
Trips to professional meetings	234 (11)
Other	59 (3)
Received any of the above gifts	920 (43)

*This table refers to the number and percentage of respondents who received each type of gift. Because faculty could receive multiple gifts, the number of recipients does not total 920, and the percentages do not total 100%. The percentages were calculated by dividing the number of recipients by the number of respondents who answered this item (2128) and multiplying the result by 100.

discretionary funds, and 66 (14%) received only trips. No respondents reported receiving support for students or other gifts alone.

Although not shown in Table 1, we found no significant difference in the percentage of faculty in each subsample who received a research-related gift. Forty-four percent of faculty in clinical departments received a gift compared with 42% of faculty in nonclinical departments and 47% of recipients of HGP funding ($P = .42$).

Males were significantly more likely than females to receive an industrial gift (45% versus 35%, $P < .001$). Also, senior faculty were more likely to receive gifts than junior faculty. Forty-eight percent of full professors received a gift compared with 41% of associate professors, 38% of assistant professors, and 29% of other faculty ($P < .001$). Half of the clinical researchers received a research-related gift compared with 36% of the preclinical researchers ($P < .001$). Also, faculty who had research grants and contracts from industry were more likely to receive research-related gifts than those without grants or contracts (70% vs 33%, $P < .001$).

Importance of Gifts

In terms of the perceived importance of these gifts to respondents' research, 13% of recipients reported that gifts from industry were "essential," 22% reported "very important," 31% reported "important," 25% reported "not very important," and 9% reported that the gifts were "not at all important" to the progress of their research. Gifts were perceived as significantly more important by preclinical researchers than clinical researchers. Seventy-one percent of preclinical researchers reported gifts were "important," "very important," or "essential" to their research compared with 64% of clinical researchers ($P = .02$).

The importance of gifts varied by type of gift received. Twenty-four percent of those who received only trips rated them as "essential," "very important," or "important" to the progress of their research. However, 75% of those who received only biomaterials, 66% of those who received only discretionary funds, and 67% of those who received only research equipment rated these gifts as "essential," "very important," or "important" to the progress of their research ($P < .001$).

Table 2. *Selected Measures of Faculty Academic Activity**

Received	No. of Publications in Last 3 y		Hours of Student Contact per Week		No. of Service Activities[†]	
a Gift	Mean (SD)	P Value	Mean (SD)	P Value	Mean(SD)	P Value
Yes	14.0 (9.7)	.002	18.0 (14.2)	<.001	2.2 (1.8)	<.001
No	10.1 (12.2)		15.7 (12.6)		1.7 (1.7)	

*Differences in means were tested using multiple regression analysis controlling for the effects due to sex, academic rank, total research funding, faculty type (clinical or preclinical researcher), and whether respondents had any research grants or contracts from industry. Means are unadjusted.
†Service indicates the number of service roles faculty hold (department chair, university-wide administrator, member of a study section or review panel, editor on the editorial board of a journal, head of a research institute, chair of a university-wide committee, officer of a professional association, or member of the board or review panel of a foundation).

Academic and Commercial Activities

On all of the dimensions measured, faculty who received gifts were significantly more productive than nonrecipients (Table 2). Faculty who received research-related gifts published significantly more articles in refereed journals in the last 3 years, had significantly more hours of student contact, and engaged in significantly more service activities than faculty who did not receive research-related gifts. These results remained even when controlling for differences due to the effects of sex, academic rank, total research funding, clinical research, and whether the respondent had any research grants or contracts from industry. There were no significant differences in the number of publications, the number of hours of student contact, or the number of service roles by type of gift received (results not shown).

Table 3 shows the commercial outcomes of research ranging from the most preliminary (applying for a patent) to the most commercially advanced (such as having a product on the market or a start-up company). On all measures, faculty who received research-related gifts were significantly more commercially productive than nonrecipients. These results remained when controlling for the effects of sex, academic rank, total research funding, type of researcher (clinical vs preclinical), whether respondents had any research grants or contracts from industry, the number of publications in peer-reviewed journals in the last 3 years, the number of hours of student contact, and the number of service roles faculty held within their university or discipline.

Table 3 also shows the measures of commercial productivity broken down by the type of gift received. The only measure of commercial productivity that differed significantly by type of gift was whether faculty reported having a product under review. Of those who received only biomaterials, 8% reported having a product under review compared with 11% of those who received only equipment, 16% of those who received only discretionary funds, and 24% of those who received only trips to professional meetings ($P = .002$).

Restrictions and Returns Associated With Gifts

More than half of all recipients thought that donors expected acknowledgment in publications (63%), that the gift not be passed on to a third party (60%), or that the gift be used

Table 3. *Commercial Outcomes of Respondents' Research by Whether Respondents Received a Gift from Industry and the Type of Gift Received**

	Applied for a Patent		Patent Issued		Patent Licensed		Trade Secret		Product Under Review		Product on the Market		Start-up Company	
	%	P Value	%	P Value	%	P Value	%	P Value	%	P Value	%	P Value	%	P Value
Received a gift														
Yes	41	<.001	23	<.001	17	<.001	12	.03	16	.02	22	<.001	13	<.001
No	23		12		8		5		7		12		6	
Type of gift†														
Equipment	32	.56	18	.53	10	.43	6	.41	11	.002	22	.74	14	.17
Biomaterials	33		15		12		9		8		16		9	
Discretionary funds	30		20		15		8		16		19		18	
Trips	24		23		18		15		24		16		11	

*Differences in proportions were tested using multiple logistic regression analysis controlling for differences due to sex, academic rank, total research funding, faculty type, receipt of research grants or contracts from industry, number of publications, hours teaching, and number of service activities.
†Comparisons among the subset of 459 gift recipients who reported receiving only 1 type of gift.

303

only for the agreed-on purposes (59%). Forty-five percent thought that donors expected that the gift not be used for any commercial application. Approximately one third thought donors expected prepublication review of articles or reports (32%), evaluation or testing of company products (30%), or that the gift not be used for commercial applications that compete with company products (29%). Twenty percent of recipients thought that donors expected a future consulting relationship, and 19% thought the company wanted ownership of all patentable research results stemming from use of the gift.

However, the restrictions and expectations of returns differed by the type of gift received (Table 4). Among those who received only equipment, the most frequently reported restrictions and expectations of returns were acknowledgment in publications (60%), evaluation and testing of company products (49%), and that the equipment not be passed on to a third party (40%). Among those who received only biomaterials, more than three fourths thought that the company expected that the biomaterial not be passed on to a third party (82%), that it not be used for commercial application (81%), that it be used only for the agreed-on purposes (78%), and that the company be acknowledged in publications (79%). Other

Table 4. *Recipients Who Reported Restrictions and Returns by Type of Gift Received**

Restrictions and Returns	Equipment Only, % (n=64)	Biomaterials Only, % (n=254)	Discretionary Funds Only, % (n=77)	Trips Only, % (n=66)	*P* Value[†]
Use only for the agreed-on purpose(s)	24	78	41	50	<.001
Acknowledgment in publications	60	79	39	26	<.001
Prepublication review of articles or reports	13	40	20	18	<.001
Coauthorship on reports or publications	2	17	8	3	<.001
Not to be used for any commercial application	20	81	14	14	<.001
Not to be used for applications that compete with company products	13	44	16	10	<.001
Not to be passed on to third parties	40	82	35	32	<.001
Ownership of all patentable results from the gift	5	32	14	7	<.001
Future consulting relationship between recipient and company	24	9	22	24	<.001
General access to university faculty and graduate students	13	4	10	10	.04
Recruitment of graduate students	3	2	1	3	.85
Evaluation and testing of company products	49	19	25	15	<.001
Training of company employees	6	1	10	7	.005
Other	5	1	4	0	.05

* In this table the numbers vary slightly among questions because of missing data: not all respondents answered all questions. The percentage of respondents who answered given questions affirmatively are represented.

[†] *P* values were calculated using χ^2 testing.

frequent restrictions and expectations of returns recipients thought were associated with gifts of biomaterials were that the biomaterial not be used for applications that compete with company products (44%), that the firm receive prepublication review of articles or reports (40%), and that the company have ownership of all patentable results from the donated biomaterial (32%). Among those who received discretionary funds, 41% believed that the company expected that the money be used for the agreed-on purpose, 39% that the company be acknowledged in publications, and 35% that the funds not be passed on to a third party. For those faculty who received only trips to meetings, the most frequently reported restrictions and expectations of returns were that the trips be used for the agreed-on purpose (50%) and that the trip not be taken by a third party (32%).

Comment

Corporate gifts are a common source of research-related resources for life scientists. Almost half of all life scientists surveyed (43%) received a gift from a company (independent of a research grant or contract), suggesting that industrial philanthropic behavior may influence a large number of life scientists. The extent of this influence may be considerable given that 66% of all recipients reported that gifts were either "important," "very important," or "essential" to the progress of their research. However, trips to professional meetings were perceived as less important than other types of research-related gifts. Also, it appears that gifts may be most influential among those faculty who conduct preclinical research.

Academic and Commercial Activities

The data presented herein suggest that gifts from industry are related to high levels of academic and commercial activities. There are several possible explanations for this finding. It may be that firms selectively provide gifts to faculty who are highly academically and commercially productive prior to receiving a gift. However, gifts may also enhance academic and commercial productivity by providing resources or exposing recipients to new perspectives on their research. Also, it may be that more commercially inclined or entrepreneurial faculty are more likely to solicit gifts from companies. Unfortunately, the design of the study does not allow us to examine these issues.

Restrictions and Returns

Our data suggest that corporate gifts may be associated with a variety of restrictions and expectations of returns. Some may be innocuous and noncontroversial. Others, however, are more problematic. Innocuous and legitimate restrictions include expecting that the gift be used for the agreed-on purpose, that it not be used for commercial applications or applications that compete with the company's products, and that the donor be acknowledged in publications stemming from use of the gift.

However, other restrictions that may be perfectly legitimate from a donor's perspective may create ethical dilemmas for recipients. Our data suggest that this is especially true of restrictions on biomaterials. While it is accepted practice for academic scientists to seek access to reagents from the acknowledged source, such a restriction may be problematic to the extent that a firm refuses to give biomaterials to other researchers interested in replicating or extending the author's research or prohibits authors from depositing it in a biomaterial bank as required by several leading journals.

Restrictions regarding a period of prepublication review present similar issues. For firms, prepublication review's a legitimate way to provide feedback on new or improved uses of a firm's biomaterial and at the same time necessary to protect its lead over competitors. As a result, academic scientists may experience delays in publication, which may be detrimental to the overall progress of research, especially in rapidly developing fields. The extent to which a period of prepublication review is problematic depends primarily on the length of time that results are withheld from the academic community. This finding is certainly cause for some concern, given that a recent study found that delays of more than 6 months were associated with industrial support of research[12] and that 70% of all gift recipients had received research funding from industry.

Our data also indicate that accepting gifts that are encumbered with restrictions regarding the ownership of patentable materials may place recipients at odds with university policies regarding intellectual property ownership. For example, we found that 32% of those who received only biomaterials thought that the donor expected ownership of all patentable results stemming from use of the gift. By accepting a gift with this restriction, without an institutionally negotiated grant or contract, faculty may be knowingly or unknowingly violating the technology transfer policies of their university.

Finally, our data suggest that industry, faculty, or both may be using the gift mechanism as a way to bypass institutional administrative structures designed to manage AIRRs. This may be most applicable to the 15% of respondents who received discretionary funds to support their research. By receiving money earmarked to support research in the form of a gift rather than as an institutionally negotiated research grant or contract faculty essentially fail to reimburse their university for overhead expenses, which is also likely to violate existing institutional policies.

Policy Implications

Problematic Restrictions and Expectations of Returns

Although there are no universally accepted rules defining a problematic restriction or expectation of return, this research suggests a set of general guidelines concerning corporate gifts. First, faculty should become familiar, if they are not already, with their institutional policies that govern gifts vs grants and contracts. Second, if existing policies regarding gifts are inadequate, academic institutions should develop through faculty new or revised policies that simultaneously encourage the sharing of resources and timely dissemination of results to the academic community and at the same time protect the legitimate interests of donors. Third, faculty should not accept any resources from a firm that expects ownership of intellectual property without an institutionally negotiated research grant or contract. Fourth, faculty bear the primary responsibility to avoid using the gift mechanism as a means to bypass existing institutional policies and administrative structures for exchanges that are more appropriately managed under the auspices of a research grant or contract.

University Regulation of Gift Relationships

Based on the data presented herein, prohibiting or heavily regulating the acceptance of direct gifts by faculty members to support their research is not warranted. Such steps may deprive researchers of resources that clearly play an important role in life sciences research and are likely to be beneficial to the advancement of scientific knowledge and its applications. However, the data do suggest that universities need to be aware of research-related gifts and monitor specific cases where expectations of return clearly pose problems for the recipient or the institution.

Limitations and Future Studies

This study has several limitations that must be considered. First, we did not attempt to verify the accuracy of recipients' perceptions of the restrictions or expectations of return associated with research-related gifts, nor did we measure whether faculty honored donors' wishes. We also have no way of knowing if or to what extent recipients' perceptions of the restrictions and expectations of return differed from that of the donors'.

Second, we examined only one kind of gift – support for individual faculty research. Gifts to institutions such as new buildings or endowed chairs may have an entirely different character than those discussed here and, therefore, these findings may not be applicable to such forms of gifts. Also, because we studied life science faculty in the 50 most research-intensive universities, these findings may not be generalizable to less research-intensive institutions.

Third, as mentioned in the "Analysis" section, because of the way the questionnaire was designed, we could analyze the effects of individual types of gifts for only a subsample of all gift recipients. The importance and expectations of return for those faculty who received multiple types of gifts may differ from those who received only 1 type of gift.

Fourth, we recognize that inferences related to the propriety receiving of research-related gifts are often subtle and situation specific and are best made on a case-by-case basis. Restrictions that appear worrisome when reported on a questionnaire may not be so in actual practice. At a minimum, expectations associated with research-related gifts deserve significantly more study and discussion in the academic community. For example, further studies should directly ask donors (in addition to recipients) what, if any, restrictions and expectations of return are associated with research-related gifts. Future studies should also examine the extent of faculty compliance with restrictions and expectations of return. Studies should investigate the effects of gifts on graduate students' and faculty members' attitudes and behaviors regarding data sharing and data withholding.

Despite these limitations, this research shows that gifts from industry to life scientists are a common and important form of academic–industrial research relationship and that at times it may be prudent for faculty members to "look a gift horse in the mouth."

This work was supported by grant HG00724-01 from the National Center for Human Genome Research of the National Institutes of Health, the National Science Foundation, and the Commonwealth Fund Task Force on Academic Health Centers.

The authors wish to acknowledge the contributions of Melissa S. Anderson, PhD, at the University of Minnesota, Nancyanne Causino, EdD, and Joel S. Weissman at the Health Policy Research and Development Unit of the Massachusetts General Hospital, and Terra Zyporin, our editorial consultant.

References

1. Caldert CC. Industry investment in university research. *Sci Technol Hum Values*. 1983;8:24–32.
2. Blumenthal D, Gluck M, Louis KS, Stoto MA, Wise D. University–industry research relationships in biotechnology: implications for the university. *Science*. 1986;232:1361–1366.

3. Cohen W, Florida R, Goe WR. *University-Industry Research Relationships in the United States.* Pittsburgh, PA: Carnegie Mellon University.

4. ———— *University-Business Partnerships: An Assessment.* London, England: Rowman & Littlefield Publishers Inc; 1994.

5. Blumenthal D, Campbell EG, Causino N, Louis KS. Participation of life science faculty in research relationships with industry. *N Engl J Med.* 1996; 335:1734–1739.

6. Waugaman PG, Porter RJ. Mechanisms of interactions between industry and the academic medical center. In: Porter RJ, Malone TE, eds. *Biomedical Research: Collaboration and Conflict of Interest.* Baltimore, MD: Johns Hopkins University Press; 1992:93–117.

7. Weinberg RA. Reflections of the current state of data and reagent exchange among biomedical researchers. In: National Academy of Sciences, ed. *Responsible Science: Ensuring the Integrity of the Research Process.* Vol 2. Washington, DC: National Academy Press; 1993:66–78.

8. National Science Foundation. *University–Industry Research Relationships: Selected Studies.* Washington, DC: National Science Foundation; 1983.

9. Rosenberg SA. Secrecy in medical research. *N Engl J Med.* 1996;335:392–394.

10. *Peterson's Guide to Graduate Programs in the Biological and Agricultural Sciences.* 28th ed. Princeton, NJ: Peterson's Guides; 1994.

11. Ahrens E. *The Crisis in Clinical Research: Overcoming Institutional Obstacles.* New York, NY: Oxford University Press Inc; 1992:51–53.

12. Blumenthal D, Campbell E, Anderson M, Causino N, Louis KS. Withholding of research results in academic life science: evidence from a national survey of faculty. *JAMA.* 1997;277:1224–1228.

Questions for Discussions

1. Which is the primary research role of the university: to foster open-ended basic research or use-inspired science?
2. How do the responsibilities and commitments of academic scientists working under a grant from a commercial enterprise differ from those of scientists employed in that company's laboratories? Do they differ from the responsibilities of academic researchers funded by the National Institutes of Health? If so, in what ways?
3. What should be the role of the university in the process of technology transfer? Should the university seek to stimulate the economy through its research?
4. Should graduate students do their dissertation research with industry funds? At industry sites? In such cases, what protections should be in place for the students?
5. You are reviewing abstracts to determine who should present at an upcoming scientific meeting. Among the submissions you read an abstract from a small company that gives data from a clinical trial suggesting that they have created a successful treatment for a serious disease. Are you free at that time to spend your personal money to buy stock in the company?

Recommended Supplement Reading

Association of American Medical Colleges. *Guidelines for Dealing with Faculty Conflicts of Commitment and Conflicts of Interests in Research.* Washington, DC: AAMC; 1990. Available at http://www.aamc.org/research/dbr/coi.htm.

Association of Academic Health Centers. *Conflicts of Interest in Academic Health Centers.* Washington, DC: AAHC; 1990.

Association of Academic Health Centers. *Conflicts of Interest in Institutional Decision Making.* Washington, DC: AAHC, 1994.

Angell M. Is academic medicine for sale? *N Engl J Med.* 2000:341:1516–1518.

Blumenthal D, Campbell EG, Causino N, Louis KS. Participation of life-science faculty in research relationships with industry. *N Engl J Med.* 1996;335:1734–1739.

Cho MK, Shohara R, Schissel A, Rennie D. Policies on faculty conflicts of interest in U.S. universities. *JAMA.* 2000;284:2203–2208.

The kept university. *Atlantic Monthly.* 2000;285:39–54.

Porter RJ, Malone TE, eds. *Biomedical Research: Collaboration and Conflict of Interest.* Baltimore, MD: The Johns Hopkins Press; 1992.

The Scientist in Society

The Scientist in Society

Interactions, Expectations, and Obligations

Ruth Ellen Bulger

Health care practitioners frequently use covenantal language when referring to responsibilities to their profession and, more recently, to their patients. Such covenants are solemn promises about how practitioners will interact with others in their profession and in society. The Hippocratic oath portrays the physician's role as promising to "use treatment to help the sick according to my ability and judgment, but never with a view to injury or wrongdoing."[1] Such oaths are still taken publicly by health practitioners when they graduate and begin clinical practice.

Scientists generally have not used covenantal language to define their responsibilities and commitments to other scientists or to the public. Scientists refer more often to advancing knowledge, seeking "objective" truth, having intellectual interests in understanding nature, and experiencing the joy of making new discoveries.

In the early 1950s, Pigman and Carmichael stated that it was timely for scientists to consider professional traditions and relate them to modern scientific work.[2] They believed that these traditions were essentially an unwritten code of professional ethics and that scientists should reconsider modern circumstances and write them into a formal code. They felt that a mere statement of principles would help, but that an extensive codification with an attempt to discipline or expose gross violations might be desirable.

This essay will argue that covenantal commitments are essential for scientists. Certain scientists have expressed such commitments, not in written codes but by perceptive and courageous stands they have taken on the social ramifications of the scientific discoveries they have made.

Hans Bethe[3] expressed ethical reservations in working on weapons development, but not on what he felt was necessary military research. During World War II, he worked on the development of radar since it did not create a new weapon, as well as on the atomic bomb because he felt that the country was in a life-or-death struggle with Nazi Germany. Yet, after the war, he refused to contribute to the development of the hydrogen bomb. He said that he saw no compelling reason to proceed with this weaponry inasmuch as there was no imminent war.

Another courageous stand was taken by Henry Beecher in 1965–66 when he chose to give a talk and write an article describing instances of what he thought were serious problems with the way in which vulnerable, unaware, and disadvantaged persons had been used in clinical research.[4] He called attention to the lack of respect that investigators expressed, by their actions, for the individuals who served as research subjects in these studies. His insights were one of the important steps that led to action by Congress in the subsequent development of the National Research Act of 1974. This law called for the appointment of the National Commission for the Protection of Human Subjects of Biomedical and Behavioral Research and the development of institutional review boards at educational institutions receiving public funds for their studies.

In 1975, in an unprecedented act of professional self-governance, a group of scientists led by Nobel laureate Paul Berg expressed concerns about the confinement of novel microbes that were being created by the new recombinant DNA laboratory technology. They met at Asilomar, California and, after much discussion, called for a moratorium on aspects of their scientific studies until certain safety requirements were met and safety was better understood.[5] Actions such as these have served to reassure the public about the social conscience of scientists and their unwillingness to put the public at risk in the name of scientific advancement. There are many other examples of scientists who have wrestled with such issues and demonstrated their dedication to each other and to the public good.

Basic Versus Applied Science

Besides having a broad and varied set of motivations for their science, other factors have contributed to the infrequent use of covenantal language by scientists. One important factor is that science has been defined and divided into the categories of basic and applied science. In 1945 Vannevar Bush, President Franklin D. Roosevelt's science adviser, studied how science had so effectively contributed to the scientific effort during World War II. Bush then wrote *Science: The Endless Frontier* in which he laid out what has become the de facto U.S. science policy for the past 50 years.[6] Bush made a distinction between basic and applied science. He proposed a peacetime science policy stressing the importance of unfettered government-supported *basic* research using autonomous, basic scientist–generated, innovative ideas. He believed that it was basic research performed without concern for practical applications that led to new knowledge because, in his opinion, practical pressures would allow applied science to "drive out the pure." Therefore, he felt that it was this pure research that deserved and required special protection and specially assured support. This opinion has recently been repeated in a report of the AAMC.[7] Bush believed in a linear model of basic research leading to applied science and then to development and production. (See also references 8 and 9.)

In an attempt to use scientific techniques to design and justify a national biomedical research policy, Comroe and Dripps[10] studied 529 key articles that described many clinical advances since the 1940s that were essential to diagnosing, preventing, or curing cardiovascular or pulmonary disease. Their study demonstrated the wide and diverse information that led to one kind of scientific advance. Comroe's and Dripps's paper is often quoted as important to understanding the truism of the unpredictability of the ultimate importance of any particular scientific study. From this observation, it is frequently concluded that a study of any particular topic a scientist might choose could lead to important scientific developments.

However, the linear understanding of scientific advancement proposed by Bush has been questioned in an important book by Donald Stokes entitled *Pasteur's Quadrant: Basic Science and Technological Development*.[8] Stokes believes that Bush's concept does not explain how science really works and must be reevaluated as a necessary step in establishing a new and improved science policy for the future of relationships among scientists, the government, and society.

Stokes asks us to consider the work of Pasteur in his studies of the germ theory of disease. Pasteur studied fundamental processes, yet his lines of inquiry were grounded in applied science such as the pasteurization of milk or immunization from disease. Stokes points out that Pasteur fit into Bush's linear model of scientific progress in two places: in the area of basic science as well as in the area of applied science. Stokes proposed folding the line in the center, forming two perpendicular axes with the *y*-axis as the increasing quest for fundamental knowledge and the *x*-axis as the increasing consideration of usefulness of the science. By dividing the space delimited by the positive *x*- and *y*-axes into four boxes (Stokes called these quadrants), Pasteur's work would be found in the upper right quadrant of the space between the two axes (demonstrating both a high value for the search of fundamental knowledge [*y*-axis] as well as being high in the category of use-inspired [*x*-axis]). Stokes calls this area Pasteur's quadrant, representing *use-inspired basic research*. The upper left quadrant would then represent *pure basic research* since it signifies work that is high in fundamental knowledge but low in the consideration of its use. Stokes named this area Bohr's quadrant. The lower right quadrant would represent *pure applied research* because the research contained here is low in fundamental knowledge and high in the consideration of its use. He named this quadrant for Thomas Edison. Stokes compares the lower left quadrant, which represents research that was neither a search for basic knowledge nor for applied use to the listing of color markings on birds in Peterson's guide.

Stokes then reanalyzed the 529 key papers from the study by Comroe and Dripps[10] according to the four quadrants. Stokes found that 37% of the publications were in Bohr's quadrant (pure basic research), 25% were in Pasteur's quadrant (both basic and applied concerns), 21% were in Edison's quadrant (purely applied), and 17% were not in any quadrant, for they represented further development of applied studies into products. Stokes concluded that Bush's assumption that basic research must be undertaken without any practical application was true for only 37% of the studies and that, for the majority of the studies, having practical applications in mind did not drive out pure research as Bush proposed. He argued that Bush's assumptions were not supported by the data and must not be allowed to impede the development of a new contract between scientists, society, and government, which he believed must be developed for the betterment of all involved.

Transferring Technology to the Private Sector for the Public's Good

One quandary that exists for scientists concerns the setting of boundaries and parameters on interactions between scientists and industry. It is the present U.S. policy that scientific discoveries that might lead to health-related new technologies need to be developed both for the good of the people's health as well as the good of the U.S. economy. Scientific advances are presently seen as an important driver of the economy, and this perception relates to the recent support for doubling the NIH budget. The FY 1999 annual licensing survey of the Association of University Technology Managers reports 417 new products developed during that year, which resulted in 270,900 jobs being supported by the advances in science and $40.9 billion in economic activity generated mainly in the United States.[11] While these are important economic issues, one must also understand the ethical issues that arise from the inherent tension between making profits and promoting societal good. These developments create a variety of conflicts of interest and conflicts of commitment for scientists, institutions, and government agencies that have not yet been dealt with in a meaningful way. (See Section X for more on such conflicts.)

Another area of concern to be addressed in a new relationship of scientists with society is how to protect the various social missions that academic health centers undertake for the country. Academic health centers (AHCs) have traditionally provided about half of the uncompensated care for those in society who can neither afford medical insurance nor pay for their own health care. Blumenthal et al.[12] have examined the social missions of AHCs and concluded that "a convincing rationale exists, we believe, for continuing to protect the social mission of academic health centers from the full force of unfettered markets." These missions include not only the patient care mission for the poor and uninsured but the added costs for training health professionals and supporting the kinds of research that competitive markets do not support since the economic benefits of certain types of scientific discoveries are uncertain during the early phases of work on many research topics.

Does Creating Knowledge Carry with It Responsibility for the Foreseeable Uses?

It is possible to maintain that the creation of knowledge should place some responsibility upon the scientist for its foreseeable uses by society. The scientists who are creating knowledge could well have better better insight into the future uses of the new information than others because they are the closest to the results and should recognize their implications before other scientists or the public do. They can also translate scientific discourse into language that the public will understand. In this process of translation and communication, answering the questions asked by the public can also illuminate issues for the scientist. Finally, society pays for much of the nation's scientific research, either through the multiplicity of funding mechanisms supported by taxes or by contributions to voluntary societies, or by purchasing the drugs or products originally developed through the support of companies.

Reiser and Bulger[13] have contended that scientists have such responsibilities for the following reasons:

1. Society has required that subjects of experiments be protected, and thus society should receive similar protections.
2. Major precedents by other scientists have established the importance of researchers' responsibility to guard individuals and society from harm caused by their creations.
3. Scientific knowledge that results from the work of researchers would not otherwise be known; thus, scientists should accept responsibility for their actions.
4. As science becomes more technical, expert advice is crucial for the public.

Although one can argue that scientists have responsibilities in all these areas, modern society is more informed about ethical issues related to new scientific developments and will demand to be partners in the ultimate decision making on how these scientific developments are to be used.

Should Scientists Have a Covenant with Society?

Many factors indicate that a new relationship among scientists, the government, and society is needed, one that might even be viewed as a kind of covenant with other scientists and society analogous to that expressed in the Hippocratic oath. If there is to be a new policy–covenant, to what issues should it extend? Is there a sufficiently canonical set of values for scientists in the United States that could be articulated as a commitment of scientists to others? Are honesty and integrity in the doing of science an issue for which there is, in fact, agreement on such a covenant? Should conducting use-inspired scientific experiments be a covenant goal and, if so, to what extent? Should economic growth be a scientific goal? Should technology transfer be a scientific goal? Is the fulfillment of basic human needs a valid goal of science policy, and, if so, how does this mesh with the capitalistic, entrepreneurial environment in which science is now immersed?

Besides the well-recognized fact that honesty, trust, and objectivity are absolutely necessary for science to progress, the Institute of Medicine's report, *Society's Choices: Social and Ethical Decision Making in Biomedicine*,[14] discusses scientists' close involvement with discovery and innovation. The report gives three reasons why scientists might have a special role in decision making concerning ethical aspects of their work. First, the openness and critical tradition within science may provide an appropriate discursive model for decision making in our pluralistic society. Second, scientists may have special insights into issues from their work that might not be readily apparent to other users and consumers of developing technology. Third, scientists might be able to separate scientific facts from areas of social negotiation. However, the report also suggests that scientists must become involved in forums that open their perceptions and assumptions to critical evaluation by others.

The underlying principles for the responsible conduct of biomedical research that might form the basis of an ethical commitment for scientists as they work toward such a statement can be grouped into the following four categories:

1. The honesty, integrity, and objectivity of the scientist that undergird the trust necessary in science;
2. The "respect for others," including research participants and subjects, the environment, and colleagues;
3. Scholarly competencies in research and transmitting its results to other scientists, students, and the public; and
4. The stewardship of resources that have been provided by society to pay for scientific endeavors.[15]

The National Science and Technology Council recently has looked at policy issues shared among government, industry, and academic institutions. The Council has published a report relating to government–industry research partnerships, the principal finding of which is that the present partnership among scientists, the government, and industry is sound and continues to serve the nation in important ways. The report articulates four well-accepted guiding principles for comment: (1) that research is an investment in the future; (2) that the link between research and education is vital; (3) that excellence is promoted when investments are guided by merit review; and (4) that research must be conducted with integrity.[16] Other than what seems to be a stance against the funding of science by lobbying for allocation of scientific resources instead of peer review, there are few original ideas that deal with the role of these partners in pressing societal concerns.

Two more penetrating statements have been published in the last few years. The Board of Directors of the American Association for the Advancement of Science (AAAS) published a statement in 1998 that challenges our present science policy:

AAAS believes that, if the United States is to respond effectively to the challenges of the 21st century, we must find ways to reorganize our science and technology enterprise to address tomorrow's needs and aspirations: maintaining global sustainability, improving human health, addressing economic disparities, understanding our place in the universe, promoting peace and security, and directing the products of technology towards the betterment of society, nationally and worldwide.

They further concluded that decisions about research and development priorities should be linked more effectively to societal goals without compromising scientific excellence and the autonomy of individual researchers.

A similar report was released by the European Commission in 1997 entitled *Society, the Endless Frontier: A European Vision of Research and Innovation Policies for the 21st Century*. It proposed a problem-driven approach directly addressing complex societal issues such as global change, ecological sustainability, genetically modified organisms, and energy and transportation systems. To achieve these aims would require extensive international collaboration in the integration of basic and applied research, new technologies and industrial processes, and socioeconomic and ethical considerations.

If it is assumed that scientists have such responsibilities to society, they might exercise them in various ways. For example, each scientist decides whether to undertake or participate in a given research project and then determines how it will be conducted. Scientists must determine and maintain the standards that will be used in all aspects of the research that they undertake, including the methods to be used, the oversight of those working in the laboratory, how data will be analyzed and interpreted, and how intellectual property will be allotted fairly. Each scientist might also choose to alert the public to foreseeable benefits and harms of the work as it progresses and stimulate and participate in the public debate on related ethical issues. Professional societies might also facilitate discussion of social and ethical issues with scientists and members of society, but societies need to distinguish clearly the positions that are self-serving from those that meet the needs of society.

Just how far does the commitment of scientists to a societal covenant extend? There is agreement among scientists on a commitment to doing research in an honest, trustworthy, competent, and ethical manner. There is a general commitment to ethical conduct in research with human volunteers and in treating animal subjects in a humane and respectful way. There is a growing awareness of the importance of educating and working with the public on scientific and ethical issues that arise from the newer developments. However, we sense less agreement on a commitment–covenant among scientists on how best to deal with pressing social issues brought about by scientific developments that might fulfill basic human needs both here and in other countries. These issues may, for some, be more a part of the individual researcher's political and economic belief systems than part of the realm of what they regard as science policy. Yet George Brown, Jr., a Congressional champion of science, maintained that the scientific community needed to keep values in mind. In an address given to the AAAS Colloquium on Science and Technology in 1992, he said,

we need a new and better vision ... Neither technology nor economics can answer questions of values. Is our path into the future to be defined by the literally mindless process of technological evolution and economic expansion or by a conscious adoption of guiding moral precepts? Progress is meaningless if we don't know where we're going. Unless we try to visualize what is beyond the horizon, we will always occupy the same shore.

References

1. Hippocratic Oath. In: *Ethics in Medicine: Historical Perspectives and Contemporary Concerns.* Reiser SJ, Dyck AJ, Curran WJ, eds. Cambridge, MA: Massachusetts Institute of Technology Press; 1977:7.
2. Pigman W, Carmichael EB. An ethical code for scientists. *Science.* 1950;111:643–647.
3. Bethe H. The ethical responsibilities of scientists: weapons development rather than military research poses the most difficult questions. *The Center Magazine.* 1983;16(5):2–5.
4. Beecher HK. Ethics and clinical research. *N Engl J Med.* 1966;274:1354–1360.
5. Berg P, Baltimore D, Brenner S, Roblin Richard O III, Singer MF. Summary statement of the Asilomar conference on recombinant DNA molecules. *Proc Natl Acad Sci USA.* 1974;71: 2593–2594.
6. Bush V. *Science – The Endless Frontier: A Report to the President on a Program for Postwar Scientific Research.* Washington, DC: The National Science Foundation; 1990.
7. Association of American Medical Colleges. *Maximizing the Investments: Principles to Guide the Federal–Academic Partnership in Biomedical and Health Sciences Research.* Washington, DC: AAMC; March 1998.
8. Stokes DE. *Pasteur's Quadrant: Basic Science and Technological Innovation.* Washington, DC: Brookings Institution Press; 1997.
9. Bulger RE. Academic health center's changing relationship with industry and the for-profit sector: Implications for academic mission, economic competitiveness, and societal needs. *New Med.* 1999;3:3–9.
10. Comroe JH, Dripps RD. Scientific basis for the support of biomedical science. *Science.* 1976;192: 105–111.
11. Pressman L, ed. *Association of University Technology Managers Licensing Survey, FY 1999– 2000.* Northbrook, Il: AUTM. Available at: www.autm.net.
12. Blumenthal D, Campbell EG, Weissman JS. The social mission of academic health centers. *JAMA.* 2000;283:373–380.
13. Reiser SJ, Bulger RE. The social responsibility of scientists. *Sci Eng Ethics.* 1997;3:137–43.
14. Bulger RE, Bobby EM, Fineberg HB, eds. *Society's Choices: Social and Ethical Decision Making in Biomedicine.* Washington, DC: Institute of Medicine, National Academy of Sciences; 1995.
15. Bulger RE. Towards a statement of the principles underlying responsible conduct in biomedical research. *Acad Med.* 1994;69:102–7.
16. National Science and Technology Council. Four proposed guiding principles for comment. *Federal Register* 64:71454, 2000.

Summary Statement of the Asilomar Conference on Recombinant DNA Molecules

Paul Berg, David Baltimore, Sydney Brenner,
Richard O. Roblin III, and Maxine F. Singer

I. Introduction and General Conclusions

This meeting was organized to review scientific progress in research on recombinant DNA molecules and to discuss appropriate ways to deal with the potential biohazards of this work. Impressive scientific achievements have already been made in this field and these techniques have a remarkable potential for furthering our understanding of fundamental biochemical processes in pro- and eukaryotic cells. The use of recombinant DNA methodology promises to revolutionize the practice of molecular biology. Although there has as yet been no practical application of the new techniques, there is every reason to believe that they will have significant practical utility in the future.

Of particular concern to the participants at the meeting was the issue of whether the pause in certain aspects of research in this area, called for by the Committee on Recombinant DNA Molecules of the National Academy of Sciences, U.S.A. in the letter published in July, 1974[*] should end; and, if so, how the scientific work could be undertaken with minimal risks to workers in laboratories, to the public at large, and to the animal and plant species sharing our ecosystems.

The new techniques, which permit combination of genetic information from very different organisms, place us in an area of biology with many unknowns. Even in the present, more limited conduct of research in this field, the evaluation of potential biohazards has proved to be extremely difficult. It is this ignorance that has compelled us to conclude that it would be wise to exercise considerable caution in performing this research. Nevertheless, the participants at the Conference agreed that most of the work on construction of recombinant DNA molecules should proceed provided that appropriate safeguards, principally biological and physical barriers adequate to contain the newly created organisms, are employed. Moreover, the standards of protection should be greater at the beginning and modified as improvements in the methodology occur and assessments of the risks change. Furthermore, it was agreed that there are certain experiments in which the potential risks are of such a serious nature that they ought not to be done with presently available containment facilities. In the longer term, serious problems may arise in the large-scale application of this methodology in industry, medicine, and agriculture. But it was also recognized that future research and experience may show

[*] Report of Committee on Recombinant DNA Molecules: "Potential Biohazards of Recombinant DNA Molecules," *Proc. Nat. Acad. Sci. USA* **71**, 2593–2594, 1974.

From *Proceedings of the National Academy of Science*, 1975, 72, 1981–1984. Summary statement of the report submitted to the Assembly of Life Sciences of the National Academy of Sciences and approved by its Executive Committee on 20 May 1975.

that many of the potential biohazards are less serious and/or less probable than we now suspect.

II. Principles Guiding the Recommendations and Conclusions

Although our assessments of the risks involved with each of the various lines of research on recombinant DNA molecules may differ, few, if any, believe that this methodology is free from any risk. Reasonable principles for dealing with these potential risks are: (*i*) that containment be made an essential consideration in the experimental design and, (*ii*) that the effectiveness of the containment should match, as closely as possible, the estimated risk. Consequently, whatever scale of risks is agreed upon, there should be a commensurate scale of containment. Estimating the risks will be difficult and intuitive at first but this will improve as we acquire additional knowledge; at each stage we shall have to match the potential risk with an appropriate level of containment. Experiments requiring large scale operations would seem to be riskier than equivalent experiments done on a small scale and, therefore, require more stringent containment procedures. The use of cloning vehicles or vectors (plasmids, phages) and bacterial hosts with a restricted capacity to multiply outside of the laboratory would reduce the potential biohazard of a particular experiment. Thus, the ways in which potential biohazards and different levels of containment are matched may vary from time to time, particularly as the containment technology is improved. The means for assessing and balancing risks with appropriate levels of containment will need to be reexamined from time to time. Hopefully, through both formal and informal channels of information within and between the nations of the world, the way in which potential biohazards and levels of containment are matched would be consistent.

Containment of potentially biohazardous agents can be achieved in several ways. The most significant contribution to limiting the spread of the recombinant DNAs is the use of biological barriers. These barriers are of two types: (*i*) fastidious bacterial hosts unable to survive in natural environments, and (*ii*) nontransmissible and equally fastidious vectors (plasmids, bacteriophages, or other viruses) able to grow only in specified hosts. Physical containment, exemplified by use of suitable hoods, or where applicable, limited access or negative pressure laboratories, provides an additional factor of safety. Particularly important is strict adherence to good microbiological practices, which to a large measure can limit the escape of organisms from the experimental situation, and thereby increase the safety of the operation. Consequently, education and training of all personnel involved in the experiments is essential to the effectiveness of all containment measures. In practice, these different means of containment will complement one another and documented substantial improvements in the ability to restrict the growth of bacterial hosts and vectors could permit modifications of the complementary physical containment requirements.

Stringent physical containment and rigorous laboratory procedures can reduce but not eliminate the possibility of spreading potentially hazardous agents. Therefore, investigators relying upon "disarmed" hosts and vectors for additional safety must rigorously test the effectiveness of these agents before accepting their validity as biological barriers.

III. Recommendations for Matching Types of Containment with Types of Experiments

No classification of experiments as to risk and no set of containment procedures can anticipate all situations. Given our present uncertainties about the hazards, the parameters proposed here are broadly conceived and meant to provide provisional guidelines for investigators and agencies concerned with research on recombinant DNAs. However, each investigator bears a responsibility for determining whether, in his particular case, special circumstances warrant a higher level of containment than is suggested here.

A. Types of Containment

1. Minimal Risk

This type of containment is intended for experiments in which the biohazards may be accurately assessed and are expected to be minimal. Such containment can be achieved by following the operating procedures recommended for clinical microbiological laboratories. Essential features of such facilities are no drinking, eating, or smoking in the laboratory, wearing laboratory coats in the work area, the use of cotton-plugged pipettes or preferably mechanical pipetting devices, and prompt disinfection of contaminated materials.

2. Low Risk

This level of containment is appropriate for experiments which generate novel biotypes but where the available information indicates that the recombinant DNA cannot alter appreciably the ecological behavior of the recipient species, increase significantly its pathogenicity, or prevent effective treatment of any resulting infections. The key features of this containment (in addition to the minimal procedures mentioned above) are a prohibition on mouth pipetting, access limited to laboratory personnel, and the use of biological safety cabinets for procedures likely to produce aerosols (e.g., blending and sonication). Though existing vectors may be used in conjunction with low risk procedures, safer vectors and hosts should be adopted as they become available.

3. Moderate Risk

Such containment facilities are intended for experiments in which there is a probability of generating an agent with a significant potential for pathogenicity or ecological disruption. The principal features of this level of containment, in addition to those of the two preceding classes, are that transfer operations should be carried out in biological safety cabinets (e.g., laminar flow hoods), gloves should be worn during the handling of infectious materials, vacuum lines must be protected by filters, and negative pressure should be maintained in the limited access laboratories. Moreover, experiments posing a moderate risk must be done only with vectors and hosts that have an appreciably impaired capacity to multiply outside of the laboratory.

4. High Risk

This level of containment is intended for experiments in which the potential for ecological disruption or pathogenicity of the modified organism could be severe and thereby pose a serious biohazard to laboratory personnel or the public. The main features of this type of facility, which was designed to contain highly infectious microbiological agents, are its isolation from other areas by air locks, a negative pressure environment, a requirement for clothing changes and showers for entering personnel, and laboratories fitted with treatment systems to inactivate or remove biological agents that may be contaminants in exhaust air and liquid and solid wastes. All persons occupying these areas should wear protective laboratory clothing and shower at each exit from the containment facility. The handling of agents should be confined to biological safety cabinets in which the exhaust air is incinerated or passed through Hepa filters. High-risk containment includes, in addition to the physical and procedural features described above, the use of rigorously tested vectors and hosts whose growth can be confined to the laboratory.

B. Types of Experiments

Accurate estimates of the risks associated with different types of experiments are difficult to obtain because of our ignorance of the probability that the anticipated dangers will manifest themselves. Nevertheless, experiments involving the construction and propagation of recombinant DNA molecules using DNAs from (*i*) prokaryotes, bacteriophages, and other plasmids, (*ii*) animal viruses, and (*iii*) eukaryotes have been characterized as minimal, low, moderate, and high risks to guide investigators in their choice of the appropriate containment. These designations should be viewed as interim assignments which will need to be revised upward or downward in the light of future experience.

The recombinant DNA molecules themselves, as distinct from cells carrying them, may be infectious to bacteria or higher organisms. DNA preparations from these experiments, particularly in large quantities, should be chemically inactivated before disposal.

1. Prokaryotes, Bacteriophages, and Bacterial Plasmids

Where the construction of recombinant DNA molecules and their propagation involves prokaryotic agents that are known to exchange genetic information naturally, the experiments can be performed in minimal risk containment facilities. Where such experiments pose a potential hazard, more stringent containment may be warranted.

Experiments involving the creation and propagation of recombinant DNA molecules from DNAs of species that ordinarily do not exchange genetic information, generate novel biotypes. Because such experiments may pose biohazards greater than those associated with the original organisms, they should be performed, at least, in low risk containment facilities. If the experiments involve either pathogenic organisms or genetic determinants that may increase the pathogenicity of the recipient species, or if the transferred DNA can confer upon the recipient organisms new metabolic activities not native to these species and thereby modify its relationship with the environment, then moderate or high risk containment should be used.

Experiments extending the range of resistance of established human pathogens to therapeutically useful antibiotics or disinfectants should be undertaken only under moderate or high risk containment, depending upon the virulence of the organism involved.

2. Animal Viruses

Experiments involving linkage of viral genomes or genome segments to prokaryotic vectors and their propagation in prokaryotic cells should be performed only with vector–host systems having demonstrably restricted growth capabilities outside the laboratory and with moderate risk containment facilities. Rigorously purified and characterized segments of non-oncogenic viral genomes or of the demonstrably non-transforming regions of onco-genic viral DNAs can be attached to presently existing vectors and propagated in moderate risk containment facilities; as safer vector–host systems become available such experiments may be performed in low risk facilities.

Experiments designed to introduce or propagate DNA from non-viral or other low risk agents in animal cells should use only low risk animal DNAs as vectors (e.g., viral, mitochondrial) and manipulations should be confined to moderate risk containment facilities.

3. Eukaryotes

The risks associated with joining random fragments of eukaryote DNA to prokaryotic DNA vectors and the propagation of these recombinant DNAs in prokaryotic hosts are the most difficult to assess.

A priori, the DNA from warm-blooded vertebrates is more likely to contain cryptic viral genomes potentially pathogenic for man than is the DNA from other eukaryotes. Consequently, attempts to clone segments of DNA from such animal and particularly primate genomes should be performed only with vector–host systems having demonstra-bly restricted growth capabilities outside the laboratory and in a moderate risk contain-ment facility. Until cloned segments of warm-blooded vertebrate DNA are completely characterized, they should continue to be maintained in the most restricted vector–host system in moderate risk containment laboratories; when such cloned segments are char-acterized, they may be propagated as suggested above for purified segments of virus genomes.

Unless the organism makes a product known to be dangerous (e.g., toxin, virus), re-combinant DNAs from cold-blooded vertebrates and all other lower eukaryotes can be con-structed and propagated with the safest vector–host system available in low risk containment facilities.

Purified DNA from any source that performs known functions and can be judged to be non-toxic, may be cloned with currently available vectors in low risk containment facilities. (Toxic here includes potentially oncogenic products or substances that might perturb normal metabolism if produced in an animal or plant by a resident microorganism.)

4. Experiments to Be Deferred

There are feasible experiments which present such serious dangers that their performance should not be undertaken at this time with the currently available vector–host systems and the presently available containment capability. These include the cloning of recombinant DNAs derived from highly pathogenic organisms (i.e., Class III, IV, and V etiologic agents as classified by the United States Department of Health, Education and Welfare), DNA containing toxin genes, and large-scale experiments (more than 10 liters of culture) using recombinant DNAs that are able to make products potentially harmful to man, animals, or plants.

IV. Implementation

In many countries steps are already being taken by national bodies to formulate codes of practice for the conduct of experiments with known or potential biohazard.* † Until these are established, we urge individual scientists to use the proposals in this document as a guide. In addition, there are some recommendations which could be immediately and directly implemented by the scientific community.

A. *Development of Safer Vectors and Hosts*

An important and encouraging accomplishment of the meeting was the realization that special bacteria and vectors which have a restricted capacity to multiply outside the laboratory can be constructed genetically, and that the use of these organisms could enhance the safety of recombinant DNA experiments by many orders of magnitude. Experiments along these lines are presently in progress and in the near future, variants of λ bacteriophage, non-transmissible plasmids, and special strains of *Escherichia coli* will become available. All of these vectors could reduce the potential biohazards by very large factors and improve the methodology as well. Other vector–host systems, particularly modified strains of *Bacillus subtilis* and their relevant bacteriophages and plasmids, may also be useful for particular purposes. Quite possibly safe and suitable vectors may be found for eukaryotic hosts such as yeast and readily cultured plant and animal cells. There is likely to be a continuous development in this area and the participants at the meeting agreed that improved vector–host systems which reduce the biohazards of recombinant DNA research will be made freely available to all interested investigators.

B. *Laboratory Procedures*

It is the clear responsibility of the principal investigator to inform the staff of the laboratory of the potential hazards of such experiments before they are initiated. Free and open discussion is necessary so that each individual participating in the experiment fully understands the nature of the experiment and any risk that might be involved. All workers must be properly trained in the containment procedures that are designed to control the hazard, including emergency actions in the event of a hazard. It is also recommended that appropriate health surveillance of all personnel, including serological monitoring, be conducted periodically.

C. *Education and Reassessment*

Research in this area will develop very quickly and the methods will be applied to many different biological problems. At any given time it is impossible to foresee the entire range of all potential experiments and make judgments on them. Therefore, it is essential to undertake a continuing reassessment of the problems in the light of new scientific knowledge. This

---

* Advisory Board for the Research Councils, "Report of the Working Party on the Experimental Manipulation of the Genetic Composition of Micro-Organisms. Presented to Parliament by the Secretary of State for Education and Science by Command of Her Majesty, January 1975." London: Her Majesty's Stationery Office, 1975, 23pp.

† National Institutes of Health Recombinant DNA Molecule Program Advisory Committee.

could be achieved by a series of annual workshops and meetings, some of which should be at the international level. There should also be courses to train individuals in the relevant methods since it is likely that the work will be taken up by laboratories which may not have had extensive experience in this area. High priority should also be given to research that could improve and evaluate the containment effectiveness of new and existing vector–host systems.

V. New Knowledge

This document represents our first assessment of the potential biohazards in the light of current knowledge. However, little is known about the survival of laboratory strains of bacteria and bacteriophages in different ecological niches in the outside world. Even less is known about whether recombinant DNA molecules will enhance or depress the survival of their vectors and hosts in nature. These questions are fundamental to the testing of any new organism that may be constructed. Research in this area needs to be undertaken and should be given high priority. In general, however, molecular biologists who may construct DNA recombinant molecules do not undertake these experiments and it will be necessary to facilitate collaborative research between them and groups skilled in the study of bacterial infection or ecological microbiology. Work should also be undertaken which would enable us to monitor the escape or dissemination of cloning vehicles and their hosts.

Nothing is known about the potential infectivity in higher organisms of phages or bacteria containing segments of eukaryotic DNA and very little about the infectivity of the DNA molecules themselves. Genetic transformation of bacteria does occur in animals, suggesting that recombinant DNA molecules can retain their biological potency in this environment. There are many questions in this area, the answers to which are essential for our assessment of the biohazards of experiments with recombinant DNA molecules. It will be necessary to ensure that this work will be planned and carried out; and it will be particularly important to have this information before large scale applications of the use of recombinant DNA molecules is attempted.

Scientific Basis for the Support of Biomedical Science

Julius H. Comroe, Jr. and Robert D. Dripps

Our project had only one goal: to demonstrate that objective, scientific techniques – instead of the present anecdotal approach – can be used to design and justify a national biomedical research policy.

Our interest in this project began in 1966 when President Lyndon Johnson said, "Presidents . . . need to show more interest in what the specific results of research are – in their lifetime, and in their administration. A great deal of *basic* research has been done . . . but I think the time has come to zero in on the targets – by trying to get our knowledge fully applied. . . . *We must make sure that no lifesaving discovery is locked up in the laboratory* [italics ours]."

The position of the Johnson Administration on basic research was bolstered by a preliminary report of a study, "Project Hindsight," commissioned by the Department of Defense and published in 1966.[1] A team of scientists and engineers analyzed retrospectively how 20 important military weapons came to be developed. Among these were weapons such as Polaris and Minuteman missiles, nuclear warheads, C–141 aircraft, the Mark 46 torpedo, and the M 102 Howitzer.

Some of the conclusions of that study were as follows. (i) The contributions of university research were minimal. (ii) Scientists contributed most effectively when their effort was mission oriented. (iii) The lag between initial discovery and final application was shortest when the scientist worked in areas targeted by his sponsor.

The President's words and the Department of Defense's report popularized a new set of terms such as research in the service of man, strategy for the cure of disease, targeted research, mission-oriented research, disease-oriented research, programmatic research, relevant research, commission-initiated research, contract-supported research, and payoff research. These phrases had a great impact on Congress and on the Office of Management and Budget and led to a sharp upsurge of contract research and commission-initiated research supported by the National Institutes of Health (NIH).

Medical and other scientists countered with carefully prepared case reports that illustrated the important contributions of basic, fundamental, undirected, non-targeted research to advances in medicine, social sciences, and physics.[2]

Since 1966 there has been a continuing debate whether the federal government would get more for its biomedical research dollars if they were used to support clinically oriented research or if they were used to support research that was not clinically oriented.

We believe that the Department of Defense's study suffered from two factors. (i) Only a preliminary report has been released (and that 9 years ago) and even it is not yet widely

From *Science*, 1976, 192, pp. 105–111. Copyright 1976 by the AAAS.

available. (ii) Some who have read it have transferred conclusions drawn from that study on development of military weapons directly to biomedical research. However, the reports of those who countered Project Hindsight also suffered from one or both of two problems. (i) Some presented single case reports and so were anecdotal or "for instance" arguments. (ii) The cases were selected by those who did the study and so were subject to their bias.

It is easy to select examples in which basic, undirected, nonclinical research led to dramatic advance in clinical medicine and equally easy to give examples in which either clinically oriented research or development was all-important. A classic example of the great importance of research completely unrelated to clinical medicine or surgery was that of Wilhelm Roentgen. While studying a basic problem in the physics of rays emitted from a Crookes' tube, he discovered x-rays that immediately became vital for precise diagnosis of many diseases and later for the treatment of some. A classic example of the importance of mission-oriented research was that of Louis Pasteur. Pasteur, originally trained as a chemist, was employed by the French government as an industrial trouble-shooter. Among the problems assigned to him were the practical ones of how to keep wine from turning to vinegar, how to cure ailing silkworms, and how to save sheep dying of anthrax and chickens dying of cholera. The solution of these practical problems led Pasteur to discover bacteria and become the founder of modern bacteriology and the father of the germ theory of disease. A classic example of the importance to medicine of development (as opposed to research) was the mass production of penicillin in the United States in the early 1940's when it was required immediately for England's war effort and later for our own.

The anecdotal or "let me give you an example" approach provides fascinating after-dinner conversation and even interesting testimony before congressional appropriations committees. However, we believe that the time has come for the nation's biomedical research policy to be based on something more substantial than a preliminary analysis of weapons development by the Department of Defense and informal let-me-give-you-an-example arguments by concerned scientists, and that Congress and the Administration should require more than for-instances from proponents or opponents of any policy for the support of medical research. We believe that the design and the broad scope of our study avoid the weaknesses of previous studies and provide and example to show how long-term policies on support of biomedical research can be developed on an objective basis.

Scope of our Study

Because the heart of our thesis is that the support of research should not be based on selected examples or anecdotes, it was mandatory that we study all of a broad field. We selected the field of cardiovascular and pulmonary diseases because these are responsible for more than half of all deaths in the United States each year and because we have some competence in evaluating research on the heart, blood vessels, and lungs, or know where to go for advice. To ensure that our study was concerned directly with the health of the nation and not with esoteric scientific discoveries, we directed our attention only to clinical advances since the early 1940's that have been directly responsible for diagnosing, preventing, or curing cardiovascular or pulmonary disease; stopping its progression, decreasing suffering, or prolonging useful life.

To avoid our own bias, we asked 40 physicians to list the advances they considered to be the most important for their patients. We then divided their selections into a cardiovascular and a pulmonary list and sent the appropriate list to 40 to 50 specialists in each field, asking

Table 1. *The Top Ten Clinical Advances in Cardiovascular and Pulmonary Medicine and Surgery in the Last 30 Years*

Cardiac surgery (including open-heart repair of congenital defects and replacement of diseased valves)

Vascular surgery (including repair or bypass of obstructions or other lesions in aorta, coronary, cerebral, renal, and limb arteries)

Drug treatment of hypertension

Medical treatment of coronary insufficiency (myocardial ischemia)

Cardiac resuscitation, defibrillation, "cardioversion" and pacing in patients with cardiac arrest, slow hearts, or serious arrhythmias

Oral diuretics (in treatment of patients with congestive heart failure or hypertension)

Intensive cardiovascular and respiratory care units (including those for postoperative care, coronary care, respiratory failure, and disorders of newborn)

Chemotherapy and antibiotics (including prevention of acute rheumatic fever and treatment of tuberculosis, pneumonias, and cardiovascular syphilis)

New diagnostic methods (for earlier and more accurate diagnosis of disease of cardiovascular and pulmonary-respiratory systems)

Prevention of poliomyelitis (especially of respiratory paralysis due to polio)

each to vote on the list and to add additional advances that they believed belonged on the list. Their votes selected the top ten advances (Table 1). With these as a starting point, we worked retrospectively to learn why and how they occurred.

With the help of 140 consultants,[3] including 46 interviewed personally, we identified the essential bodies of knowledge that had to be developed before each of the ten clinical advances could reach its current state of achievement. To make clear what we mean by this, let us consider cardiac surgery.

When general anesthesia was first put to use in 1846, the practice of surgery exploded in many directions, except for thoracic surgery. Cardiac surgery did not take off until almost 100 years later, and John Gibbon did not perform the first successful operation on an open heart with complete cardiopulmonary bypass apparatus until 108 years after the first use of ether anesthesia. What held back cardiac surgery? What had to be known before a surgeon could predictably and successfully repair cardiac defects? First of all, the surgeon required precise preoperative diagnosis in every patient whose heart needed repair. That required selective angiocardiography which, in turn, required the earlier discovery of cardiac catheterization, which required the still earlier discovery of x-rays. But the surgeon also needed an artificial heart–lung apparatus (pump-oxygenator) to take over the function of the patient's heart and lungs while he stopped the patient's heart in order to open and repair it. For pumps, this required a design that would not damage blood; for oxygenators, this required basic knowledge of the exchange of O_2 and CO_2 between gas and blood. However, even a perfect pump-oxygenator would be useless if the blood in it clotted. Thus, the cardiac surgeon had to await the discovery and purification of a potent, nontoxic anticoagulant – heparin.

These are just a few examples; obviously Gibbon needed many more essential bodies of knowledge. Table 2 lists 25 that we believe he needed in 1954 before he could perform open-heart surgery with confidence in the result; we list all of these because some, such

Table 2. *Essential Bodies of Knowledge Required for Successful Open-Heart Surgery*

Preoperative diagnosis of cardiac defects
Anatomic and clinical
Physiologic: electrocardiography, other noninvasive tests
Physiologic: cardiac catheterization
Radiologic: selective angiocardiography

Preoperative care and preparation
Blood groups and typing; blood-preservation; blood banks
Nutrition
Assessment of cardiac, pulmonary, renal, hepatic, and brain function
Management of heart failure

Intraoperative management
Asepsis
Monitoring ECG, blood pressure, heart rate, EEG, and blood O_2, CO_2, and pH
Anesthesia and neuromuscular blocking agents
Hypothermia and survival of ischemic organs
Ventilation of open thorax
Anticoagulants
Pump-oxygenator
Elective cardiac arrest; defibrillation
Transfusions; fluid and electrolytes; acid–base balance
Surgical instruments and materials
Surgical techniques and operations

Postoperative care
Relief of pain
General principles of intensive care; recording and warning systems
Management of infection
Diagnosis and management of circulatory failure
Diagnosis and management of other postoperative complications
Wound healing

as antibiotics, are so commonplace in 1976 that we forget that even they once had to be discovered! For the ten advances, we identified 137 essential bodies of knowledge.

The knowledge essential for these advances has accumulated over decades or centuries from the lifetime work of many thousands of scientists. It was clearly impossible for us to read all of their publications to determine how and why the research of each was done. But, because we were determined to avoid the let-me-give-you-an-example approach, we did examine about 4000 published articles. Of these, we identified about 2500 specific scientific reports that were particularly important to the development of one or more of the 137 essential bodies of knowledge. We arranged these chronologically in 137 tables. From these, with the advice of consultants, we then selected more than 500 essential or key articles for careful study.

Why did we spend several years collecting and reading thousands of articles and arranging more than 2500 of these in 137 chronological tables before doing our final analysis? There were several reasons.

1) It was essential that we have tangible evidence that our selections came from painstaking, scholarly review and not from the imperfect memories of a group of scientists at a cocktail party.

2) The chronological lists facilitate analysis of lags between initial discovery and clinical application (to be reported elsewhere).

3) They emphasize to the reader that scientific advance requires far more work than that reported by the discoverer or by those who wrote key articles essential for his discovery. We believe that a major defect in education in science in high school and colleges is the perpetuation of the one person = one discovery myth (for example, Marconi = wireless; Edison = electric light) and that this is partly responsible for the anecdotal approach to national science policy. Without a long chronologic tabulation, such as the electrocardiography (ECG) list in Table 3, some might consider that Einthoven in 1903 invented the ECG in its 1976 form, without help from those who preceded or followed him. Chronological tables provide specific evidence for policy-makers that scientists earlier and later than the discoverer have always been essential to each discovery and its full development. A defect in tables is that they can convey only a bit of the message, because even a long list includes only a small fraction of the good, original research that helped to move us away from complete ignorance toward full knowledge.

Definition of a Key Article

1) It had an important effect on the direction of subsequent research and development, which, in turn, proved to be important for clinical advance in one or more of the ten clinical advances under study.

2) It reported new data, new ways of looking at old data, a new concept or hypothesis, a new method, new drug, new apparatus, or a new technique that either was essential for full development of one or more of the clinical advances (or necessary bodies of knowledge) or greatly accelerated it. The key article might report basic laboratory investigation, clinical investigation, development of apparatus or essential components, synthesis of data and ideas of others, or wholly theoretical work.

3) A study is not a key study (even if it won the Nobel Prize for its author) if it has not yet served directly or indirectly as a step toward solving one of the ten clinical advances.

4) An article is a key article if it described the final step in the clinical advance, even though it was an inevitable step requiring no unusual imagination, creativity, or special competence (for example, first person to report on a new drug in humans even though basic work on animals had been done and results in humans were largely predictable).[4]

Selection and Analysis of Key Articles

Because these key articles formed the basis of our analysis, we devoted considerable thought to their selection. We realized that bias in selecting them could invalidate our study and that their careful review by consultants was essential. At the same time, experience with pilot studies showed us that scientists are rarely unanimous in voting that Jones's discovery is more important than Smith's. Sometimes this is because of justified differences in judgment; sometimes it is because there is no one article that can be singled out from many in a steady advance with many equal contributors. We solved this problem for the purposes of this study (though not for election of individual scientists to a "Hall of Fame") by first selecting

Table 3. *Chronological Events in the Development of Electrocardiography. The Scientists' Names that Are Printed in Boldface Type Indicate Key Articles*

Year of Discovery	Scientist	Event and Publication
B.C.	Ancients	Early manifestations of electricity: electric fish, rubbed amber, lodestone, terrestrial lightning
1660	von Guericke	First electricity machine (friction of glass and hand) [*Experimenta Nova Magdeburgica* (Jansson, Amsterdam, 1672), book 4, p. 147]
1745	von Kleist	Charge from electricity machine stored in glass bottle and delivered as static electric shock [Letter to Dr. Lieberkühn, 4 November 1745; J. G. Krüger, *Geschichte der Erde* (Luderwaldischen, Halle, 1746)]
1745–1750	Musschenbroek	Electricity stored in Leyden jar; shocks killed small animals [*Introductio ad Philosophiam Naturalem* (Luchtmans, Leyden, 1762), pp. 477–1132]
1752	**Franklin**	Kite and key used to charge Leyden jar from lightning; identity of lightning and electricity proved [*Philos. Trans. R. Soc. London* **47**, 565 (1751–1752)]
1756–1757	Caldani	Nerve and muscle excited by discharge from Leyden jar [*Institutiones Physiologicae* (Pezzana, Venice, 1786)]
1780	**Galvani**	Stimulation of nerve by Leyden jar and "electricity machine" caused identical muscle contraction [*Bononiensi Scientiarum et Artium Instituto Atque Academia Commentarii* **7**, 363 (1791)]
1786	**Galvani**	Concept of animal electricity [*Bononiensi Scientiarum et Artium Instituto Atque Academia Commentarii* **7**, 363 (1791)]
1791	**Galvani**	Contraction of heart muscle produced by discharge from electric eel; contraction of muscle caused by injury current [*Dell'uso e dell'attività dell'arco conduttóre nelle contrazioni dei muscoli* (Tommaso d'Aquino, Bologna, 1794)]
1800	Volta	Electricity generated by dissimilar metals; voltaic pile or battery [*Philos. Trans. R. Soc. London Part 2* **90**, 403 (1800)]
1839	Purkinje	Purkinje's fibers in the cardiac ventricles [*De Musculari Cordis Structura* (Friedlaender, Bratislava, 1839)]
1842	**Matteucci**	Muscle contracts if its nerve is laid across another contracting muscle [see Dumas, *C. R. Acad. Sci.* **15**, 797 (1842)]
1843	DuBois-Reymond	Action current in nerve as well as muscle [*Untersuchungen über Thierische Elektrizität* (Reimer, Berlin, 1848–49)]
1852	Stannius	Ligatures demonstrating specific conduction paths in heart [*Arch. Anat. Physiol. Wiss. Med.* p. 85 (1852)]
1856	Kölliker and Müller	Frog muscle contraction used as indicator of cardiac currents [*Verh. Phys.-Med. Ges. Würzberg* **6**, 428 (1856)]

Table 3. *(continued)*

Year of Discovery	Scientist	Event and Publication
1875	Lippmann	Use of capillary electrometer [*Ann. Chim. Phys. Ser. 5* **5**, 494 (1875)]
1876	Marey	Refractory period in early cardiac systole [*Physiol. Exp. Trav. Lab. Marey* **2**, 63 (1876)]
1878	Engelmann	Studied electrical excitation of isolated frog heart [*Pflügers Arch.* **17**, 68 (1878)]
1879–1880	**Burdon-Sanderson and Page**	First ECG in intact animals (frogs) [*J. Physiol.* **2**, 384 (1879–1880)]
1883	Gaskell	Sequence of contraction from sinus venosus to atria to ventricles [*J. Physiol.* **4**, 43 (1883)]
1887	**Waller**	First human ECG using Lippmann's capillary electrometer [*J. Physiol.* **8**, 229 (1887)]
1887	McWilliam	Noted fibrillary contractions of heart [*J. Physiol.* **8**, 296 (1887)]
1893	**His**	Atrioventricular bundle [*Arbeit. Med. Klin. Leipzig.* **14**, 14 (1893)]
1893	Kent	Atrioventricular bundle [*J. Physiol.* **14**, 233 (1893)]
1897	Ader	Thread or string galvanometer [*C. R. Acad. Sci.* **124**, 1440 (1897)]
1903	**Einthoven**	Sensitive string galvanometer for measuring human ECG; telemetry of ECG signals [*Pflügers Arch.* **99**, 472 (1903)]
1906	Tawara	Atrioventricular node [*Das Reizleitungssystem des Säugetierherzens* (Fischer, Jena, 1906)]
1907	Keith and Flack	Sinoatrial node, mammals [*J. Anat. Physiol.* **41**, 172 (1907)]
1908	Mackenzie	Polygraph, venous pulse and arrhythmias [*Diseases of the Heart* (Frowde, London, 1908)]
1909–1920	**Lewis**	ECG and arrhythmias in man (numerous articles in *Heart*, a magazine he founded)
1913	Einthoven, Fahr, de Waart	Equilateral triangle theory of ECG [*Arch. Ges. Physiol.* **150**, 275 (1913)]
1914	Garrey	Mechanisms of flutter and fibrillation; "circus" movements [*Am. J. Physiol.* **33**, 397 (1914)]
1915	Lewis and Rothschild	Excitation wave in dog heart [*Philos. Trans. R. Soc. London Ser. B* **206**, 181 (1915)]
1918	Smith	ECG changes after ligating a branch of coronary artery in dogs [*Arch. Int. Med.* **22**, 8 (1918)]
1926	Rothberger	Arrhythmias in man [in *Handbuch der Normalen und Pathologischen Physiologie* (Springer, Berlin, 1926), vol. 7]
1927	Wenckebach and Winterberg	Arrhythmias in man [*Die unregelmässige Herztätigkeit* (Engelmann, Leipzig, 1927)]
1930	**Wilson**	Laws of distribution of potential differences in solid conductors; modern theory of ECG [*Am. Heart J.* **5**, 599 (1930)]

Table 3. *(continued)*

Year of Discovery	Scientist	Event and Publication
1939	Hodgkin and Huxley	Transmembrane action potential recorded in giant axone of squid [*Nature (London)* **144,** 710 (1939)]
1946 1949	Graham and Gerard } Ling and Gerard	First measurement of transmembrane potential in skeletal muscle with intracellular microelectrodes [*J. Cell. Comp. Physiol.* **28,** 99 (1946); *ibid.* **34,** 383 (1949)]
1949	Coraboeuf and Weidmann	Intracellular electrode to record mammalian cardiac potentials [*C. R. Seances Soc. Biol. Paris* **143,** 1329 (1949)]
1951	**Draper and Weidmann**	Intracellular electrode used to measure transmembrane potentials of heart muscle cells [*J. Physiol.* **115,** 74 (1951)]
1958	Alanís, González, López	Electrical activity of bundle of His [*J. Physiol.* **142,** 127 (1958)]
1960	Giraud, Peuch, Latour	Electrical activity of bundle of His in man [*Bull. Acad. Natl. Med. Paris* **144,** 363 (1960)]
1967–1968	**Scherlag** *et al.*	Recording from bundle of His by cardiac catheter in man [*J. Appl. Physiol.* **22,** 584 (1967); *ibid.* **25,** 425 (1968)]
1967	Watson, Emslie-Smith, Lowe	Recording from bundle of His in patient undergoing cardiac catheterization [*Am. Heart J.* **74,** 66 (1967)]

key articles in 42 of our tables and then sending the same tables (with no clue to our choices) to reviewers for their independent selection. We then analyzed the articles that we had selected to determine the goal of the investigators and repeated the same process for the articles selected by our reviewers. Although there was not complete agreement on the selection of individual key articles, there was almost exact agreement on the type of articles selected. Thus the percentage of key articles reporting research that was not clinically oriented was almost identical in their selections and in ours (Table 4). Because our interest was in determining the type of research reported in key articles (for example, clinically oriented research or that which was not clinically oriented) rather than in identifying specific scientists and their reports, we believe that the agreement on type, based on a sample of more than 50 percent of our key articles, justifies our extending it to the whole group.[5]

Once the key articles were selected, we re-read and analyzed each article to determine the answers to the following questions. (i) How many key studies were clinically oriented? How many were not directed toward the solution of a clinical problem? (ii) How many key articles reported basic research? Other kinds of research? Development or engineering?

Was the Key Research Clinically Oriented?

To eliminate uncertainty about our definitions, in this section we avoid classifying research as clinical investigation, basic research, fundamental studies, directed or undirected research, or targeted or nontargeted research. Instead, we use only two terms; (i) clinically oriented research, and (ii) research that was not clinically oriented.

Table 4. *Goal of Authors of Key Articles as Selected by Reviewers and by Us from the Same 42 Tables*

Key Articles Selected by	Number of Articles	Goal Was not Clinically Oriented	Goal Was Clinically Oriented	Percent of Total not Clinically Oriented
Reviewers	494*	189*	305*	38.3
Us	267	101	166	37.8

*Total number of key articles selected by reviewers is higher than number selected by us because (i) the reviewers on the average selected 8.4 key articles per table and we selected on the average only 6.7 for these 42 tables; and (ii) we sent some tables to more than one reviewer.

We define research as clinically oriented, even if it was performed entirely on animals, tissues, cells, or subcellular particles, if the author mentions even briefly an interest in diagnosis, treatment, or prevention of a clinical disorder or in explaining the basic mechanisms of a sign or symptom of the disease itself. Thus the Nobel Prize–winning research of Enders, Weller, and Robbins on extraneural culture of poliovirus in vitro was classified as clinically oriented because the team expressed an interest in multiplication of poliovirus outside the nervous system (for example, in the patient's gastrointestinal tract).

We define research as not clinically oriented if the author neither state nor suggest any direct or indirect bearing that their research might have on a clinical disorder of humans, even though their work later helped to clarify some aspect of it. An article can be classified as not clinically oriented even if the research is done on a human (for example, Oliver's administration of an adrenal extract, later known as epinephrine, to his son in 1895 to see whether it would narrow the diameter of his radial artery).

Each article was classified as one or the other without consideration of earlier or later work of the same investigator and without being influenced by later stories (written or verbal) of "Why I did my research." The results of classifying 529 key articles into these two categories are shown in Table 5.

These data strongly support our contention that those concerned with preserving or changing national biomedical science policy should disregard anecdotal "evidence" no matter how convincingly the case is presented. Table 5 shows that someone looking for evidence to defend any position on the support of research can get it by choosing the right clinical advance as his example or his for-instance. If one picks vascular surgery or antibiotics or poliomyelitis, one can "prove" that clinically oriented research deserves major support; if one selects hypertension or oral diuretics or new diagnostic tests, one can "prove" that research that is not clinically oriented deserves major support.

The most important figure in Table 5 is that, for cardiovascular and pulmonary advances as a whole, 41 percent of all work judged to be essential or crucial for later clinical advances was not clinically oriented at the time of the research; 41 percent of the investigators, when they did their work, expressed no interest in a clinical problem – their goal was knowledge for the sake of knowledge. These data indicate clearly that planning for future clinical advances must include generous support for innovative and imaginative research that bears no discernible relation to a clinical problem at the time of peer review. Because of many unknown factors (for example, ratio of clinical as compared to non-clinical scientists who

Table 5. *Goal of Authors of 529 Key Articles that Later were Judged to be Essential for a Clinical Advance*

Clinical Advance	Clinically Oriented	Not Clinically Oriented	Total	Percent of Total not Clinically Oriented
Cardiac surgery	53	35	88	39.8
Vascular surgery	40	8	48	16.7
Hypertension	35	44	79	55.7
Coronary insufficiency	44	21	65	32.3
Cardiac resuscitation	24	16	40	40.0
Oral diuretics	19	24	43	55.8
Intensive care	*	*	*	*
Antibiotics	40	13	53	24.5
New diagnostic methods	41	53	94	56.4
Poliomyelitis	16	3	19	15.8
Total	312	217	529	41.0

*A key article is assigned to only one advance even though it may have been essential to more than one. Because practically every key article in intensive care was also essential to other advances, these articles were assigned elsewhere (for example, to cardiac or vascular surgery, coronary insufficiency, resuscitation, or antibiotics).

do not produce key articles to those who do; relative costs of supporting one type of scientist versus the other), we cannot translate "generous support" into a percentage of NIH's budget for extramural programs. Nor can we transfer conclusions from a study of cardiovascular and pulmonary research to other research fields, such as cancer research. But the conclusion seems inescapable that programs to identify and then to provide long-term support for creative individuals or groups (judged more likely than others to produce key research) should be expanded.

Was the Key Research Basic or Not?

Earlier, we avoided using the term basic research. We must now use it and define what we mean by it. We classify research as basic when the investigator, in addition to observing, describing, or measuring, attempts to determine the mechanisms responsible for the observed effects; with our definition, basic research can be on healthy or sick people, on animals, tissues, cells, or subcellular components. Our definition differs from the layman's (and some scientists') concept that research is more and more basic when the unit investigated is smaller and smaller; further, it allows that work on small units, such as cells, need not be basic if it is purely descriptive. It steers clear of whether the research was initiated by the investigator or by a commission, whether it was undirected or directed, whether supported by grant or by contract, because who initiated, directed, or supported the research has nothing to do with whether it is basic.

We analyzed each key article to determine how each investigator carried out his research and put each article in one or more of six categories.

1) Basic research unrelated to the solution of a clinical problem.
2) Basic research related to the solution of a clinical problem.

The clinical relationship was obvious when the investigator studied basic mechanisms of disease in patients; when it was not obvious, we depended on the investigator's statement, no matter how brief, that he initiated his research to gain further insights to the diagnosis, treatment, or prevention of human disease.

Two examples will clarify the difference between categories 1 and 2. When Landsteiner discovered human blood groups in 1900 he was investigating a basic problem in immunology and had no thought of the importance of his discovery to the transfusion of blood; this was clearly basic research unrelated at the time to the solution of a clinical problem (category 1). When Landsteiner, in 1909, found that a nonbacterial material (a virus) caused poliomyelitis in monkeys, this again was basic research but, since it was clearly related to a clinical problem, it fits category 2.

3) Studies not concerned with basic biological, chemical, or physical mechanisms.

These include purely descriptive studies (for example, description of a new disease, such as Stokes–Adams disease, without an investigation of the mechanism); an important observation that initially required no research (inhalation of ether causes anesthesia); a new procedure that required no research (cardiac catheterization); a new operation on humans that first required only perfecting surgical techniques in animals; and clinical tests of a new diuretic, antibiotic, or antihypertensive drug in humans without measurements designed to determine its mechanism of action.

4) Review and critical analysis of published work and synthesis of new concepts (without new experimental data).
5) Developmental work or engineering to create, improve, or perfect apparatus or a technique for research use.
6) Developmental work or engineering to create, improve, or perfect apparatus or a technique for use in diagnosis or care of patients.

The difference between categories 5 and 6 can be clarified by an example. Bayliss and Müller developed a roller-pump in 1929 to solve a problem in basic cardiac physiology; we classify this under category 5 even though later, as the DeBakey pump, it had widespread clinical use. The Drinker respirator (iron lung), developed for clinical use, we classify under category 6.

The results of classifying 529 key articles into these six categories are shown in Table 6. Note that of 567 entires, 209 are in category 1 and 141 in category 2; the total of studies in basic research, either unrelated or related to a clinical problem, was 350, or 61.7 percent of the total number of entries. Other types of clinically oriented studies (some inevitable once the basic research was done)[4] accounted for 21.2 percent of the total; development and engineering (much of it inevitable once the basic research was done)[4] accounted for 15.3 percent; synthesis accounted for less than 2 percent. Basic research therefore was responsible for almost three times as many key articles as other types of research and almost twice as many as non-basic research and development combined.

Table 6. *Types of Research Reported in 529 Key Articles*

Type	Basic: Not Clinically Oriented	Basic: Clinically Oriented	Not Basic	Review and Synthesis	Development: Research	Development: Clinical	Total
Cardiac surgery	34	23	19	0	3	11	90
Vascular surgery	9	7	14	3	0	21	54
Hypertension	42	16	21	2	0	0	81
Coronary insufficiency	21	20	22	1	1	3	68
Cardiac resuscitation	16	11	9	0	0	6	42
Oral diuretics	23	13	6	1	0	0	43
Intensive care	*	*	*	*	*	*	*
Antibiotics	12	18	21	1	0	2	54
New diagnostic methods	49	21	5	2	17	22	116
Poliomyelitis	3	12	3	0	1	0	19
Total	209	141	120	10	22	65	567[†]
Percent of total	36.8	24.9	21.2	1.8	3.9	11.4	—

*Because practically every key article in intensive care was also essential to other advances, these articles were assigned elsewhere (for example, to cardiac or vascular surgery, coronary insufficiency, resuscitation, or antibiotics).

[†]The total number of entries in the six categories (567) exceeds the total in Table 5 (529) by 38 entries. This is because some key articles fit into more than one category here, particularly when articles reporting development of new apparatus also reported research using it; no article in Table 5 was classified more than once.

Objectivity of Our Study

Research on the process of discovery is unusually difficult in that the data come from judgments and decisions and not from physical measurements. Further, no matter how many consultants participate in the judgments and no matter how distinguished each is, to be a consultant each must be an expert in his field of knowledge (we cannot ask clergy, lawyers, or ethicists to determine which were the key advances leading to the prevention of poliomyelitis), and as such, each is likely to have some bias.

In the case of our study, its objectivity is strengthened by the fact that, although the data and conclusions emphasize the importance of nonclinically oriented research and of basic research for clinical advance, only 26 percent of our consultants and only 24 percent of advisers on key articles were basic scientists.[3,5]

In the long run, data and conclusions from any single study should stand, fall, or be modified not by anecdotes or gut reactions, but by confirmation or refutation by better studies with improved design and more objective methods. We believe that a $2 billion industry might well put more of its annual budget into research on improving its main product, which in this case is discovery and its application.

Summary and Conclusions

There has been much expert testimony before congressional committees and much national debate on the relative value of targeted in contrast to nontargeted and of applied in contrast to basic biomedical research. Most of it has been based on anecdotal evidence and little or none on an objective analysis of research in broad fields of medicine and surgery. This is understandable because for-instances are easy to come by, whereas research on research is unusually difficult and time consuming. Because we believe that national biomedical science policy should be based on research on the nature of discovery and its application, we have devoted several years to analyzing how and why lifesaving advances have come about in cardiovascular and pulmonary diseases. The advances that we studied were open-heart surgery, blood vessel surgery, treatment of hypertension, management of coronary artery disease, prevention of poliomyelitis, chemotherapy of tuberculosis and acute rheumatic fever, cardiac resuscitation and cardiac pacemakers, oral diuretics (for treatment of high blood pressure or of congestive heart failure), intensive care units, and new diagnostic methods. We screened more than 4000 scientific articles published in these fields, selected 2500 of these for further consideration, and then analyzed 529 of those that we (and 140 consultants) considered to be essential for the clinical advances.

Our analysis showed the following. (i) Of 529 key articles, 41 percent of all work judged to be essential for later clinical advance was not clinically oriented at the time it was done; the scientists responsible for these key articles sought knowledge for the sake of knowledge. (ii) Of the 529 articles, 61.7 percent described basic research (defined as research to determine mechanisms by which living organisms – including humans – function, or mechanisms by which drugs act); 21.2 percent reported other types of research; 15.3 percent were concerned with development of new apparatus, techniques, operations, or procedures; and 1.8 percent were review articles or reported synthesis of the data of others. Our data show that clinical advance requires different types of research and development and not one to the exclusion of another. Thus the problem is not either-or, but a question of how much support to one type and how much to another. Our data compel us to conclude (i) that a generous portion of the nation's biomedical research dollars should be used to identify and then to provide long-term support for creative scientists whose main goal is to learn how living organisms function, without regard to the immediate relation of their research to specific human diseases, and (ii) that basic research, as we have defined it, pays off in terms of key discoveries almost twice as handsomely as other types of research and development combined.

We believe that much more research needs to be done on the nature of research and its application so that data from objective studies can be applied to all aspects of biomedical research. Because the very nature of research on research, particularly if it is prospective rather than retrospective, requires long periods of time, we recommend that an independent, highly competent group be established with ample, long-term support to conduct and support retrospective and prospective research on the nature of scientific discovery, to analyze the causes of long and short lags between discovery and clinical application and to suggest and test means of decreasing long lags, and to evaluate present and proposed mechanisms for the support of biomedical research and development.

References and Notes

1. C. W. Sherwin and R. S. Isenson, *First Interim Report on Project Hindsight* (Office of Director of Defense Research and Engineering, Washington, D.C., 30 June 1966, revised 13 October 1966).
2. J. A. Shannon, in *Research in the Service of Man: Biomedical Knowledge, Development and Use* (Document 55, U.S. Senate, 90th Congress, 1st session, 1967), pp. 72–85; M. B. Visscher, in *Applied Science and Technological Progress* (National Academy of Sciences Report, Washington,

D.C., 1967), pp. 185–206; *Technology in Retrospect and Critical Events in Science* (National Science Foundation, Washington, D.C., 1968), prepared by Illinois Institute of Technology; K. W. Deutsch, J. Platt, D. Senghass, *Science* **171,** 450 (1971); G. Holton, *Grad. J.* 9, 397 (1973); *Interactions of Science and Technology in the Innovative Process: Some Case Studies* (National Science Foundation Report NSF C667, Washington, D.C., 1973), prepared by Battelle Laboratories; E. H. Kone and H. J. Jordan, Eds., *The Greatest Adventure: Basic Research That Shapes Our Lives* (Rockefeller Univ. Press, New York, 1974).

3. Of these, 70 were clinicians, 37 were basic medical scientists, and 33 were engineers, science administrators (in industry, government, or universities), or science writers.

4. Some consultants did not designate such contributions as key articles. We did, however, because we knew of a number of instances in which the final step was "inevitable" but no one seemed willing to take it (for example, vascular surgery was inevitable by 1910 but was not applied until 1939).

5. Bias could also enter into our selection of reviewers of tables. Thirty-two reviewers were physicians, surgeons, or medical or surgical specialists; 10 were basic medical scientists. All were highly knowledgeable in the field that they reviewed.

6. Supported by contract 1–HO–1–2327 from the National Heart and Lung Institute and grants from the Commonwealth Fund and the Burroughs Wellcome Fund.

Genetics and Human Malleability

W. French Anderson

Just how much can, and should we change human nature. . .by genetic engineering? Our response to that hinges on the answers to three further questions: (1) What *can* we do now? Or more precisely, what *are* we doing now in the area of human genetic engineering? (2) What *will* we be able to do? In other words, what technical advances are we likely to achieve over the next five to ten years? (3) What *should* we do? I will argue that a line can be drawn and should be drawn to use gene transfer only for the treatment of serious disease and not for any other purpose. Gene transfer should never be undertaken in an attempt to enhance or "improve" human beings.

What Can We Do?

In 1980 John Fletcher and I published a paper in the *New England Journal of Medicine* in which we delineated what would be necessary before it would be ethical to carry out human gene therapy.[1] As with any other new therapeutic procedure, the fundamental principle is that it should be determined in advance that the probable benefits outweigh the probable risks. We analyzed the risk–benefit determination for somatic cell gene therapy and proposed three questions that need to have been answered from prior animal expermentation: Can the new gene be inserted stably into the correct target cells? Will the new gene be expressed that is, function) in the cells at an appropriate level? Will the new gene harm the cell or the animal? These criteria are very similar to those required before use of any new therapeutic procedure, surgical operation, or drug. They simply require that the new treatment should get to the area of disease, correct it, and do more good than harm.

A great deal of scientific progress has occurred in the nine years since that paper was published. The technology does now exist for inserting genes into some types of target cells.[2] The procedure being used is called "retroviral-mediated gene transfer." In brief, a disabled murine retrovirus serves as a delivery vehicle for transporting a gene into a population of cells that have been removed from a patient. The gene-engineered cells are then returned to the patient.

The first clinical application of this procedure was approved by the National Institutes of Health and the Food and Drug Administration on January 19, 1989.[3] Our protocol received the most thorough prior review of any clinical protocol in history: It was approved only after being reviewed fifteen times by seven different regulatory bodies. In the end it received unanimous approval from every one of those committees. But the simple fact that the NIH and FDA, as well as the public, felt that the protocol needed such extensive review demonstrates that the concept of gene therapy raises serious concerns.

From *The Hastings Center Report*, 1990, 20, (Jan.–Feb.) pp. 21–24. Reproduced by permission.

We can answer our initial question, What can we do now in the area of human genetic engineering?, by examining this approved clinical protocol. Gene transfer is used to mark cancer-fighting cells in the body as a way of better understanding a new form of cancer therapy. The cancer-fighting cells are called TIL (tumor-infiltrating-lymphocytes), and are isolated from a patient's own tumor, grown up to a large number, and then given back to the patient along with one of the body's immune growth factors, a molecule called interleukin 2 (IL–2). The procedure, developed by Steven Rosenberg of the NIH, is known to help about half the patients treated.[4]

The difficulty is that there is at present no way to study the TIL once they are returned to the patient to determine why they work when they do work (that is, kill cancer cells), and why they do not work when they do not work. The goal of the gene transfer protocol was to put a label on the infused TIL, that is, to mark these cells so that they could be studied in blood and tumor specimens from the patient over time.

The TIL were marked with a vector (called N2) containing a bacterial gene that could be easily identified through recombinant DNA techniques. Our protocol was called, therefore, the N2–TIL Human Gene Transfer Clinical Protocol. The first patient received gene-marked TIL on May 22, 1989. Five patients have now received marked cells. No side effects or problems have thus far arisen from the gene transfer portion of the therapy. Useful data on the fate of the gene-marked TIL are being obtained.

But what was done that was new? Simply, a single gene was inserted into a population of cells that had been obtained from a patient's body. There are an estimated 100,000 genes in every human cell. Therefore the actual addition of material was extremely minute, nothing to correspond to the fears expressed by some that human beings would be "reengineered." Nonetheless, a functioning piece of genetic material was successfully inserted into human cells and the gene-engineered cells did survive in human patients.

What Will We Be Able to Do?

Although only one clinical protocol is presently being conducted, it is clear that there are several applications for gene transfer that probably will be carried out over the next five to ten years. Many genetic diseases that are caused by a defect in a single gene should be treatable, such as ADA deficiency (a severe immune deficiency disease of children), sickle cell anemia, hemophilia, and Gaucher disease. Some types of cancer, viral diseases such as AIDS, and some forms of cardiovascular disease are targets for treatment by gene therapy. In addition, germline gene therapy, that is, the insertion of a gene into the reproductive cells of a patient, will probably be technically possible in the foreseeable future. My position on the ethics of germline gene therapy is published elsewhere.[5]

But successful somatic cell gene therapy also opens the door for enhancement genetic engineering, that is, for supplying a specific characteristic that individuals might want for themselves (somatic cell engineering) or their children (germline engineering) which would not involve the treatment of a disease. The most obvious example at the moment would be the insertion of a growth hormone gene into a normal child in the hope that this would make the child grow larger. Should parents be allowed to choose (if the science should ever make it possible) whatever useful characteristics they wish for their children?

What Should We Do?

A line can and should be drawn between somatic cell gene therapy and enhancement genetic engineering.[6] Our society has repeatedly demonstrated that it can draw a line in biomedical research when necessary. The Belmont Report illustrates how guidelines were formulated to delineate ethical from unethical clinical research and to distinguish clinical research from clinical practice. Our responsibility is to determine how and where to draw lines with respect to genetic engineering.

Somatic cell gene therapy for the treatment of severe disease is considered ethical because it can be supported by the fundamental moral principle of beneficence: It would relieve human suffering. Gene therapy would be, therefore, a moral good. Under what circumstances would human genetic engineering not be a moral good? In the broadest sense, when it detracts from, rather than contributes to, the dignity of man. Whether viewed from a theological perspective or a secular humanist one, the justification for drawing a line is founded on the argument that, beyond the line, human values that our society considers important for the dignity of man would be significantly threatened.

Somatic cell enhancement engineering would threaten important human values in two ways: It could be medically hazardous, in that the risks could exceed the potential benefits and the procedure therefore cause harm. And it would be morally precarious, in that it would require moral decisions our society is not now prepared to make, and it could lead to an increase in inequality and discriminatory practices.

Medicine is a very inexact science. We understand roughly how a simple gene works and that there are many thousands of housekeeping genes, that is, genes that do the job of running a cell. We predict that there are genes which make regulatory messages that are involved in the overall control and regulation of the many housekeeping genes. Yet we have only limited understanding of how a body organ develops into the size and shape it does. We know many things about how the central nervous system works – for example, we are beginning to comprehend how molecules are involved in electric circuits, in memory storage, in transmission of signals. But we are a long way from understanding thought and consciousness. And we are even further from understanding the spiritual side of our existence.

Even though we do not understand how a thinking, loving, interacting organism can be derived from its molecules, we are approaching the time when we can change some of those molecules. Might there be genes that influence the brain's organization or structure or metabolism or circuitry in some way so as to allow abstract thinking, contemplation of good and evil, fear of death, awe of a 'God'? What if in our innocent attempts to improve our genetic make-up we alter one or more of those genes? Could we test for the alteration? Certainly not at present. If we caused a problem that would affect the individual or his or her offspring, could we repair the damage? Certainly not at present. Every parent who has several children knows that some babies accept and give more affection than others, in the same environment. Do genes control this? What if these genes were accidentally altered? How would we even know if such a gene were altered?

My concern is that, at this point in the development of our culture's scientific expertise, we might be like the young boy who loves to take things apart. He is bright enough to disassemble a watch, and maybe even bright enough to get it back together again so that it works. But what if he tries to "improve" it? Maybe put on bigger hands so that the time can be read more easily. But if the hands are too heavy for the mechanism, the watch will run slowly, erratically, or not at all. The boy can understand what is visible, but he cannot comprehend the precise engineering calculations that determined exactly how strong each spring should be, why the gears interact in the ways that they do, etc. Attempts on his part to improve the watch will probably only harm it. We are now able to provide a new gene so that a property involved in a human life would be changed, for example, a growth hormone gene. If we were to do so simply because we could, I fear we would be like that young boy who changed the watch's hands. We, too, do not really understand what makes the object we are tinkering with tick.

In summary, it could be harmful to insert a gene into humans. In somatic cell gene therapy for an already existing disease the potential benefits could outweigh the risks. In enhancement engineering, however, the risk would be greater while the benefits would be considerably less clear.

Yet even aside from the medical risks, somatic cell enhancement engineering should not be performed because it would be morally precarious. Let us assume that there were no medical risks at all from somatic cell enhancement engineering. There would still be reasons for objecting to this procedure. To illustrate, let us consider some examples. What if a human gene were cloned that could produce a brain chemical resulting in markedly increased memory capacity in monkeys after gene transfer? Should a person be allowed to receive such a gene on request? Should a pubescent adolescent whose parents are both five feet tall be provided with a growth hormone gene on request? Should a worker who is continually exposed to an industrial toxin receive a gene to give him resistance on his, or his employer's request?

These scenarios suggest three problems that would be difficult to resolve: What genes should be provided; who should receive a gene; and, how to prevent discrimination against individuals who do or do not receive a gene.

We allow that it would be ethically appropriate to use somatic cell gene therapy for treatment of serious disease. But what distinguishes a serious disease from a "minor" disease from cultural "discomfort"? What is suffering? What is significant suffering? Does the absence of growth hormone that results in a growth limitation to two feet in height represent a genetic disease? What about a limitation to a height of four feet, to five feet? Each observer might draw the lines between serious disease, minor disease, and genetic variation differently. But all can agree that there are extreme cases that produce significant suffering and premature death. Here then is where an initial line should be drawn for determining what genes should be provided: treatment of serious disease.

If the position is established that only patients suffering from serious diseases are candidates for gene insertion, then the issues of patient selection are no different than in other medical situations: the determination is based on medical need within a supply and demand framework. But if the use of gene transfer extends to allow a normal individual to acquire, for example, a memory-enhancing gene, profound problems would result. On what basis is the decision made to allow one individual to receive the gene but not another: Should it go to those best able to benefit society (the smartest already?) To those most in need (those with low intelligence? But how low? Will enhancing memory help a mentally retarded child?)? To those chosen by a lottery? To those who can afford to pay? As long as our society lacks a significant consensus about these answers, the best way to make equitable decisions in this case should be to base them on the seriousness of the objective medical need, rather than on the personal wishes or resources of an individual.

Discrimination can occur in many forms. If individuals are carriers of a disease (for example, sickle cell anemia), would they be pressured to be treated? Would they have difficulty in obtaining health insurance unless they agreed to be treated? These are ethical issues raised also by genetic screening and by the Human Genome project. But the concerns would become even more trouble-some if there were the possibility for "correction" by the use of human genetic engineering.

Finally, we must face the issue of eugenics, the attempt to make hereditary "improvements." The abuse of power that societies have historically demonstrated in the pursuit of eugenic goals is well documented.[7] Might we slide into a new age of eugenic thinking by starting with small "improvements"? It would be difficult, if not impossible, to determine where to draw a line once enhancement engineering had begun. Therefore, gene transfer should be used only for the treatment of serious disease and not for putative improvements.

Our society is comfortable with the use of genetic engineering to treat individuals with serious disease. On medical and ethical grounds we should draw a line excluding any form of enhancement engineering. We should not step over the line that delineates treatment from enhancement.

References

1. W. French Anderson and John C. Fletcher, "Gene Therapy in Human Beings: When Is It Ethical to Begin?," *New England Journal of Medicine* 303:22 (1980), 1293–97.
2. See also W. French Anderson, "Prospects for Human Gene Therapy," *Science*, 26 October 1984. 401–409; T. Friedman, "Progress towards Human Gene Therapy," *Science*, 16 June 1989, 1275–81.
3. J. Wyngaarden, "Human Gene Transfer Protocol," *Federal Register* (1989), vol. 54, no. 47, pp. 10508–10510.
4. Steven A. Rosenberg *et al.*, "Use of Tumor-Infiltrating Lymphocytes and Interleukin–2 in the Immunotherapy of Patients with Metastatic Melanoma," *New England Journal of Medicine* 319:25 (1988), 1676–80.
5. W. French Anderson, "Human Gene Therapy: Scientific and Ethical Considerations," *Journal of Medicine and Philosophy* 10 (1985):275–91.
6. W. French Anderson, "Human Gene Therapy: Why Draw a Line?," *Journal of Medicine and Philosophy* 14 (1989), 68–93.
7. See, for example, Kenneth M. Ludmerer, *Genetics and American Society* (Baltimore, MD: The Johns Hopkins University Press, 1972), and Daniel J. Kevles, *In the Name of Eugenics* (New York: Alfred A. Knopf, 1985).

Questions for Discussion

1. As a scientist, do you feel that you have a responsibility to covenant with society? If so, in what areas of your work does this covenant apply (choice of research topic, how you do your science, how you relate to the public)? How do you plan to carry out your personal commitment to society?

2. What responsibility (if any) do scientific investigators have to ensure that the public understands their work? In what ways is science education beneficial to society and scientists alike? What are the consequences of scientific illiteracy?

3. If you recognize that the results of your research pose risks to the public welfare, what responsibilities do you have to work with relevant organizations and institutions in society to prevent or resolve potential problems?

4. In choosing questions for research, do you consider whether specific work has potential for application outside the laboratory or is more fundamental? If so, how does this information affect your choices and actions?

Recommended Supplemental Reading

Chalk R, ed. *Science, Technology, and Society*. Washington, DC: American Association for the Advancement of Science; 1988.

de Cerreño ALC, Keynan A (eds.). Scientific cooperation, state conflict: The roles of scientists in mitigating international discord. *Ann NY Acad Sci.* 1999;866:1–281

Miller DK. Scientific societies and public responsibilities. *Ann NY Acad Med.* 1971;196:247–255.

Nelkin D. *Selling Science: How the Press Covers Science and Technology*, 2d ed. New York: W.H. Freeman & Co.; 1995.

Cases for Discussion

Using Cases in the Study of Ethics

Elizabeth Heitman

Analysis and discussion of cases are essential in the study of ethics. Ethics courses in many professional programs, particularly in the health sciences, use the case method to illustrate the scope of ethical issues in the field and to teach a structured system for ethical decision making in practice. The case method is based on the formal examination of realistic scenarios that students might encounter in their own work. Scenarios must be general enough for students to analyze from their own knowledge, experience, and imagination but also detailed enough to provide meaningful ethical choices.

Case discussion is best accomplished in a small group setting in which everyone has an opportunity to participate. It is often beneficial for the instructor to read the case aloud rather than relying on students to read it individually. Hearing the story as a group rather than reading it silently helps students to engage each other and the instructor and moves the group more smoothly into discussion. Reading the case aloud also reduces the likelihood that individual readers will accidentally skip parts of the text.

The goals of case discussion are to determine an ethical resolution to the problem(s) raised in the case and to define one or more courses of action for achieving that resolution. Although discussion can be quite creative, analysis of the case should be systematic – much like the study and analysis of a scientific problem. Using a formal, stepwise procedure can be particularly helpful for students and others just beginning to use the case method, and following a structured protocol can ensure that the relevant practical information and ethical considerations are identified and addressed. The fundamental steps in case analysis are outlined below.

Step 1: *Recognize and identify the ethical issues and specific ethical problems in the case.*

The first step in any discussion is for the group to *identify the ethical questions* that the case raises. The recognition of ethical issues requires some familiarity with the ethical norms of the field and an ability to articulate them, and the phrasing of questions may reflect important assumptions and biases that need to be discussed as part of the later analysis. Often, however, ethical issues evoke emotional responses – particularly anger, frustration, and indignation that something "isn't right." It is the instructor's responsibility to help the group learn to translate these reactions into more objective observations and logical reasoning as they formulate statements of the ethical issues.

The instructor may choose to expand some questions or break others into simpler components, or encourage students to do so. Initially questions should be identified *without* attempting to answer or analyze them until several have been spelled out. The questions can be written on a blackboard, or a student can serve as recorder for the group. The instructor may ask the group to prioritize the individual issues or group them by levels of importance before proceeding to the step of fact finding.

Step 2: *Identify key facts, establish important definitions, and gather other necessary information.*

As in research, it is essential to get the facts of a case before attempting to evaluate it. Gathering information and clarifying the meaning of events can resolve many ethical conflicts. As part of the discussion, students should try to identify what information is and is not available and how needed information can be gained. Some important factual issues to consider include:

- Who are the main parties in the case? What are their respective roles and relationships, and how do these affect their actions and responsibilities?
- What are the relevant scientific, social, and financial facts of the matter? Which facts (if any) are in dispute? What information is missing?
- How do the relevant parties interpret the facts of the case? Do they understand central concepts and their respective roles in the same way? Why do they believe the problem exists?
- When did events important to the situation occur, what events are likely in the near future, and when does a decision need to be made to address the identified problems?

The instructor may opt to discuss each of these points before examining the specific ethical issues identified in step 1 or may begin with the ethical issues, addressing the factual questions that pertain to each in turn. Later in the discussion, it can be instructive to consider how changing certain facts or circumstances can alter both the analysis and the recommended course of action. Additionally, uncertainty about some issues is almost always a part of ethical decision making, and case discussion offers the opportunity for students to practice making decisions without complete knowledge of the context or details of a problematic situation.

Step 3: *Identify professional ethical principles, standards of practice, and law relevant to the ethical issues of the case.*

In identifying the ethical issues that the case raises, even beginning students can often draw on known or presumed standards of practice and formal statements of ethical principles. A number of scientific organizations have published formal codes of ethics and statements on specific ethical issues in the past decade, and case discussion provides an opportunity to consider the application of these statements in practice. Cases also help students to examine the practical meaning of more general ethical standards, such as "research must serve the public interest."

Because scientists are trained to look for concrete answers, students may be frustrated to discover that applying formal codes and policy statements seldom provides satisfactorily comprehensive answers to a case's practical questions. Similarly, some cases may raise legal issues that cannot be answered definitively, especially in new areas of research for which adequate law has not yet been developed. In such situations, both ethical guidelines and the law should be used as references for constructing a plan of action that conforms to broader ethical principles. Discussion should also consider how specific standards relate to other important norms and values, whether there is any hierarchy among them, and why.

At times, authoritative ethical guidelines, and even laws, may appear to conflict, and mutually exclusive actions may seem to be mandated by equally persuasive ethical arguments. Such a situation is known as a *dilemma*. By definition, a dilemma cannot be resolved by analytic methods – some ethical value must always be compromised. True ethical dilemmas are not common in scientific research. However, many ethical issues pose dilemmas for social policy. As in the case of laboratory research with animals, what might appear to be a straightforward ethical decision for a single researcher can become a significant debate when addressed by members of a multicultural society who adhere to a wide array of competing values. Because the focus of the case method is practical ethical decision making, it is important to address the specific ethical questions of the case before moving to discuss its implications for social policy.

Step 4: *Identify the possible alternative courses of action, the ethical arguments for and against their implementation, and their likely outcomes.*

Once the ethical issues are identified and the facts of the case are known, the discussion should identify the courses of action that are both reasonable and possible under the circumstances. In establishing a best-case scenario and the steps most likely to achieve it, students can consider their ethical goals and the most important standards of professional behavior to follow in achieving them. In real life, it may not be possible to achieve the ideal resolution to an ethical problem, or a solution may be possible only with significant sacrifice. Thus, other acceptable middle ground scenarios and how to achieve them should be explored as well. Because action based on even the most careful ethical analysis may have a disastrous outcome if essential information is not available or unforeseeable circumstances arise, it may be instructive to identify a worst-case scenario and consider how to prevent it. For each situation, students should explore the ethical rationale for their suggested actions, project the likely effects of their actions, and consider how the unintended consequences of seemingly ethical behavior might raise new problems.

Step 5: *Choose the course that is best supported by the preceding analysis.*

Ethical analysis in professional life leads to decision and action. Although ethical decision making in the protected environment of the classroom does not require the moral courage needed to act on one's convictions, the ability to take a considered position is a skill that can be improved through regular case discussion. Each participant should be encouraged to select a preferred course of action and articulate why it is the best option.

In many situations, the choice among a number of alternatives will be unanimous. However, minority opinions should be respected, both as a matter of procedure and as a cornerstone of professional collegiality. In practice researchers may feel compelled to compromise their own judgment when they are in the minority – especially in the face of institutional definitions of ethical standards and regulatory compliance. While scientists are not subject to the threats of legal liability that affect other professions, researchers are increasingly held accountable for their individual actions apart from institutional responses. Ultimately, researchers' professional integrity depends not only on their adherence to standards of good science but also on their actions being consistent with their personal ethical commitments.

Step 6: *Evaluate the actions taken and their subsequent outcome.*

Just as even the most elegant scientific hypothesis must be tested experimentally, the value of any ethical analysis is determined by evaluating its outcomes. Whenever possible, it is important to examine the events that occur after the implementation of a considered ethical judgment. By evaluating the outcomes of ethical decision making, it may be possible to see how certain actions lead to specific results, while other variables are shown to have unexpected influence. Deliberate reflection on causes and effects increases the likely reproducibility of desired outcomes in ethics just as in science. Cases from the history of science, or cases drawn from events in the professional life of instructors, are thus often more valuable for comprehensive discussion than published case studies precisely because their outcome is known and can be evaluated in the light of the students' analysis and recommendations. Where it is not possible to know the outcome of a case, whether because it is fictional or ongoing, the reasoned projection of likely consequences becomes more important.

Sources of Case Studies

Case studies in research ethics are now available in a variety of publications (1) and many professional journals include news stories and case presentations that can be used in ethics education. Resources are also available to help faculty frame events in their own work as cases (2). As noted earlier, faculty members' cases are particularly valuable teaching tools because the instructor's personal knowledge of the context and details of the case can give depth to the discussion. Whenever a real case is used for teaching purposes, however, the presenter must be careful to change the names of key figures and any identifying details that would compromise the confidentiality of the persons involved.

The cases included here are intended to illustrate different aspects of each chapter's main topic and were written specifically for use with the accompanying readings. These cases are fictional, although most are based on events from the editors' professional careers. Due to the logistical difficulty of providing information on the outcome of these cases without unduly influencing their discussion, the narrative of each case stops at the point at which a decision and action are required. Course instructors are welcome to modify these cases to adapt them to the specific needs of their students.

References

1. Schrag B, ed. *Research Ethics: Cases and Commentaries.* Vol. I–IV (revised). Bloomington, IN: GREE; 2000.
2. Naumes W, Naumes MJ. *The Art and Craft of Case Writing.* Thousand Oaks, CA: Sage Publications; 1999.

The Roots of Honor and Integrity in Science

Case 1

For several years, the Student Governance Association (SGA) of Midstates University has debated drafting an honor code for all academic work. The need for an honor code had been discussed for almost a decade, but the effort to draft a code gained renewed momentum following a well-publicized episode of organized cheating in the introductory biochemistry class. Still, nothing has actually been written in the 3 years since the cheating scandal.

The Pasteur Society, an honor society of students in the life sciences, has always been a strong advocate for a university-wide honor code. Its members have been frustrated with the SGA's ongoing debate and decide to compose their own code of ethics for students in sciences. They hope that a multidisciplinary code of ethics for science students can serve as a basis for a university honor code, but they also want the document to speak primarily to the needs and values of students in scientific research.

How should the Pasteur Society proceed with its plan to draft a code of ethics for multi-disciplinary science students, and what values and issues should the code address?

Case 2

For several years, the Student Governance Association (SGA) of Midstates University has debated drafting an honor code for all academic work. The need for an honor code had been discussed for almost a decade, but the effort to draft a code gained renewed momentum following a well-publicized episode of organized cheating in the introductory biochemistry class. Still, nothing has actually been written in the 3 years since the cheating scandal.

The faculty of the Division of Natural Sciences quickly grew impatient with the SGA's debate. Last semester the dean appointed a faculty committee to prepare a set of comprehensive rules for academic honesty in all divisional courses. The committee's first draft meets with general faculty approval and is sent back to the committee for only minor revisions.

Professor Spindler is concerned that, while the rules are straightforward, they do not convey the professional and collegial tone essential to fostering ethical behavior among scientists. She challenges her colleagues to draft an accompanying statement of values in science to provide a foundation for the new procedural rules. Among the issues that she insists must be addressed are the nature of the student–teacher relationship in science and how science faculty should convey the ethical standards of their related disciplines to students. The dean appoints Professor Spindler to chair a committee to draft such a document for release with the new rules on academic honesty.

What should such a statement of professional and ethical values include, and how should it distinguish the ethics of teaching in science from the ethics of research in general?

The Responsible Conduct of Research

Case 1

Dr. Lowery is the director of an advanced tumor biology class with several instructors. For the final exam, Dr. Lowery gave a 48-hour, open-book, take-home test with one question from each instructor. She told the students that they could make use of any nonhuman resource in answering the questions but that they *must not* collaborate or receive help from anyone in or outside of the course.

Each instructor graded the answers to his or her question. Dr. Jarvis reported to Dr. Lowery that two students, Mason and Gwen, had turned in answers to his question that were suspiciously similar, including two full sentences that were identical. Dr. Lowery reviewed the answers and agreed that there were indeed significant reasons to suspect that Mason and Gwen had collaborated. She also noted that they had both done very well in the course and would earn A's with good performances on the final exam.

Dr. Lowery called Dr. Jarvis, Gwen, and Mason to her office to discuss the situation. She showed the two students their answers, with the identical passages highlighted, and asked them to explain how the similarities could have occurred. After some hesitation, Gwen stated that she and Mason had *not* collaborated. Rather, she explained, they had both copied the identical passages from the same reference in the *Journal of Biological Chemistry*. Mason supported her statement. Both Gwen and Mason said they felt that there was nothing wrong in copying the passages from the journal because the test had been open book.

After several minutes of discussion about the concept of plagiarism and the need to cite quoted material even in an exam, Mason admitted that Gwen had told him about the journal article. When asked to explain why they had talked about the exam after explicitly being told not to, the students replied that the examination question "was very hard."

How should the students' actions be judged?

Case 2

Near the end of the academic year, the Awards Committee at Urban University Graduate School of the Health Sciences meets to consider the nominees for merit-based scholarships for the coming year. Each committee member agrees to take several student portfolios to review for discussion at a meeting the next week. Committee member Dr. Porter, an associate professor in statistics, reviews her assigned portfolios immediately so that she can return to preparing a talk on the role of statisticians in the detection of research fraud. Her top choice is Philip Abbott, a psychologist who has taken a leave of absence from his position at the state's main university to pursue a master's degree in epidemiology. His academic performance has been uniformly excellent, and he has received nominations for a scholarship from several faculty members.

After finishing her review of the scholarship candidates, Dr. Porter logs on to the Web site of the Office of Research Integrity to see whether it offers any information about statisticians and misconduct. She downloads several years' worth of the ORI newsletter, looking for stories that she might use as examples. Unexpectedly, she comes across the headline "Abbott Fired for 4 Counts of Misconduct" and is shocked to read that 2 years earlier Dr. Philip Abbott had been investigated on charges of falsifying research data and had been fired from his university job. His lawsuit challenging the charges and his firing is still pending.

Dr. Porter is uncertain what to do with this information. It appears from his portfolio that Dr. Abbott is a model student. Still, she knows that the literature on academic misconduct suggests that seemingly excellent students may cheat to maintain their outstanding academic records. As a member of the school's Admissions Committee, Dr. Porter is certain that Dr. Abbott's application for the epidemiology master's program did not tell the whole story about his work history. However, she wonders whether his recent success is a sign that he has been rehabilitated.

How should Dr. Porter respond to her discovery that Dr. Abbott has been found guilty of research misconduct at another institution?

The Ethics of Authorship and Publication

Case 1

Dr. Warren is the editor of *Biomedical Methodologies*, an 8-year old quarterly journal with an international readership and pool of authors. Dr. Warren has just sent an issue's final proofs to press when he receives an e-mail from Dr. Hannah, one of the issue's authors. Dr. Hannah is a rising star in her field. Her paper compares three variations on a particular research method as used in the United States and two European centers. Dr. Hannah collected her European data from the published literature while working as a visiting fellow in two prominent research institutes. In both settings she worked with little supervision or collaboration, but she established good personal relationships with the other researchers there.

Dr. Hannah wants to make a late correction to her article, adding four more authors. A few weeks before she had enthusiastically sent copies of her author's proofs to the directors of the two European labs where she had worked. That morning, however, Dr. Hannah received a stern letter from the director of the second facility informing her that sharing authorship credit was the norm in his country. Dr. Hannah now fears that she erred seriously in not listing both center directors and her two office mates as authors despite their having had almost no role in designing the project and none in writing the paper. She is worried that any future European collaboration depends on adding their names to the paper.

The journal's policy is that authors take responsibility for assigning authorship, yet Dr. Hannah acknowledges that her attribution will be false. She has also cited the paper elsewhere as hers alone – "forthcoming" in the journal. Practically, the entire article will have to be reset to add four names and their affiliations, adding potentially significant expense and delay to its publication.

Should Dr. Warren add the additional names to the title page?

Case 2

Members of the Grand Old State University (GOSU) Biology Department had recently submitted a large, complex program project grant to the National Institutes of Science, and Professor Kane, chair of the Biology Department at Competitive State University (CSU), was part of the site visit team. Professor Kane was impressed by the department's research in support of the grant application. GOSU researchers reported that one particularly exciting patch clamp study using frog skin had recently been accepted for publication in the *American Journal of Biology*. It demonstrated a new single-channel protein that actively transported a specific molecule that had been found polluting the water in local streams. This transport proved toxic to the skin cells. The article speculated that this newly discovered channel might be involved with the recent death of frogs in the region.

When Professor Kane returned to CSU, he mentioned this work and the forthcoming article to Dr. Tristan and his graduate student Yazmin, who were working on a similar patch clamp system. That afternoon, Dr. Tristan asked Yazmin to see if she could repeat the results that Professor Kane had described. Knowing the details of the work at GOSU, Yazmin had no trouble repeating the experiment, and she wrote it up for Dr. Tristan. The next Monday Yazmin was dismayed when Dr. Tristan showed her a Brief Report that he had written using her patch clamp data. He intended to submit it to the *Aquatic Pathobiology Journal* with both of them as authors. The *Aquatic Pathobiology Journal* was edited by one of

Dr. Tristan's friends and typically had a short turnaround time before publication. Dr. Tristan expressed confidence that they could beat the GOSU team's study into print.

When Yazmin had initially repeated the GOSU patch clamp experiment, she had had no intention to use the data for publication. Yet now she was reluctant to confront her PI about his unauthorized knowledge of the GOSU study and was somewhat eager to get her name on this easy paper directly related to her own research.

How should Yazmin respond to Dr. Tristan's plans for publication?

Research with Human Beings

Case 1

Dr. Moss, a parasitologist, Dr. Pushkin, a pharmacologist, and Dr. Inez, an internist specializing in infectious diseases are collaborating on a prophylactic drug against infection with *Giardia*, a water-borne organism that causes gastrointestinal distress and diarrhea in humans. *Giardia* is a significant public health problem in many countries without adequate water treatment facilities. In the United States it commonly affects children in day-care centers and their families as well as campers and hikers who drink water from mountain streams. Treatment is available for *Giardia* infection, but it too can cause intestinal distress in some people; for a small portion of the population this medication can have more severe side effects with nausea and vomiting. The researchers hope to produce a drug for short-term use that could be taken once a day beginning 24 hours before possible exposure.

The team has completed the Phase I test establishing the maximum tolerated (toxic) dose of their drug and is ready to begin Phase II testing for effectiveness. They plan to have a multiarm, randomized controlled trial to determine the most effective dosage and schedule. Subjects would be given either the drug or the placebo followed 24 hours later by water either seeded with *Giardia* or not.

The team is eager to test the drug in a group similar to the U.S. population at greatest risk for infection. They hope to recruit normal adult volunteers. How should their need for subjects be advertised, and to whom? What should the study's informed consent document say about the project?

Case 2

Dr. Pham is a geneticist researching genetic factors in heart disease together with Dr. Jacob, a cardiologist who treats a large number of patients with a family history of heart disease. Many of Dr. Jacob's patients have served as research subjects for Dr. Pham's work, providing not only family history and extensive interview information but also tissue samples for genetic screening.

Dr. Pham's team is very close to identifying what they believe is an important genetic marker for early-onset heart disease. They are planning a large-scale research project in which patients with a family history of heart disease would complete a comprehensive health survey and then be screened for the potential genetic marker. When the individual patient has completed the survey and screening, as many of his or her family members as can be recruited will also be given the survey and screening.

In drafting the informed consent documents for the research protocol, Drs. Pham and Jacob consider the many possible demands that they might receive for information stemming from this project. If the genetic marker turns out to be important, many people may want to know about their genetic makeup and future risk. Although all personal identifiers will be coded for the study, the research data will reveal which participants have the marker and which do not. Dr. Jacob would like to know his patients' genetic status as early as possible to provide the most appropriate preventive care for them individually. But Dr. Pham is concerned that they won't really know the meaning of the genetic marker for several years, and he is hesitant to reveal it to anyone. Changing governmental regulations about the disclosure of genetic research data make him even more cautious.

Drs. Pham and Jacob want to resolve as many of these issues as possible before the actual research begins and to ensure that patients and their family members truly understand the nature of the study before they agree to take part in it. How can they minimize the negative social impact of the information they discover while maximizing its scientific and clinical value?

Ethics in Epidemiologic Research

Case 1

South Central University (SCU) Health Science Center has a growing interdisciplinary research program involving its medical school, graduate school, school of public health, and three teaching hospitals. Collaboration among clinicians, laboratory scientists, and epidemiologists has resulted in the identification of previously unknown biological markers for skin cancer, gall bladder disease, and cataracts. Other collaborative projects have characterized previously unrecognized populations at high risk for specific adverse events in surgery and postoperative intensive care.

SCU's vice president for research is enthusiastic about the epidemiologic work behind these recent successes. He has proposed creating a comprehensive clinical database that would make vital information available to university researchers. The database would include medical records data and data from pathologic and genetic analysis of blood and tissue obtained from patients in the course of clinical care. As part of the project, tissue samples would also be banked for future study.

SCU's IRB has expressed concern that this use of patient data and tissue will require revision of its informed consent policies for epidemiologic research. Several researchers have expressed frustration that the informed consent requirements for clinical research unnecessarily complicate epidemiologic studies involving no additional intervention or risk of physical or psychosocial harm.

The vice president for research proposes adding a disclosure statement about the University's research activities to the general consent form for treatment that patients sign upon admission to the hospital. Thus, patients would be informed that their medical records might be reviewed by researchers in the same way that they might be by their insurance company or quality assurance analysts. Likewise, just as the surgical consent form includes the patient's authorization for the hospital to use tissue obtained from surgical procedures, the general consent form could include the patient's authorization for banking and genetic analysis of other tissue.

By making consent to epidemiologic research part of the standard admissions procedure, both patients and researchers would be spared the bother and bureaucratic delay of executing multiple consent forms. And because the IRB would still review every study, patients would be protected from any negative ethical consequences of specific research projects.

How should the university's hospitals and IRB respond to this proposal?

Case 2

Dr. Boynton is an epidemiologist with the state's birth defects registry who has been tracking the rate of extremely premature delivery (less than 28 weeks' gestation) for more than a decade. Dr. Moore, a senior pathologist at Augustus Medical University (AMU), has a substantial record of research on placental malformation and premature birth. Together they are planning a prospective study of the relationship between premature delivery and the presence of cocaine, methamphetamine, marijuana, nicotine, and alcohol in the placenta.

Initially Dr. Moore will screen samples of placental tissue from all births under 28 weeks' gestation that occur in the 10 hospitals that account for 65% of the state's extremely premature deliveries. Samples will be tested for the presence of the drugs of interest and their metabolites. Dr. Boynton will use birth certificate registry data to code the samples according to the age, race, parity, and residential zip code of the mother and the gestational age of the fetus at delivery. After coding, no personal identifiers will be linked with the data.

This project is being funded by the governor's campaign against drug abuse. It is intended to serve as the first step in a larger project to reduce the incidence of severe prematurity by reducing the use of illicit drugs, alcohol, and tobacco by pregnant women.

The project will require review by the IRBs at AMU and the state health department as well as the approval of the individual hospitals' research committees. Because the project relies exclusively on placental tissue samples and standard birth registry data, the researchers do not plan to inform the individual pregnant women about the study either before or after they deliver. How should the IRB respond to the proposed study?

The Humane Care and Use of Animals in Research

Case 1

Dr. Katz is the director of the animal facilities for an academic medical center in a large city. Dr. Katz is recognized nationally for promoting strict standards for the humane use of animals in research. His policies have also reduced the number of animals needed for individual studies and improved the validity and applicability of those studies. Dr. Katz's careful management has kept his institution's animal facilities well run and the animals well cared for.

One of Dr. Katz's few critics is a member of city council. Councilwoman Nates insists that the city's policy of selling pound animals for research victimizes family pets and the people who love them. She has made a formal proposal to abolish the practice.

Under a contract with the city, Dr. Katz gets roughly 20 dogs a year from the city pound. He selects healthy animals from those that are scheduled to be euthanized (via the gas chamber), and the university pays the city a small processing fee to cover the cost of the animal's housing at the pound. Some pound dogs are used for training in recovery surgery and others in longer-term physiology studies. About half of the dogs are adopted when the study ends. The rest are euthanized by anesthesia overdose. Pound animals cost less than purpose-bred animals, but Dr. Katz believes that using pound animals in research saves animal life as well. Dogs picked up by the city are euthanized if their owners do not claim them within 5 days.

Are Dr. Katz's animal procurement practices ethically sound? How should the city council respond to Councilwoman Nates' proposition?

Case 2

James is a second-year doctoral student working in Dr. Olden's lab at Underfunded Private University (UPU). During a poster session at a professional meeting, he strikes up a conversation with a postdoc from Progressive Medical University (PMU) about their experience with a particular rat model. James is surprised to hear that the postdoc is concerned about preventing discomfort for the rats during a procedure that James had always been told was painless. The postdoc seems equally surprised when James talks about his use of a procedure that is prohibited at CMU because of the distress it causes the animals.

After several minutes of discussion, James confesses that he is sometimes uncomfortable working with rats. Although he learned some of his rat technique from Dr. Olden at the beginning of his program, he has had to teach himself several procedures as his research has progressed. Because no one he knows uses these procedures, James hasn't had anyone at UPU to ask for help. Dr. Olden has repeatedly reassured him that his techniques are satisfactory and that much of his growth as a scientist will come from figuring out how to do things himself. Still, James has been distressed at the number of rats he has used trying to get his methods right and the time and money his self-training has cost the lab.

The postdoc expresses sympathy for James's situation but insists that James needs to find someone to help him get his methods up to standard if he wants his project to work. He maintains that if Dr. Olden won't ensure that his students have appropriate skills in animal research for the projects they undertake, it is up to James to see that he gets the proper training elsewhere.

How should James respond (both short-term and long-term) to the postdoc's implication that his animal research techniques are inadequate?

Management of and Access to Scientific Data

Case 1

Joseph is a second-year doctoral student in microbiology who entered the program with a master's degree from his native country. He works in a large lab with several other students, fellows, and technicians. Their PI travels frequently, and Carol, a senior technician, is in charge of almost all of the lab's day-to-day activities.

Joseph originally expected a close working relationship with his new adviser, and was disappointed that they seldom saw each other. He was also surprised that Carol wanted to review his work every week. She routinely examined his notebooks and questioned his methods, results, analysis, and plans for future experiments. Carol seldom gave feedback other than short critical notes like "this can't be right." After several weeks, Joseph asked Carol whether she was unhappy with his work. Carol replied that she was not dissatisfied but rather that she was responsible for the students when the PI was away. She found that reviewing students' lab notebooks was the best way to measure their progress. None of the other students complained, but Joseph resented having his worked checked by a technician, and her supervision felt like an invasion of his privacy.

One afternoon, in the middle of a complex experiment, Joseph had an idea for a new procedure that he outlined in a mix of his native language and English. Later that week, when Carol reviewed his notebook, she said nothing about the strange notation. Joseph recognized that he could maintain some privacy by taking notes in his native language.

Now at the end of the year, Joseph keeps roughly half of his records in his native language with enough basic documentation in English to satisfy Carol that he is making progress.

Are Joseph's record-keeping methods acceptable?

Case 2

Darlene is an advanced graduate student at State Land-grant University. She is about to finish her dissertation on the cloning of a gene and the biological actions of the protein it produces. A manuscript describing her results has already been accepted for publication in a competitive journal. When Darlene started graduate work at State, she had elected to work with Dr. Goforth because his laboratory was well supported by NIH funds, he had an impressive publications record, and he had supervised several Ph.D. students who had gone on to good academic positions. Darlene has always gotten along well with Dr. Goforth and is sorry to be leaving his lab.

Darlene has been offered a postdoctoral fellowship at another university. Her future mentor has requested that she bring samples of various biological reagents that she had produced during her doctoral training so that they could continue to develop her research in this area. However, when Darlene asked Dr. Goforth about how best to take the samples with her, Dr. Goforth not only refused to let her have samples but also told Darlene that she had to leave her computerized database and laboratory notebooks at State as well. Darlene was so stunned by this response that she couldn't even think to ask why.

How can Darlene ethically retain access to dissertation research data and the biological tools that have been the foundation of her work? How should she respond to Dr. Goforth's refusal to let her take essential data and materials with her?

The Work of the Academic Scientist

Case 1

Sean is a fourth-year graduate student in Dr. Murray's research group who is purifying a newly discovered enzyme from beef heart. Both he and Dr. Murray think this enzyme should be important to the metabolic integrity of the heart.

Dr. Murray encourages her students to communicate openly with other researchers and to present their work at meetings whenever possible. When Sean presented his dissertation work in a 10-minute talk at a regional meeting, he received good comments from several members of the audience. One listener, Dr. Frank, invited Sean to dinner that night to talk about their common research interests. Over dinner Dr. Frank asked Sean many questions about his work with Dr. Murray. True to Dr. Murray's philosophy, Sean talked openly with Dr. Frank. When dinner was over, Sean told Dr. Frank that he had enjoyed their conversation and looked forward to an ongoing professional exchange.

Three months later, Sean learned that Dr. Frank had published a paper in *Online Biological Notes* about a very similar enzyme from sheep lung. Although the purification reported by Dr. Frank was less extensive than the one that Sean had accomplished, Dr. Frank's paper reported some kinetic properties of the sheep lung enzyme that were to have been a major part of Sean's dissertation.

Sean is devastated and afraid that his dissertation research has been wasted. How should Sean proceed with his dissertation? What should Sean tell Dr. Murray about Dr. Frank's article?

Case 2

Marie and Leon are second-year graduate students working under Dr. Ortega, a prominent scientist whose research team includes several trainees at various points in their studies. The lab has a very collegial atmosphere that Marie and Leon enjoy. They typically have worked under the supervision of Charles, a postdoctoral fellow who will take a tenure-track position at another university at the end of the year.

One morning, the newspaper carries a front-page story that a researcher from the university's medical school is under investigation for scientific misconduct. No one in the lab can talk about anything else as they try to figure out from the article what could have happened. Charles, Marie, and Leon identify a number of errors in the reporter's discussion of the basic science behind the case. Charles is adamant that researchers need to support each other and science itself against uneducated lay critics, and he is eager to dispute the article. Together the three draft a letter to the editor of the newspaper pointing out the problems with the original story and disagreeing with the reporter's conclusions about the medical school researcher's actions.

Before mailing the letter, they take it to show Dr. Ortega. Surprisingly, Dr. Ortega is very critical of the letter and their desire to respond to the newspaper article. "You're right that the article is very misleading, but I can't let you submit this," says Dr. Ortega. "Everything that is sent out of this lab for publication reflects on me, this department, and this university. We can't get involved in this mess or it will look as if we know something about the guy's work. We don't really know what he was doing, and I don't even understand that much about the field. But once the press gets your letter, there will be no end to the calls, and we may all be treated like suspects. I'm sorry, but this is for the authorities to sort out."

How should the three trainees respond to the newspaper article in light of their advisor's objections?

The Scientist and Industry

Case 1

Dr. Richards is an assistant professor in the Department of Biochemistry at Small State University (SSU). Now in his third year at SSU, Dr. Richards is concerned that he won't have enough funded research to earn promotion and tenure. He has begun some promising theoretical work and is collaborating on a biochemistry textbook for nurses, but he has not been able to obtain grant funding for bench research.

A potential answer to Dr. Richards' worries appears unexpectedly when a collaborator on the nursing textbook introduces him to a representative from BioLife Pharmaceuticals, a small but successful local biotech company. BioLife is looking for researchers to conduct preliminary tests on a protein that they hope will become the basis of a new wound-healing medication.

BioLife's representative offers Dr. Richards a 2-year contract. He would work collaboratively with one of BioLife's founders at first but would work independently on the bulk of the project. BioLife's representative assures Dr. Richards that he will be free to publish the results of his research, after review by his collaborator, and that the company will even provide him with secretarial and editorial assistance to facilitate publication in appropriate journals. If the initial phase of the research is successful, BioLife would extend

Dr. Richards' contract for 3 more years, and his responsibility would grow to include monthly trips to San Diego, Seattle, and Atlanta to help plan a multicenter, phase I drug trial.

Dr. Richards is very excited. BioLife's proposal offers him the opportunity to work on something that is both interesting and self-supporting. The project will require lab assistants, so Dr. Richards would be able to provide employment for several of his promising undergraduates as well as research opportunities for graduate students. And with meaningful research under way, he might even be able to ask for a teaching assistant for his undergraduate class.

What should Dr. Richards consider before accepting BioLife's offer?

Case 2

Deborah is a doctoral candidate in chemical engineering who has completed her dissertation and is scheduled to graduate in May. Deborah's dissertation is based on research begun by her adviser, Dr. Boudreaux, a decade ago with funding from a manufacturer of artificial heart valves. Her work examines the interaction between surface coatings used on specific valves and the formation of blood clots.

Deborah completed her research in October and finished writing the text of her dissertation in December. The contract between Dr. Boudreaux and the valve company gives the company 90 days for prepublication review of all research publications. Dr. Boudreaux has always ensured that students finish their work well in advance of graduation to allow time for the company's review. However, for as long as anyone can remember the company has returned theses and dissertations in under a month with no comments or questions. Deborah confidently sends her dissertation off in time to enjoy Christmas break.

In January Deborah and her adviser set a March defense date and submit the necessary university paperwork for her to graduate. But in early February they receive word that the company wants more time to consider Deborah's findings. The company representative reminds Dr. Boudreaux that the contract provides for a 90-day extension of the review period when the publication discusses potentially patentable discoveries. Neither Dr. Boudreaux nor Deborah can imagine what potentially patentable discovery might be discussed in her dissertation. Deborah is horrified to think that she might not be able to graduate in May and is worried that she might lose the postdoctoral fellowship that she had planned to take in July.

How should Deborah and Dr. Boudreaux deal with this unexpected setback?

The Scientist in Society

Case 1

Dr. Chen is a senior immunologist whose research focuses on genetically modified vegetables that contain vaccine-like properties in their peel. Dr. Chen is also active in international efforts to vaccinate children in developing countries, where he works with the private aid project "Immunize Today: Prosper Tomorrow" (ITPT).

Dr. Chen left academics a decade ago to form a company specializing in "nutraceuticals," food plants with specific medicinal value. Within 5 years, his company was bought by TransNational Seed Company, an agricultural biotech firm specializing in genetically enhanced cereal crops resistant to insects, disease, and drought. Since that time, the company's patents on its plants and methods have reaped billions of dollars. In the developing countries where TransNational Seed Co. has donated or sold enhanced seeds, nutritional status has improved wherever the plants have been grown. However, natural food activists have accused TransNational Seed Co. of designing "self-neutering" plants, thus ensuring an ongoing market for their product by preventing farmers from harvesting seeds.

While Dr. Chen has grown rich personally, he remains much more interested in the social mission of his science than in profit. In his home laboratory garden he has developed a vaccine-carrying potato that he hopes to patent in ITPT's name. Concerned that the TransNational Seed Co.'s board will attempt to claim rights to this development, Dr. Chen is prepared to sabotage the testing that would confirm the potatoes' immune-enhancing effects.

How should Dr. Chen make his case about the social responsibility of TransNational Seed company in the patenting and distribution of the new potato?

Case 2

The science faculty at Western State University (WSU) are a close-knit group of researchers and teachers who enjoy strong professional collegiality. Despite its large student body, WSU's community has a small-town atmosphere in which everyone knows everyone and many professors' families are friends as well as neighbors.

For the past month, several members of the biology faculty have been concerned about rumors that the state school board may eliminate the subject of evolution from the science curriculum of the state's public middle and high schools. The local newspaper has reported that vocal proponents of both creationism and evolution have harassed school board members about the upcoming selection of science textbooks. Under this public pressure, the school board president has suggested that it might be best simply to avoid the subject of humanity's origins altogether. She points out that schools in other states have simply stopped teaching about human reproduction because of public controversy over what to teach and when.

When the school board formally proposes dropping evolution from the public middle and high school curriculum, the WSU science faculty convene a lunchtime meeting to discuss what practical action they might take as concerned scientists, educators, taxpayers, and parents. However, before long some of the faculty begin to question each others' religious beliefs and commitment to science. Two faculty members begin a loud debate over the appropriate role of religious texts in scholarship, and another questions the intelligence of anyone who would take most religious teachings seriously. The meeting breaks up with bad feelings all around and none of the original goals accomplished.

Should the WSU faculty try again to coordinate a response to the school board's proposal? What sort of response would be appropriate?

Index